NAIL THE BOARDS !
THE ULTIMATE INTERNAL MEDICINE REVIEW FOR BOARD EXAMS

D1129421

Bradley D. Mittman, M.D.

SECOND EDITION

FRONTRUNNERS BOARD REVIEW, INC.
39 Lyon St.
Valley Stream, NY 11580

PREFACE

This review is ideal for medical students & residents who are looking for the ultimate board review book for the **USMLE Steps 2 & 3**. Students who are preparing for these exams and are thinking about a residency in medicine, as well as internal medicine residents will ALSO be *way ahead* of the game when it comes time to sit for their medicine boards, that one last boards you'll take in your third year of medicine residency. This book is concise, thorough, and **fully-outlined**, so you will clearly see the relationship between the concepts you'll have to know. It also features tons of *great* **MNEMONICS** you'll thank your lucky stars for. Speaking of stars, we know you'll appreciate our ample use of formatting, especially the use of **STARRED ITEMS** ✪ to help call attention to *particularly* important material. You should know that this book is an excellent *companion* to the Frontrunners' Internal Medicine Q&A Review: Self-Assessment & Board Review, which features <u>over 1200 Q&A</u> to prepare you for battle. At the same time these resources are outstanding study aids for medical students, residents, internists, and other health care professionals who simply want the *best* no-nonsense review of internal medicine. Originally designed as the syllabus for the Frontrunners Internal Medicine Board Review Course, which continues to be held in New York, this book remains today much of the same core material for the board review course, which has seen unparalleled pass rates among its students on the boards. Over the years, we've been blessed with tons of questions and answers from the boards that have been voluntarily submitted by physicians, who have gone on to pass the boards, in their effort to help those "soldiers left behind"! The course has been widely and enthusiastically received for its unconventional, no-nonsense approach to the review of internal medicine. Unfortunately, thousands of physicians, wanting to be board-certified, are simply unable to attend a formal board review course due to time or geographic constraints. For those physicians especially this book will be a welcome review.

All major subsections of the exam have been represented with each section bearing its own chapter. Aren't you tired of reading and rereading (or even falling asleep!) amid long-winded paragraphs from standard textbooks that never make it clear what's important to know for the exam? So were we, and that's how this syllabus came into being. This book is completely outlined, so that the relationship between concepts is crystal clear—no more guessing! You'll also find tons of key mnemonics you'll *definitely* be using on your exam, along with <u>contributive formatting through the use of bolds, underlining, italics, boxed-in points, and of course, the starred items to help call attention to *particularly* important material</u>, although we would like to think that everything in here is important. Moreover, the thorough and realistically designed *Index section* will make your look-ups a whole lot easier.

Having said all this, we also realize that there are individuals who have, over the years, grown weary of tedious self-study and who want to take advantage of a sit-down, "feed-me" style of board review, with all the same core material, slides, cases, and more, even if the syllabus can come to them. For this reason we continue to offer our formal board review courses, which include: 1) the **WEEKEND MARATHON board review courses**, typically a few weeks before the exam—ideal for most physicians who can only spare a weekend; that weekend, however, covers 16 hours of highly intensive review and is not for the faint of heart; and 2) our more detailed 4-month board review course for more local physicians. For details/registration on any of our internal medicine board review courses *or* to order the Frontrunners' Internal Medicine Q&A Review: Self-Assessment & Board Review, call us at **866-MDBOARDs**.

We're confident that you'll find this an outstanding resource for your upcoming board exam as well as your day-to-day practice of internal medicine. But however you plan to use this book, our greatest hope is that we help you achieve your goals AND show you the easiest way there!

With best wishes for you,

Bradley D. Mittman, MD

Bradley D. Mittman, MD
FRONTRUNNERS BOARD REVIEW, INC.

• NOTICE •

The book is not intended to serve as a complete or standard textbook of internal medicine nor any subspecialties, but rather as a resource to assist the physician in his or her review specifically for the boards. It is in no way intended to be used as the sole reference for one's study or practice of internal medicine nor any subspecialties. Neither the author nor the publisher can be held accountable for any student's or students' individual board scores. Medicine is an ever-changing science. As new research and clinical experience broaden our knowledge, changes in the treatment and drug therapy are required. The author and publisher of this work have checked with sources believed to be reliable in their efforts to provide information that is complete and generally in accord with the standards accepted at the time of publication. However, in view of the possibility of human error or changes in medical sciences, neither the author nor the publisher nor any other party who has been involved in the preparation or publication of this work warrants that the information contained herein is in every respect accurate or complete, and they are not responsible for any errors or omissions or for the results obtained from use of such information. Readers are encouraged to confirm the information contained herein with other sources. This is particularly true insofar as drug selection and dosage are concerned. The reader is urged to check the package insert for each drug for any change in indications or contraindications, dosage, warnings, precautions, or drug-drug interactions.

Dedication

To Andre without whom this work might never have come to be. "You're my star, and when I'm far, you're not alone, 'cause your heart's my home."--Lenny Kravitz

TABLE OF CONTENTS:

1. <u>HEMATOLOGY</u>

Commonly Asked Material:

1. Know the similarities and differences between **<u>Waldenstrom's Macroglobulinemia</u>** and Multiple Myeloma.

- <u>Waldenstrom's</u>, remember, is a lymphoproliferative disorder of excess IgM production, yielding presentations of either *splenomegaly and anemia, or hyperviscosity-related symptoms*, such as headache, chest pain, SOB, fatigue, and lethargy. Remember, rouleaux formation here too (not just multiple myeloma). Management of Waldenstrom's includes *plasmapheresis to ↓ blood viscosity* and intermittent *chemo with agents such as cyclophosphamide and chlorambucil as needed*.

- The *terms* "monoclonal gammopathies", "paraproteinemias", and "plasma cell dyscrasias" are often used interchangeably to describe disorders such as multiple myeloma and Waldenstrom's macroglobulinemia.

SIMILARITIES AND DIFFERENCES BETWEEN WALDENSTROM'S MACROGLOBULINEMIA (WM) AND MULTIPLE MYELOMA (MM)	
<u>**SIMILARITIES**</u>	<u>**DIFFERENCES**</u>
1. Bone marrow dyscrasia and *hyperviscosity-related symptoms* 2. Serum M component (monoclonal IgM paraprotein; "<u>M spike</u>") > 3g/dL on SPEP) 3. Patients present with *weakness and fatigue* (largely due to anemia 2° to bone marrow infiltration by plasma cells), and *recurrent infections* (deficiency of normal antibodies and impaired neutrophil function) 4. *<u>Normocytic, normochromic anemia; rouleaux</u>* formation	1. *Lymphadenopathy/ hepato/splenomegaly* more common in WM 2. *Rouleaux formation* and a positive Coombs' test are much more common in WM 3. *Epistaxis, visual disturbances, and neurologic symptoms* (e.g. peripheral neuropathy, dizziness, headache, and transient paresis) are much more common in WM; 4. No bone lesions or hypercalcemia in WM (re: *plasmacytoma* in MM) 5. *Renal disease* is uncommon in WM.

2. Can **<u>Pernicious Anemia</u>** lead to malignancy?

- Yes, the disease develops into malignancy in **10%** of cases.

3. Recognize a classic case of **TTP** (Thrombotic Thrombocytopenic Purpura) and know the initial management:
   - Remember: "**F.A.T. R.N.**" ✪ to recall the classic pentad of presenting signs and symptoms:

     Fever

     Anemia (microangiopathic hemolytic anemia); hemolysis→ *schistocytes*

     Thrombocytopenia

     Renal findings

     Neurologic findings

   - Etiology: 90% are idiopathic; most of the rest are seen with pregnancy and OCPs
   - Coombs *negative*
   - Treatment of choice is plasmapheresis, using FFP plasma exchange. Monitor platelet counts, LDH, and peripheral smears for schistocytes for response to treatment. Generally speaking, in TTP platelet transfusions should be avoided because they can precipitate thrombotic events.

4. Be able to recognize a Schistocyte/**Schistocytes** on a peripheral blood smear and know the entire DDx

   > ✪ **AGN, ARF, DIC, HTN, Pulm HTN, HUS, PAN, SLE, TTP, HELLP syndrome, and preeclampsia**→all of these can give microangiopathic hemolytic anemia (**Coombs negative**)→which in turn gives *schistocytes*. Microangiopathic hemolytic anemia also often results in *platelet destruction* due to microvascular shearing, and of course, many of these disorders also reveal thrombocytopenia (eg DIC, HUS/TTP, SLE, HELLP)

5. Remember, in evaluating patients with **normocytic anemias**, ✓ the absolute reticulocyte count first to see if the patient is simply not making enough at the marrow *versus* hemolysing or hemorrhaging.

6. Know the laboratories you could find in a **hemolytic anemia** → *Reticulocytosis and fragmented red cells* on the peripheral blood smear; *elevated indirect*, i.e. unconjugated, bilirubin, (no greater than 4 to 5 mg/dL unless comorbid liver disease is present); *decreased haptoglobin* (binds the protein or globin part of hemoglobin and that complex is cleared within minutes by the lymphoreticular system); *positive urine hemosiderin test* (iron loss as hemoglobin or hemosiderin in the urine); and *↑LDH*. (Interestingly, the combination of an increased serum LDH and a reduced haptoglobin is 90 percent specific for diagnosing hemolysis, while the combination of a normal serum LDH and a serum haptoglobin greater than 25 mg/dL is 92 percent sensitive for ruling out hemolysis). The *smear* too, of course, can provide a number of clues: Spherocytes, Schistocytes, and Sickle cells (and obviously reticulocytes) may be indicative of hemolysis.

7. Know the management of **autoimmune hemolytic anemia** → steroids; consider splenectomy for refractory cases; blood transfusions as appropriate.

HEMATOLOGY

8. Know **AUTOIMMUNE HEMOLYSIS**

- You order a **Coombs test** (also known as D.A.T. or Direct Antiglobulin Test) when you suspect AHA. Accordingly, a positive Coombs test means the hemolytic anemia is *immune*. The term "direct", as in "His Direct Coombs test was positive" implies detection of antibodies *directly* on the RBC membrane. The following chart is useful in helping you distinguish features of warm (70%) vs. cold (15%) antibodies. The remainder of the antibodies are drug-induced (so-called "Coombs-negative AHA").

Coomb's positive Autoimmune Hemolysis:

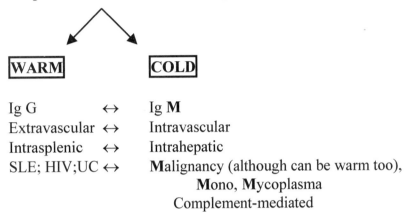

WARM		**COLD**
Ig G	↔	Ig **M**
Extravascular	↔	Intravascular
Intrasplenic	↔	Intrahepatic
SLE; HIV;UC	↔	**M**alignancy (although can be warm too), **M**ono, **M**ycoplasma Complement-mediated

- One might remember: "**M**mmm, **cold** beer. My **Compliments** to your bar." (beer→intrahepatic)

- *See Figure 1 Appendix: Hemolytic Anemia--Algorithm*

9. **HEREDITARY SPHEROCYTOSIS**

   a. The most common red cell *membrane disorder* causing hemolysis *in whites*. (Other membrane disorders that can result in hemolysis *in general* include hereditary elliptocytosis, spur cell anemia as seen in severe liver disease, and PNH.)

   b. Patients usually present with:
      i. A *positive family history* of mild anemia and splenectomy may be found.
      ii. *Spherocytes* on peripheral blood smear
      iii. *Negative Coombs'* test
      iv. An *osmotic fragility* test can confirm the diagnosis

   c. The molecular defect is defective or deficient **ankyrin** (protein that links the RBC membrane to the cytoskeleton)

   d. Concomitant *parvovirus infection can yield aplastic crisis*.

   e. *Splenectomy for symptomatic* cases

10. **G6PD DEFICIENCY**

    ➤ The most common red cell *enzyme* deficiency associated with hemolytic anemia.

    ➤ Specific medications in G6PD-deficient individuals may result in *methemoglobin formation*, where the iron in heme is oxidized from Fe^{2+} to Fe^{3+}) with subsequent hemolysis. Early on these patients may appear blue, yet have a normal arterial pO2. Medications that can do this include → *antimalarials, sulfa drugs, probenicid, and methylene blue*.

    ➤ Red cell G6PD levels can be measured for diagnosis. *Note,* however → *levels should not be measured during or shortly after a hemolytic episode because* the older red cells containing decreased levels of G6PD will already have lysed, leaving only the younger cells containing higher levels, yielding falsely normal levels.

11. *Know to order a Peripheral Blood Smear in someone who presents with thrombocytopenia (<150) for the first time.*

    ➤ The peripheral blood smear is valuable for two main reasons here: 1) in order to R/O plt *clumping* (which can give you falsely lower platelet counts; and 2) if platelets are truly low on the PBS, a bone marrow biopsy will be needed to *check for megakaryocytes* (platelet precursors), which, if elevated, generally implies peripheral platelet loss/consumption, and, if low, imply underproduction of platelets by the bone marrow.

12. Be able to recognize **Fe-Deficiency Anemia** on a peripheral blood smear. Remember the central pallor combined with an erythrocyte size *less than* the size of a surrounding normal lymphocyte nucleus.

13. **CHRONIC GRANULOMATOUS DISEASE**

    a. *Deficient superoxide anion production* by neutrophils leads to defective oxidative metabolism and consequent *inability to kill engulfed microorganisms*.

    b. Patients may present with *recurrent lymphadenitis*, hepatic abscesses, or osteomyelitis, with a positive *family history of frequent infections*

    c. Diagnosis → *nitroblue tetrazolium test* (superoxide from normal phagocytes converts yellow tetrazolium dye to blue)

14. **CML:**

    a. A number of different chemotherapeutic agents have been employed to treat patients with CML. The most commonly utilized agents include hydroxyurea (HU) and busulfan (BU). Up to 90 percent of patients will have a hematologic remission with these agents. However, treatment with either drug is not curative, does not prolong overall survival, and only rarely results in attainment of a cytogenetic response. Accordingly, such chemotherapy must be considered palliative.

b. Alpha interferon offers several advantages over hydroxyurea and busulfan:
    i. Higher rate of karyotypic response
    ii. A longer median time to progression of CML (accelerated phase or blast crisis)
    iii. Improved median survival

    However, IFNa therapy is associated with significant toxicities that include fever, chills, and flu-like symptoms in the majority of treated patients.

c. **Be able to recognize a CML CBC differential:**
    i. Leukocytosis >100,000 common; <10% blasts in chronic phase
    ii. Granulocytes seen in all stages of maturation with basophilia and eosinophilia
    iii. Platelets often > 400,000

d. **Know the CML translocation:**
    i. The Philadelphia chromosome (**t 9,22**) is the hallmark of the disease
    ii. The Philadelphia chromosome carries a ***good*** prognosis, as opposed to AML (poor prognosis)
    iii. ✪ This ***translocation*** results in the formation of a **chimeric bcr-abl gene** resulting in:
        a)) Maturation block (granulocytes) as noted above on the peripheral blood smear
        b)) Blast crisis

e. **Know when the CML patient who would benefit from a bone marrow transplant** (BMT)
    ✓ Allogeneic BMT should be performed during the chronic phase, within the first 6-12 months in patients < 55 y.o. who have an HLA-identical match or an identical twin.

15. Understand the indication for ***autologous*** BMT

    ✓ It is used preferred when the patient's bone marrow is normal and we want to remove the marrow and spare it from the highly bone marrow-toxic chemotherapeutic regimens of such cancers as germ cell tumors and breast cancer, after which regimens the patient's original normal marrow may be returned to the patient without having suffered the toxicity.

16. **TREATMENT OF BLOOD PRODUCT** →   **IN ORDER TO PREVENT**

TREATMENT OF BLOOD PRODUCT	IN ORDER TO PREVENT
• Washed/frozen RBCs	Febrile/allergic reactions
• Irradiation	GVHD (Graft vs. Host Disease)
• 3rd generation filter (leukocyte depleted)	CMV

17. Be able to differentiate coagulation disorders from defects in platelet function:

    • **Coagulation disorders**: These are characterized by joint, soft tissue and organ bleeding.

    • **Defects in platelet function**: These are characterized by purpura (petechiae and ecchymoses) of the skin and hemorrhage from mucous membranes.

18. Know the **indications for FFP** (fresh frozen plasma)

    i. FFP has all blood factors except 5 & 8, so can use for most everything, except must use cryoprecipitate for Hemophilia A

    ii. **Useful in multiple coagulation disorders:**
- ✓ Anticoagulation overdose
- ✓ Liver disease
- ✓ Massive transfusion
- ✓ DIC
- ✓ Plasmaphereses
- ✓ Vit K deficiency

    See Figure 3 (Appendix): *Intrinsic & Extrinsic Clotting Cascade*

19. Recognize a case of **Delayed Transfusion Reaction:** i.e. 3-5 days after receiving a transfusion of packed red blood cells, the patient returns to the hospital with **scleral icterus, malaise, fatigue, elevated LDH**, etc.

    a. Incidence: F>M
    b. Cause: Antibody in the *recipient vs. foreign-donor serum proteins*. The recipient's plasma already contains antibody before the transfusion because of previous transfusion, or previous pregnancy.
    c. *Coombs test is +*
    d. 1/3rd of these reactions are asymptomatic. The rest may show *Fever/Chills/Jaundice/Anemia*
    e. **Treatment**…
        i. IV fluids
        ii. Antihistamines
        iii. Monitor Hgb and urine output

20. Know that **recurrent abortions may be seen in**:

    a. *Anticardiolipin syndrome*
    b. *Lupus anticoagulant*
    c. *Fibrinogen disorders*
    d. *Factor 13 deficiency*

21. Be able to recognize **atypical lymphocytes**, *associated with mononucleosis*, on a peripheral blood smear.

22. Recognize a classic case of **H.A.T.T. (Heparin Associated Thrombocytopenia with Thrombosis)**

    a Heparin may enhance platelet aggregation, causing:
        1. Decrease platelet count
        2. Thrombosis (venous > arterial)

b. The mechanism is immunologic, with heparin-specific Ig G and antibodies vs. the platelet-heparin complex

c. **<u>Develops 3-15 days after initiating the heparin, with a median time of 10 days</u>** after initiation.

d. The treatment is to stop the heparin ASAP.

e. Because of HATT, a CBC should be checked QD in patients on heparin, with special attention to the platelets.

HEMATOLOGY NOTES

✪ IMPORTANT CELL TYPES ON PERIPHERAL BLOOD SMEAR:

- **Ringed sideroblasts**→alcohol is the #1 cause of acquired sideroblastic anemia

- **Spherocytes**→autoimmune hemolytic anemia; hereditary spherocytosis

- **Atypical (reactive) lymphocyte**→infectious mono

- **Basophilic stippling** → *thalassemia*, arsenic, lead poisoning, sickle cell, megaloblastic and sideroblastic anemias; ribosomal precipitates cause the stippling.

- **Target cells**→ *thalassemia*, jaundice/hepatitis, post-splenectomy; G6PD deficiency (Heinz bodies too); HbC and HbSC disease

- **Stomatocytes**→acute alcoholism; hereditary hemolytic anemia

- **Acanthocytes** (<u>spur</u> cells)→<u>liver</u> disease

- <u>**Burr**</u> cells→<u>Uremia</u>; if you confuse spur and burr cells, you may choose to recall that in advanced uremia, the concentration of urea in sweat may be so high that, after evaporation, a fine white powder can be found on the skin surface, so-called "<u>uremic frost</u>", so burr goes with uremia!

- **Heinz bodies (aka bite cells)**→G6PD deficiency predisposes to oxidative chemical insult and subsequent *Coombs-positive* hemolysis; **Italian & African-American** men. Key culprits include antimalarials; sulfonamides; dapsone; nitrofurantoin; nitrites; Heinz bodies represent precipitation of denatured hemoglobin in the cytoplasm.

- **Howell-Jolly bodies** → Solitary circular black dots seen at the margins of RBCs. They represent large DNA fragments; seen post-splenectomy and in hyposplenism.

- **Schistocytes** (aka **helmet cells**) (from any cause of microangiopathic hemolytic anemia—see DDx above in question section)→*Coombs test is negative*

- **Auer rods**→PML (Promyelocytic leukemia=<u>AML M3</u> subtype); if you have to have AML, hope to see Auer rods, since M3 carries the best prognosis 2° to potential for cure with <u>ATRA</u> (all-transretinoic acid); however, in actuality, you can also see Auer rods in types M1-M3; remember <u>DIC</u> in association with PML.

- **Hairy cells**→Hairy cell leukemia (curable with 2-CDA); these cells are said to have a "fried egg" appearance.

HYPOCHROMIC, MICROCYTIC Anemias ("A LIT MIC", as in a light microscopy)
  - ➤ A nemia of Chronic Disease
  - ➤ L ead poisoining
  - ➤ I ron deficiency
  - ➤ T halassemia; thyroid ($\downarrow$)

MACROCYTIC Anemias ("B. HERS")

- **B** $_{12}$ (and folate)
- **H** ypothyroidism
- **E** toh
- **R** eticulocytosis
- **S** ideroblastosis

NORMOCYTIC, NORMOCHROMIC ("*Losing it, Lysing, Low production*")

- Losing it: Acute hemorrhage
- Lysing it: Acute hemolysis (eg HUS, TTP)
- Low production: Aplastic anemia; pure RBC aplasia; myelofibrosis; CRF*

  * Erythropoiesis is ↓ in CRF, usually secondary to the effects of retained toxins on the bone marrow as well as to diminished endogenous epo levels by the diseased kidneys.

A COMPARISON OF THE MAJOR HYPOCHROMIC MICROCYTIC ANEMIAS:

Disease	MCV	RBCs	RDW	TIBC	FE	*FERRITIN*
FE DEFICIENCY	↓	↓	↑	↑	↓	↓
ACD	NL/↓	↓	NL	↓	↓	**NL**
THALASSEMIA	↓	↑	NL/↑	NL	NL/↑	NL/↑

MCV/RBC is another indicator that is often used to distinguish thalassemia and Fe def anemias:
- ✓ A ratio < 13 suggests thalassemia
- ✓ ≥13 suggests Fe deficiency anemia.

ANEMIA OF CHRONIC DISEASE

- A hypoproliferative anemia in which red cell precursors are deficient in their uptake and utilization of iron.
- **Associated with** the **3C's**: Chronic infections (e.g., osteomyelitis); Connective tissue diseases (e.g., rheumatoid arthritis and SLE); and Carcinomas
- Note the importance of RDW, TIBC and ferritin in differentiating iron deficiency anemia from ACD.

THALASSEMIA

- Defective globin chain synthesis, therefore defective Hgb
- Can affect the alpha or the beta chains, and can be minor (heterozygous) or major (homozygous)
- *Beta thalassemia* (2 genes) can be either heterozygous ("trait"), showing microcytosis with mild or no anemia, or homozygous, showing severe anemia
- *Alpha thalassemia* involves 4 genes. If only one is affected, the disease is usually silent. If 2 genes are affected, see microcytosis. A 3 gene defect yields Hgb H disease. Defects in all 4 genes yields hydrops fetalis.
- B. thalassemia: look for ↑ **Hgb A2** on Hgb electropheresis (normal 2.5%; 5% in B Thal major and minor)
- B. thal. **major**
    - ✪ Look for ↑ **Fetal Hgb** (normal < 1%; 50% in Thal major; 2-3% in Thal minor)
        - B. thalassemia major rarely survives to adulthood without BMT
- Electropheresis is normal in alpha thalassemia
- *B. thalassemia minor is the predominant thalassemia seen in adults*
- presents asymptomatically with a microcytic-hypochromic anemia

ERYTHROPOETIN LEVELS

- Re: there is an inverse relationship between the epo level and the Hgb (or Hct). Regulation is linked to an oxygen sensor.

↓ Epo level	↑ Epo level
P. Vera	Pure RBC aplasia
R.A.	Fe deficiency
HIV	Tumors (esp renal)
	High altitude

VITAMIN B12 DEFICIENCY

1. KEY FEATURES:

    a) *Hypersegmented neutrophils*; important sign as often appear before the:

        (1) **Macrocytosis**; or
        (2) **Anemia (megaloblastic)**, which can also result from folate deficiency

    b) ↑ *Serum MMA* (methylmalonic acid) level; ↑ serum gastrin levels.

    c) *Schilling test* is done to see if the B12 deficiency is due to *lack of Intrinsic Factor* (i.e. Pernicious Anemia), *malabsorption at the terminal ileum*, or *bacterial overgrowth*. You measure levels of radioactive B12 in a 24h urine.

There are **3 parts to the Schilling test:**

- Part 1: give 500 mg <u>PO</u> of cobalt-radiolabeled B12 and <u>check the urine</u>. If the level < 5% in the urine, **then B12 absorption is abnormal and proceed to Part 2.**

- Part 2: <u>retest after adding Intrinsic Factor</u>: if the patient puts out > 5% in the urine, then it was because they were initially lacking in I.F., and the dx is **Pernicious Anemia**. If < 5% shows up in the urine, then the problem was not lack of I.F., but is either **malabsorption at the terminal ileum** or **bacterial overgrowth**.

- Part 3: <u>retest after a course of antibiotics</u>, **testing for bacterial overgrowth of the small bowel**, as in disorders such as blind loop syndrome and scleroderma.

d) *Pernicious anemia*

  (1) The #1 cause of Vitamin B12 deficiency
  (2) Check **anti-intrinsic factor (IF) antibodies** in the serum for diagnosis (in 60% of patients)
  (3) **Antiparietal cell antibody** (in 90% of patients), but specificity is low
  (4) Check TFTs as thyroid disorders, also ↑ incidence of hyper or Hypothyroidism (other autoimmine disorders)
  (5) ↑ risk of gastric malignancy, so consider direct visualization and biopsy with endoscopy

e) *Neurologic findings*

  (1) Ataxic gait 2° to degeneration of the posterior columns
  (2) Dementia
  (3) Seizures

2. TYPICAL ORDER of events in B12 deficiency…

  a) Serum homocysteine and MMA ↑

  b) Serum B12 ↓

  c) MCV ↑ but still normal; hypersegmented neutrophils seen

  d) MCV ↑ beyond normal

  e) Anemia develops

  f) Symptoms seen

✪ Note that while this is the *usual* sequence of events, patients symptomatic with B12 deficiency *need not have* abnormal MCV or Hct ! This is frequently asked.

FOLATE DEFICIENCY

1. Usually secondary to poor PO intake (some elderly; dementia); alcoholics; malnutrition
2. *Megaloblastic* anemia as per vit B12 deficiency
3. As opposed to vit B12, however, *no neurologic complications.*

ALCOHOLISM

1. #1 cause of acquired sideroblastic anemia
2. Can see ↑ MCV (may be 2° to folate defiency)
3. Often see ↑ PT 2° to ↓ production of clotting factors 2° to liver disease

PNH (PAROXYSMAL NOCTURNAL HEMOGLOBINURIA)

1. **PNH** is a **result of** an acquired stem cell dysfunction that renders the patient at increased risk for complement-mediated cell lysis. RBCs, WBCs, and platelets are unusually sensitive to complement; Coombs' test is negative.

2. *Hemolytic anemia:* hemolysis is intravascular, yielding hemoglobinemia and hemoglobinuria (see next section for more on these).

3. Leukemia (**AML**) develops in 5-10%

4. *Aplastic anemia* is an important complication to remember for the exam

5. Dx: **Flow cytometry** has largely replaced Ham's test, is much more sensitive and specific, and directly checks for so-called "PNH cells," i.e., GPI-AP-deficient cells, or deficiency in certain anchor proteins on the cell surface that therefore predisposes to hypersensitivity to complement-mediated lysis with subsequent cytopenias.

6. One should think about ordering **flow cytometry in any of the following situations:**
   a. Unexplained hemolytic anemia or hemoglobinuria (not hematuria);
   b. Unexplained cytopenias, especially with any suggestions of intravascular hemolysis (e.g., low haptoglobin, elevated LDH, hemosiderinuria, or, of course, hemoglobinemia and/or hemoglobinuria);
   c. History of aplastic anemia, even if in "remission"; and
   d. Unexplained thromboembolic disorders, *especially* the Budd-Chiari syndrome.

7. 50% of deaths due to PNH are associated with *venous thromboembolism*, including Hepatic Vein Thrombosis (**Budd-Chiari Syndrome** is the major cause of death), and another 25% will die from **hemorrhage** (i.e., from thrombocytopenia due to aplastic anemia)—sounds a little like H.A.T.T. (Heparin Associated Thrombocytopenia with Thrombosis) with the combination of thrombosis and thrombocytopenia (or even DIC for that matter).

8. The various treatment options include thrombolytics/anticoagulation as appropriate, androgens, immunosuppressive, and BMT.

HEMATOLOGY

HAPTOGLOBIN, HEMOSIDERIN, HEMOGLOBINURIA, HEMOSIDERINURIA !

> Remember, after RBC lysis, the carrier protein **haptoglobin** binds Hgb; the hemoglobin-haptoglobin complex is rapidly removed by the liver, leading to a reduction in plasma haptoglobin. *If* the haptoglobin-binding capacity of the plasma is *exceeded*, free hemoglobin is left to pass through the glomeruli on its own. If this happens, the filtered hemoglobin is reabsorbed by the proximal tubule, where it is broken down, and the heme iron becomes incorporated into storage proteins (ferritin and **hemosiderin**). Staining the sediment with Prussian blue can help ✓ for the presence of hemosiderin in the urine. A positive stain indicates that a significant amount of circulating free hemoglobin has been filtered by the kidneys. Hemosiderin usually appears 3 to 4 days after the onset of hemoglobinuria. So, in summary, for severe lysis, there's **Lysis → Hgb-Haptoglobin complex → Hgburia → Hemosiderinuria**

HEMOLYTIC UREMIC SYNDROME (HUS)

1. ✪ Similar to TTP, except w/o the Fever or Neurologic involvement (F**AT R**N without the F or N)

2. Management in adults, however, is the same as for TTP

3. *Hemorrhagic colitis* 2° to **E coli 0157H7** (tainted beef)

4. The most worrisome complication of E coli 0157H7 and most frequently involves children under the age of 5 to 10 years. HUS is the most common cause of acute renal failure in children in the United States.

SICKLE CELL ANEMIA

1. 8% of blacks carry the Sickle cell **trait;**

2. Patients with sickle cell **trait** often have painless **hematuria** and may be associated with pyelonephritis in pregnancy; there is **no anemia, no ↑ risk of infections, no ↑ mortality;** those with "trait" also have difficulty concentrating their urine (hypo/isosthenuria). They have no pain crises.

3. Long-term exchange transfusion in SS anemia useful in patients with **cerebrovascular complications.**

4. **Treatment→** Prevention; Hydration; Analgesia; Exchange Transfusions as appropriate to decrease the Hgb S to <30%) ; *hydrea* is used to ↓ risk of complications.

5. **Pathophysiology**→Acute crises are due to recurrent obstruction of the microcirculation by intravascular sickling, caused by diminished oxygen delivery→more sickling→worse oxygen delivery→etc.

6. **Atypical symptoms** may suggest→pneumonia; pulmonary infarction; acute pyelonephritis; or cholecystitis. Remember, infections are the #1 cause of death in SS disease.

7. **5 MAIN CRISES ✪ :**

   a. **Vaso-occlusive("painful" or "infarctive" crisis)**

      i) Most frequent type of crisis
      ii) 2° to microvascular obstruction from sickled cells which starts the cycle of tissue hypoxia that in turn causes more sickling.
      iii) Seen in long bones, chest, and abdomen
      iv) Causes autosplenectomy

   b. **Aplastic Crisis**

      i) Bone marrow suppression 2° to infections (usually viral)
      ii) Because of the short RBC lifespan, even brief periods of suppression may have a significant effect on Hgb level
      iii) Usually follows a febrile illness and lasts 5-10 days

   c. **Megaloblastic Crisis**

      i) Usually due to folate deficiency, esp in late pregancy
      ii) Associated with ↑MCV and ↓Hgb

   d. **Sequestration Crisis**

      i) Pooling of RBCs in the spleen, seen primarily in young children

   e. **Hemolytic Crisis**

      i) Usually 2° to infection or drugs→ ↑retic count, ↑unconjugated bili, and jaundice
      ii) Especially in patients with G6PD deficiency, hereditary spherocytosis, and mycoplasma pneumonia

8. <u>**Avascular necrosis**</u> a common complication; remember to order the MRI if you suspect it!

9. **Renal complications**→**papillary necrosis;** <u>**hyposthenuria**</u> (inability to concentrate the urine; nocturia; enuresis); focal segmental glomerulonephropathy;

10. **Priapism** also common

11. ✪ **Pulmonary** Crisis: <u>**Acute Chest Syndrome**</u> causes 20% of SS deaths: look for Fever, Chest pain, Tachypnea, ↑WBC count, and pulmonary infarcts; in adults sickling here is usually unaccompanied by infection.

CLL (Chronic Lymphocytic Leukemia)

1. **#1** malignancy in the U.S. and #1 form of leukemia ≥60 yo; 90% of pts are > 50 yo; CLL is characterized by malignant B lymphocytes.

2. **Fever** should always be presumed 2° to infection and not the leukemia (except for *Richter's transformation to Large Cell Lymphoma, which carries a poor prognosis*)

3. ↓ **Gamma globulins** (re: CLL is a disease of B cells) predispose to infection. Of those with infection, half have low gamma globulins

4. Other **complications**→Autoimmune hemolytic anemia; thrombocytopenia; ↑incidence of solid tumors of the lung and skin; AML

5. A poor prognosticator is **lymphocyte doubling time** in < 1 year

6. ✪ Staging: **RAI CLASSIFICATION**:

   Stage 0:   Lymphocytosis only
   Stage 1:   "   + Lymphadenopathy
   Stage 2:   "   +   "   +   Splenomegaly

   --
   Stage 3:   "   **+ Anemia**
   Stage 4:   "   **+ Thrombocytopenia**

7. ✪ Remember it's important to know the Rai stage since <u>treatment does not prolong survival</u> in stages I or II, and is generally **reserved for Stage 3 and 4 only**! *Management* of Rai 3 (+ anemia) and Rai 4 (+ thrombocytopenia) includes <u>chlorambucil ± prednisone</u>. For patients who relapse, <u>fludarabine</u> is often used.

8. **Treatment for CLL includes** observation if the patient is asymptomatic. Oral alkylating agent chemotherapy with or without prednisone is commonly employed if the patient is symptomatic with fever, night sweats, fatigue, or massive splenomegaly.

9. **Gamma globulin therapy** may be given prophylactically even if the patient has never had infection, as long as his Ig G is <0.3 g/dl.

10. **Patients with CLL have an increased incidence of autoimmune diseases, particularly** autoimmune hemolytic anemia, but ITP and pure red cell aplasia are seen as well.

11. The **median survival time** for CLL is 5 years from the onset of treatment.

HAIRY CELL LEUKEMIA

1. Represents < 2% of all leukemia; cytopenias/splenomegaly predominate; essentially a B cell dz.

2. **Hairy cells ("fried egg" appearance)** with cytoplasmic projections seen on blood smears

3. **TRAP +** (stain positively to tartrate-resistant acid phosphatase)

4. **Dry TAP** on bone marrow aspiration (consistent with the pancytopenia often seen)

5. ✪ Neutropenia→infections (these infections are different as they tend to be **atypical mycobacterial and other ususual infections, like toxoplasmosis, legionella, and nocardia**)→these infections are the primary cause of mortality in HCL.

6. ✪ **2-CDA** (2-Chlorodeoxyadenosine) **is the treatment** of choice, producing complete remission in 85%-88% of patients after a single continuous 7day IV infusion; a longer unmaintained disease-free state can be achieved with fludarabine.

LYMPHOPROLIFERATIVE DISORDERS: $\underline{4}$ Important Ones: "C$_a$LL 4 H$_e$LP"
(disorders of clonal expansion of lymphocytes): (maybe you'd like an onc consult?!)

CLL
Hairy cell leukemia
Lymphoma (e.g., Hodgkin's disease, and NHL)
Plasma cell dyscrasias (hyperproliferation of immunoglobulin by plasma cells)
> Multiple myeloma, MGUS, Waldenstrom's macroglobulinemia, primary amyloidosis, and cryoglobulinemia.

MULTIPLE MYELOMA ✪ *(for more details on MM and MGUS, see Oncology)*

1. **≥10% plasma cells found in the bone marrow** { **< 10% in MGUS** (Monoclonal Gammopathy of Undetermined Significance) }

2. **M protein→ < 3 g/dl in MGUS; > 3 in MM;**

3. **In MGUS**, there is absence of lytic lesions, anemia, hypercalcemia, renal insufficiency, and little to no Bence Jones proteinuria, and these patients commonly develop **malignant transformation** into MM, amyloidosis, macroglobulinemia, or a related lymphoproliferative process (approximately 15 % at 10 years and 25 % at 15 years). Approximately 25% of patients go onto develop multiple myeloma. Periodic monitoring of MGUS patients is therefore important.

4. In diagnosing multiple myeloma, 80-90% of cases are detected using SPEP (*serum* protein electropheresis); *the remainder, which secrete only light chains,* can be diagnosed with a **UPEP** (*urine* PEP).

5. Clinical features→<u>bone pain (#1 symptom)</u>; renal insufficiency; <u>hypercalcemia</u>; weakness/fatigue; **spinal cord compression; pneumococcal infection**.

6. Normochromic normocytic anemia

7. Xrays→"***punched out*" <u>lytic lesions</u>; osteoporosis; pathologic **fractures**

8. Because it is not curable, tx should be delayed until evidence of progression seen.

AML (Acute Myelogenous Leukemia=Acute Nonlymphocytic Leukemia, ANLL)

1. Remember, the **<u>Philadelphia</u>** chromosome (t 9,22), carries a ***worse* prognosis** here (**as opposed to CML**)

2. **In differentiating AML from ALL histochemically**, remember, ALL stains positive for Periodic acid-Schiff stain (PAS) and is associated with *TdT enzyme*. Myeloid leukemias stain positive for myeloperoxidase. Flow cytometry, however, is considered the gold standard.

3. As we noted earlier, all of the following are critical to know: **<u>Auer rods</u>**→PML (Promyelocytic leukemia=**<u>AML M3</u> subtype**). The important **(t15,17) translocation** renders PML very sensitive to and potentially curable with **<u>ATRA</u>** (all-transretinoic acid). Remember also **<u>DIC</u>** in association with PML. Auer rods are classically associated with M3 (but can also be seen in M1 and M2).

4. Age <40 yo and achieving complete remission after first cycle of Idarubicin (or Daunarubicin) + AraC (Cytarabine) carry good prognosis.

5. Median age of patients with AML is 65 yo

6. Platelet transfusions are required throughout the course of treatment.

7. Recommendations:
   - *If patient <55yo →consider BMT in 1st remission if poor prognostic; BMT in early relapse or 2nd remission if no poor prognostics.*

AML Response to Chemo Alone:

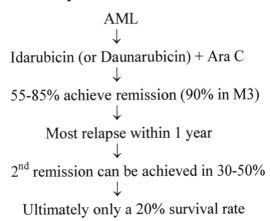

AML
↓
Idarubicin (or Daunarubicin) + Ara C
↓
55-85% achieve remission (90% in M3)
↓
Most relapse within 1 year
↓
2nd remission can be achieved in 30-50%
↓
Ultimately only a 20% survival rate

For acute leukemic patients who present with **WBC >100,000** the initial complication of greatest concern is cerebral hemorrhage. For patients with **leukemic meningitis or leukostasis with neurologic findings**, <u>emergency treatment</u> ✪ includes:

1. **Leukopheresis**
2. **Cranial irradiation**
3. **Hydroxyurea**

Acute leukemic patients with **Tumor Lysis Syndrome** should be managed with hydration, allopurinol, and alkalinization of the urine. Look for ↑K, ↑uric acid, ↑phos, lactic acidosis, and hyp**o**calcemia.

ALL (Acute Lymphoblastic Leukemia)

1. More common in **children** (who have complete remission rates of >90%)

2. 1/3 of patients present with **bleeding**

3. Bone pain/LN/HM/SM are more common in ALL (3/4 patients) than AML (1/2 of patients)

4. **CALLa antigen** is a **good** prognosticator

THE MYELOPROLIFERATIVE DISORDERS :

The four disorders—ALL can lead to AML!

			LAP Score
1.	**CML**	↑WBCs	↓
2.	**Myelofibrosis**	↑Fibrosis	↑
3.	**P. Vera**	↑RBCs	↑
4.	**Essential Thrombocythemia**	↑Platelets	↑

➢ *Other disorders with ↓ LAP scores* include: PNH, aplastic anemia, and Wilson's

➢ **SPLENOMEGALY** is common in **ALL 4 TYPES**.

Let's examine each of the main myeloproliferative disorders one by one…

---

1. CML

- An acquired defect of clonal origin that is the result of a translocation.

- **Philadelphia chromosome** (t 9,22) is the hallmark:

  - *Translocation causes a bcr-abl chimeric gene →results in premature termination of granulocyte maturation and also results in blast crisis.*

- **The only *low* LAP score among the four myeloproliferative disorders** shown

- *Don't confuse with a* **LEUKEMOID REACTION**, where you can see an increase in the WBC count to $> 25 \times 10^9$/L, secondary to another condition. In contrast to a leukemoid reaction, in CML, the WBC is usually > 100,000, LAP level is ↓ (high in leukemoid); the spleen is usually enlarged; bone marrow is panhypocellular (vs. myeloid hyperplasia only in leukemoid); and, of course the presence of the Philadelphia chromosome (translocation; 90% of cases).

- **CBC→WBC>100,000; granulocytes found in all stages of maturation**; platelets typically >400,000.

- Marked leukocytosis (**>300,000**) may cause **leukostasis**, manifesting as **blurred vision, respiratory distress, priapism**, etc.

- Good prognosis→ small spleen size and 0%-10% circulating blasts
- Poor prognosis: age>45 and platelet<70,000
- ↑ Vit B12, as with P. Vera

- **CHRONIC PHASE:**

  - ☞ *<10% blasts in blood and bone marrow*
  - ☞ *2-3 years in duration*

- **TREATMENT:**
  - ➢ **Allo BMT is the treatment of choice** and is the only curative regimen, *not* conventional chemo.
    - ◆ **Should be performed in the chronic phase , within the 1ˢᵗ 6-12 months in patients <55 yo who have an HLA-identical match or an identical twin.**

    - ◆ Survival is 63% at 3 years

  - ➢ However, **3 agents commonly used in the initial tx of CML** are:
    1. Hydroxyurea—tx of choice for high blast counts and leukostasis; safe in thrombocytopenia; continued maintenance tx is important.
    2. Busulfan
    3. Alpha interferon— works by suppressing the Philadelphia chromosome

> ➤ Hydroxyurea is not only for sickle cell anemia and the leukostasis of CML, but is also used for marked thrombocytosis (> 700,000) in order to decrease the risk of thrombosis.

> ➤ Remember the **_COMPLICATIONS of BMT_** in general:

    1. *Early*:
        a. **GVHD****
            i. Skin→rash
            ii. GI →diarrhea; liver pathology
            iii. CMV infection
        b. **V.O.D. (Veno-occlusive disease)**
            i. Hepatomegaly
            ii. Ascites
            iii. Jaundice

    ** Following BMT, methotrexate and cylosporine can be used to help prevent GVHD (immune prophylaxis)

    2. *Late:*
        a. HSV, VZV
        b. PCP
        c. Chronic GVHD

> ➤ **MGMT OF "BLAST CRISIS"**→ allopurinol, fluids, hydroxyurea, cranial radiation, and leukocyte apheresis.

> ➤ **CHRONIC phase→ACCELERATED phase ("BLAST CRISIS") when ≥ 20% BLASTS**

---

2. MYELOFIBROSIS

a. Due to hyperproliferation of **fibroblasts**

b. **SPLENOMEGALY** *always* **present**

c. Hypocellular marrow 2° replacement of marrow by fibrosis leads to *pancytopenia*

d. **'TEARDROP' CELLS**

e. *Leukoerythroblastic* peripheral blood smear (nucleated RBCs, early myeloid forms, including blasts) in 96%; large, abnormal platelets

f. There is no specific therapy for idiopathic myelofibrosis. Treatment includes *supportive care* with transfusions, growth factors, and antibiotics as needed. Hydroxyurea, splenectomy, and radiation therapy can *palliate* symptomatic splenomegaly

---

3. POLYCYTHEMIA VERA ---Everything is ↑ *except* the Epo level !

- As its name suggests, P Vera is a clonal disorder involving a multipotent hematopoietic progenitor cell in which there is overproduction of phenotypically normal red cells, granulocytes, and platelets in the absence of a recognizable physiologic stimulus. Patients therefore may show erythrocytosis, leukocytosis, and thrombocytosis; splenomegaly common (75%).

- **Splenomegaly** can lead to hemolysis→ ↑LDH

- Uncontrolled erythrocytosis can lead to neurologic symptoms, such as headache, blurred vision, dizziness, vertigo, paresthesias, focal weakness and a variety of other complications including Budd-Chiari Syndrome as well as intravascular thrombosis in heart, brain, and lungs. **Thrombotic complications** are, in fact, *the major cause of death* in P Vera.

- **↑ LAP** score is used to differentiate it from other forms of erythrocytosis (stress, anoxic, tumor)

- **↓ Epo** level (remember the inverse correlation with Hgb/Hct).

- With the exception of **aquagenic pruritus**, no symptoms distinguish polycythemia vera from other causes of erythrocytosis.

- **Diagnostic criteria**: ↑RBC mass + arterial Oxygen sat>92% + either (splenomegaly or at least 2 of the following):

    1. WBC >12,000 (white count elevated in 2/3rds of cases)
    2. Platelets > 400,000 --may treat with Anegralide, hydrea, or alpha interferon, or even P32 (thrombocytosis in half of cases)
    3. ↑LAP
    4. ↑B12 (re: seen in CML too)

- Notice, nowhere in these criteria do you see a high Hgb or Hct listed. However, this is actually how this disorder most often comes to attention. Remember the first step in approaching a high Hct is to obtain a **RBC mass (↑)**

- **TREATMENT** is **phlebotomy** q 2-4 months if asymptomatic. The goal is to keep the Hct below 45 men and 42 in women.

    - Supplement phlebotomy with hydroxyurea (starting dose 15 to 20 mg/kg per day) in patients who are at high-risk for thrombosis (age over 70, prior thrombosis, platelet count >1,500,000/μL, presence of cardiovascular risk factors). Aspirin may be used for those who fail hydroxyurea.

    - Anagrelide (starting dose 0.5 mg four times per day) is used mainly to manage thrombocytosis in patients refractory to other treatments. It must be given with caution in patients with known or suspected heart disease, which may limit its utility in the elderly.

- <u>Myelosuppressive therapy</u> [traditionally with phosphorus-32 (32P) or an alkylating agent such as busulfan, cyclophosphamide, or chlorambucil], when combined with phlebotomy, reduces the incidence of thrombosis, but increases the risk of AML, lymphoma, gastrointestinal, and skin malignancies.

4. ESSENTIAL THROMBOCYTHEMIA :

> A clonal stem cell disorder
> The median age at diagnosis is 60 years

> *A persistent and otherwise unexplained elevation in platelet count, in a non-splenectomized patient with normal serum ferritin and C-reactive protein levels, suggests a diagnosis of ET.*

> **DIAGNOSTIC CRITERIA** (*need all*):

- Platelet count >600,000/μL (>1,000,000/μL for entering therapeutic protocols)

- Megakaryocytic hyperplasia on bone marrow aspiration and biopsy

- Absence of the Philadelphia chromosome

- Absence of infection, inflammation, and other causes for reactive thrombocytosis

- Normal red blood cell (RBC) mass or a hemoglobin concentration <13 g/dL

- Presence of stainable iron in a bone marrow aspiration or ≤1 g/dL increase in hemoglobin concentration after a 1 month trial of oral iron therapy.

> **TREATMENT OPTIONS**
- At present, <u>anagrelide</u> is a reasonable alternative for patients who do not tolerate <u>hydroxyurea</u> or for whom long-term therapy is planned and a concern regarding drug leukemogenicity exists.
- Alpha interferon controls the thrombocytosis associated with any myeloproliferative disorder including ET
- <u>Alpha interferon</u> may also be considered for controlling thrombocytosis in patients failing both hydroxyurea and anagrelide
- <u>Low-dose ASA</u> may be safe and possibly effective in preventing thrombosis in ET. It is especially effective in treating the vasomotor symptoms of ET and PV, such as acral paresthesias and erythromelalgia (burning pain in the feet or hands accompanied by erythema, pallor or cyanosis, in the presence of palpable pulses) **Erythromelalgia** and the associated symptom of **acral paresthesias** are considered to be **pathognomonic microvascular thrombotic complications in PV and essential thrombocythemia**, and are associated with platelet counts above 400,000/μL. Erythromelalgia is associated with platelet consumption and platelet thrombi in the microvasculature. Symptoms respond dramatically to **aspirin** in low doses.

VON WILLEBRAND'S DISEASE

1. The #1 inherited bleeding disorder

2. vWF performs two critical functions in hemostasis: it acts as a bridging molecule for normal platelet adhesion and aggregation, and it acts as a carrier for factor VIII in the circulation, increasing the half-life of factor VIII five-fold. It is manufactured by megakaryocytes (platelet precursor cells) and endothelial cells.

3. vWD is secondary to a <u>congenital deficiency of vWF, factor 8: ag,</u> which results in low platelet adhesion. This <u>defect in platelet adhesion</u> can be tested for using: **<u>Ristocetin aggregation</u>** assay: normally, platelets will aggregate in the presence of ristocetin; in vWD, the platelets do not.

4. Diagnosis
   a. vWF may be decreased in either <u>number or function</u>

   b. **<u>vWF is important in platelet aggregation (thus the prolonged bleeding time)</u>**

   c. The low factor VIII concentration in vWD is due, at least in part, to the decreased levels of vWF, since vWF normally protects factor VIII from proteolytic inactivation by activated protein C and its cofactor protein S and prolongs its half-life in the circulation five-fold. **PTT** *usually* ↑ (normal in some patients).

5. Treatment:
   ✓ For **MILD bleeds** → **<u>dDAVP</u>** (desmopressin), a synthetic vasopressin analogue that stimulates release of stored factor 8: ag multimers from endothelium;
   ✓ For **more SEVERE bleeds** → <u>factor 8 concentrates</u> or **cryoprecipitate** (rich in factor 8 and vWF)

DIC (Disseminated Intravascular Coagulopathy)

1. A *"<u>consumptive coagulopathy</u>"* characterized by microvascular clotting secondary to thrombin deposition.
2. Carries a 50-80% mortality
3. **<u>Platelet aggregation results in *thrombocytopenia,* ↓ fibrinogen, and ↑ D-dimers</u>**

4. *↑PT, PTT,* and thrombin time

5. ↓ Platelet counts and fibrinogen

6. Classic complication of **<u>PML (*AML type M3,* promyelocytic</u>)** ✪

7. *<u>Schistocytes</u>* seen secondary to the microvascular obstruction

8. Thrombosis > bleeding

9. <u>**Sepsis is the #1 cause**</u>

10. Malignancy is the #2 cause

11. <u>**As opposed to liver disease, DIC produces a much greater thrombocytopenia and Factors 7 and 10 are normal in DIC**</u>.

12. Heparin only indicated with evidence of fibrin deposition and thrombosis.

CONDITIONS ASSOCIATED WITH AN ISOLATED ↑PT

1. Vitamin K deficiency

2. Factor VII deficiency

3. Coumadin.

Deficiencies of factor X V, II, and fibrinogen are associated with an ↑PT and PTT, since they are all part of the final common pathway (see figure 3 appendix)

DDx of an ↑PTT:

Congenital:

➢ Dysfibrinogenemia (↑PT too)

➢ Hemophilia A, B

➢ VWD

Acquired:

➢ DIC (↑PT too)

➢ Heparin

➢ Lupus anticoagulant

SELECTIVE DDx of an ↑ BLEEDING TIME
1. Aspirin, NSAIDs
2. Defects of platelet aggregation VWD Bernard-Soulier syndrome Glansmann's
3. Paraproteinemia
4. Myeloproliferative disorders
5. DIC
6. Uremia (defective platelet release)
7. Afibrinogenemia

8. Thrombocytopenia (<90,000 cells/μL)
    - **↓ Production***
        - Aplastic anemia
        - Megaloblastic anemia
        - Myelophthistic disorder (replacement of normal bone marrow with metastatic tumor or infection)
    - **↑ Peripheral Destruction***
        - AIDS
        - DIC
        - HUS, TTP
        - Immune-mediated
            - Drugs (eg PCN)
            - ITP
            - SLE
        - Severe septicemia

    * *Can differentiate between these 2 by checking the smear of B.M. biopsy for megakaryocytes (platelet precursors): low if ↓ production; ↑ if peripheral destruction.*

DDX OF BLEEDING DIATHESIS WITH ALL NORMAL ROUTINE PARAMETERS
(normal bleeding time, normal platelet count, and normal PT and PTT)

- ➤ vWD
- ➤ Factor XIII deficiency
- ➤ Hyperfibrinolysis
- ➤ Collagen vascular disorders

FACTOR XII DEFICIENCY
- ➤ **The most common genetic reason for an elevated PTT**
- ➤ **No treatment is necessary since Factor XII deficiency <u>does not cause bleeding</u>.**

not to be confused with...

FACTOR XIII DEFICIENCY ✪

1. **All routing <u>clotting tests are normal</u>; however, →** the *<u>urease clot solubility</u>* test (clot stability assay) is **positive,** since the absence of fibrin crosslinking causes a clot to lyse much more rapidly in 5 molar urea.
2. **Think of this disease when the patient has DELAYED POST-OP BLEEDING** *24 to 36 hours after surgery* or trauma (e.g. after dental work when patient returns home and gums bleed later that night) --since the initial <u>clot is mechanically weak</u>—*and poor wound healing.* Interestingly, it's very much the <u>opposite</u> of Factor XII deficiency in fact (where you saw coags elevated but no bleeding)
3. **<u>FFP</u> is the treatment.**

HYPERCOAGUABLE STATES

ANTITHROMIN III DEFICIENCY:

- ➤ Remember, AT III is a natural anticoagulant that acts at factors 12, 11, 9, and thrombin.
- ➤ *Renal vein thrombosis* is a classic thrombotic complication
- ➤ *Acquired AT deficiency is seen in*:

  - ☞ Liver disease*
  - ☞ DIC*
  - ☞ OCP use**
  - ☞ Pregnancy**
  - ☞ *Nephrotic syndrome* (AT III is one of the proteins lost!)**

    - * These may also lead to ↓ *activity* of proteins C and S.
    - ** These may also lead to ↓ protein S *levels*

FACTOR V LEIDEN DEFICIENCY ✪

- ➤ Also known as **activated protein C (aPC) resistance** because a specific mutation in the factor V gene (called factor V Leiden) makes factor V resistant to degradation by activated protein C.

- ➤ *Terminology*--Causes 90% of cases of APC or Activated Protein C resistance. APC resistance and Factor V Leiden should not be used synonymously, since pregnancy, OCP use, select antiphospholipid antibodies, and other factor V point mutations account for the *other* 10% of cases of APC resistance.

- ➤ *Prevalence and Risk:*

  - ✓ *Accounts for 30-50% of patients with "idiopathic" venous thrombosis and 20-30% of cases of DVT in patients <45yo*; present in 2-5% of the general population!

  - ✓ Factor V Leiden + OCP use → 35-fold relative risk of DVT (OCP use alone confers a 4-fold relative risk of DVT). So, don't forget (!) to look for this disease in women who develop **DVT while on OCPs or while pregnant, i.e. in addition to the usual studies of Protein C & S, etc.**

  - ✓ APC resistance accounts for approximately one third of cases of "idiopathic" DVTs.

  - ✓ The *most common* inherited thrombogenic disorder
    - • Heterozygosity→confers a 7-fold ↑ lifetime risk of DVT
    - • Homozygosity →confers an 80-fold ↑ risk

- ➤ **Screen** for this by ordering an *APC ratio, a clotting-based assay*
  - ☞ Can **confirm** the presence of factor V Leiden through *molecular-based assays* for the factor.

ACTIVATED PROTEIN C (aPC) and PROTEIN S

➤ Protein C and S degrade factors 8 & 5.

➤ Remember, adults with heterozygous protein C *or* S deficiencies may experience *__warfarin-induced skin necrosis__* shortly after starting warfarin without concomitant heparin therapy. This complication results from the short half-life of Protein C which warfarin accelerates, causing rapid depletion and a paradoxical worsening of the hypercoaguable state.

➤ In addition, testing for these 3 cannot be reliably performed during an acute even because levels fluctuate during active thrombosis. If indicated, testing for these can be done 3 weeks after anticoagulant therapy has been d/c'd.

PROTEIN S DEFICIENCY:
☞ More common than protein C deficiency or AT III deficiency.
☞ A vitamin K-dependent factor that is **required for activated *protein C* anticoagulant activity**. Remember, **activated protein C functions as an anticoagulant by destroying factors 5 and 8** (with the help of protein S).

PROTEIN C DEFICIENCY—Remember, because of its role in destroying factors 5 and 8, a deficiency in Protein C (or S for that matter) will result in a hypercoaguable state. In patients with protein C deficiency, a potential therapeutic complication is the development of *__warfarin-induced skin necrosis__*. This cx results from the short half-life of Protein C which warfarin accelerates, causing rapid depletion and a paradoxical worsening of the hypercoaguable state. For this reason, protein C deficient patients should receive *__heparin first__*. Note also that because proteins C and S *are vitamin-K dependent*, a proper diagnosis of protein C or S def cannot be made if the patient is vit-K deficient.

AFIBRINOGENEMIA & DYSFIBRINOGENEMIA

➤ **Thrombin time & reptilase time** is useful in diagnosing **afibrinogenemia & dysfibrinogenemia** (and also DIC).

➤ If both the thrombin time and reptilase time are prolonged, it points to one of these.

PROTHROMBIN 20210

➤ Autosomal dominant disorder reflecting a guanine to adenine base substitution in the prothrombin gene, resulting in ↑ prothrombin activity and an ↑ risk of venous and arterial thrombosis.

➤ This mutation is only slightly less prevalent in the general population than factor V Leiden.

HYPERHOMOCYSTINEMIA

- $\uparrow$ homocysteine levels have been associated with both arterial & venous thrombosis
- Hyperhomocystinemia (> 15 μmol/L)
    - May be inherited or acquired
    - *Associated disorders*:
        - Dietary deficiencies of folate , B6, or B12
        - CRF
        - Pernicioius anemia
        - Hypothyroidism

- Foods rich in *folate, B12, & B6 lower plasma homocysteine* levels
    - Numerous randomized, placebo-controlled studies are underway, however, to see if there is actually a link between lowering the homocysteine concentration and reduced mortality.
    - *Until* these studies are completed the AHA recommends that a patient with homocysteine levels > 10μmol/L should undergo dietary modification to ensure they are getting the RDA for folate (400μg), B6 (2mg), and B12 (2.5μg)→recheck homocysteine level in 1 month→if still high, vitamin supplements→recheck in 1 more month.

TROUSSEAU'S SYNDROME

- Migratory venous or arterial thrombophlebitis associated with mucinous adenocarcinomas (eg prostate) and myeloproliferative disorders
- Due to the development of a cysteine protease that activates Factor X
- Approximately 15 percent of patients who develop DVT or PE have a diagnosis of cancer.
- The most common cancers associated with thromboembolic episodes include lung, pancreatic, gastrointestinal, breast, ovarian, and genitourinary cancers, lymphomas, and brain tumors.

APPROACH TO AN ELEVATED PT or PTT

- A "*mixing study*" or ""*1 to 1 dilution test*" ✪ can be done in order to see if the patient is lacking in a particular clotting factor **or** if a factor inhibitor is present. Essentially, where patient serum is mixed with control serum (that should have all the appropriate clotting factors), *then the patient's PTT should normalize or "correct" if s/he was deficient in a particular factor* (that the control patient's serum provided). *If it doesn't correct, then a factor inhibitor is present* (e.g. factor VIII inhibitor, lupus anticoagulant, anticardiolipin antibody that could increase the PTT).

    - ✪ **PT/PTT CORRECTS:**   Evaluate for FACTOR DEFICIENCIES or vWD. Measure **FACTOR V** to distinguish between 2 common causes of acquired factor deficiencies, namely **liver disease** *versus* **vitamin K deficiency,** *since factor V is independent of vitamin K.* (Of course, you could just choose to give vitamin K and see if the PT or PTT normalizes!):

- ➢ **If Factor V is low,** then there is **hepatic** dysfunction; if it's normal, vitamin K deficiency is present.

- ➢ *Remember "1972" to help remind you of which factors are vitamin K-dependent: that is, Factor 10, 9, 7, and 2 (as well as protein C & S).*

- ✪ **PT/PTT FAILS TO CORRECT,** factor inhibitors, such as <u>FACTOR VIII INHIBITOR</u> and <u>ANTIPHOSPHOLIPID ANTIBODIES</u> (e.g. lupus anticoagulant and anticardiolipin antibodies—*described below*) should be ruled out. The next step is to **add a source of phospholipid** to the mixed plasma. Correction of the PTT suggests the presence of antiphospholipid antibodies.

  - ➢ If the PTT <u>STILL</u> does not correct, the Bethesda assay is performed to rule out *Factor VIII inhibitor*. Alternatively, the *Russell Viper Venom Time* can be checked (prolonged in the presence of antiphospholipid antibody) . In RVVT the venom bypasses factor V to activate factor X, but still needs phospholipid to work.

    - ☞ The sudden presence of *large hematomas or extensive ecchymoses in an elderly individual without significant trauma* or known bleeding disorder should always raise the clinical suspicion of acquired **factor VIII inhibitor.**

      versus…

    - ☞ Patients with **antiphospholipid antibodies,** on the other hand, tend to present with *thrombotic* rather than bleeding episodes.

- ✪ <u>**KEY ANTIPHOSPHOLIPID SYNDROMES**</u> (*factor inhibitors* which ↑ PTT)

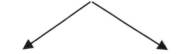

Lupus Anticoagulant　　　　**Anticardiolipin Antibody**
(This is a *pro*coagulant!)

ANTIPHOSPHOLIPID ANTIBODY SYNDROME

- ➢ *Since antiphospholipid antibodies include lupus anticoagulant and anti-cardiolipin antibodies, either of these can lead to antiphospholipid antibody syndrome.*

- ➢ These antibodies, <u>cross react with</u> several negatively-charged phospholipids, accounting for many of the clinical findings.

- ➢ *Remember lupus 'ANTI-coagulant' is actually a 'PRO-coagulant', as clearly seen in this syndrome since it predisposes to DVT and arterial thrombosis*

➤ CLINICAL MANIFESTATIONS ✪
  1. **Recurrent spontaneous abortions**
  2. **Thrombocytopenia**
  3. **Neurologic events**
  4. **Venous thromboses**
  5. **Arterial Thromboses**
       a) CVA; recurrent TIAs
       b) Extremity gangrene
       c) Visceral infarction
  6. **Livedo Reticularis**
  7. **↑ PTT**
  8. **False + VDRL**

➤ Can be 1° or 2°
  ■ **2° causes:**
      o Autoimmune diseases, eg **SLE**, RA
      o Drugs (eg antibiotics, procainamide, hydralazine)
      o Viral infections (Hep C, HIV, syphilis)
      o Lymphoma

COMMON DDX OF LUPUS ANTICOAGULANT
  1. SLE
  2. ITP
  3. RA
  4. AIDS
  5. *Drugs*: dilantin, hydralazine, quinidine, procainamide

✪ CRYOPRECIPITATE VS. FRESH FROZEN PLASMA:

	KEY INDICATIONS	**FACTORS**
FFP	Multiple clotting deficiencies, DIC, severe liver disease, coumadin overdose	All factors (but relatively remember high volume load)
CRYOPRECIPITATE	Hemophilia A, vWD, DIC, Factor 13 deficiency	vWF, 8, 13, fibrinogen

WARFARIN

  1. Use **INR 2.5-3.5 for the following** important scenarios:
     ➤ *Recurrent DVT or prior thrombolembolism*
     ➤ *Prevention of recurrent MI*
     ➤ *Prosthetic heart valve*
     ➤ *Mitral stenosis*
     ➤ *Persistent atrial thrombus on TEE*

2. Afib, routine DVT, CVA, and most medical and surgical thromboembolic states→ shoot for **INR 2.0-3.0**

3. Contraindicated in pregnancy because of the risk of teratogenesis (nasal hypoplasia; CNS abnormalities)

4. Re: Metronidazole and Sulfonamides: $\uparrow$ warfarin level
   Barbiturates, Carbamazapine, and Rifampin: $\downarrow$ warfarin level

LOW MOLECULAR-WEIGHT Heparin- - ADVANTAGES Over Conventional Heparin:

1. *Precludes daily   PTT* determination
2. *More predictable* response
3. *Better safety* profile (eg less thrombocytopenia)
4. Ease of administration
5. And, of course, less time in the hospital (following a regimen such as the one shown below for enoxaparin, most patients are admitted to the hospital for observation *overnight*, and discharged the next morning.)

OUTPATIENT DVT MANAGEMENT with Enoxaparin (a Low Molecular Weight Heparin):

1. If patient is appropriate for outpatient therapy[1] , arrange instruction in self-injection thru a home health nurse.
2. Educate about the side effects of LMWH and signs/symptoms of a PE
3. Dosing of enoxaparin is **1mg/kg SC q 12h**
4. Oral anticoagulation with warfarin is started at the same time, with a 5 mg loading dose daily for two days with further dosing adjusted to keep the INR between 2 and 3. There should be an **overlap for at least 5 days** between LMW heparin and warfarin, and LMW heparin should not be discontinued before day five even if the INR is in the therapeutic range. The initial rise in the INR induced by warfarin primarily reflects its effect on factor VII, which has the shortest plasma half-life. However, the full antithrombotic effect of warfarin requires a reduction in factor X and prothrombin levels, which occurs at four to five days.
5. **Continue warfarin for 3-6 months**, but consider long-term treatment with warfarin if this is a 2nd episode of DVT.

[1.] *Patient should not have any of the following*:
   a. Active PUD
   b. Concurrent symptomatic PE
   c. Current active bleeding
   d. Familial bleeding disorder
   e. Inability to use LMWH because of some coexistant disease
   f. Known deficiency of AT III, Protein C, or Protein S
   g. Noncompliance
   h. Pregnancy
   i. ≥ 2 prior episodes of DVT or PE

> The new AHA guidelines on **Low-Molecular-Weight Heparins** (e.g. Lovenox®= enoxaparin, Fragmin®=dalteparin, Innohep®=tinzaparin) recommend _LMW heparins as FIRST-LINE for prevention and treatment of venous thromboembolism (VTE) and even unstable angina as an alternative to heparin._

INDICATION	MODERN OPTIONS
Preventing VTE: Total Hip Replacement or abdominal surgery)	Lovenox or Fragmin
Preventing VTE: Knee Surgery and medical patients at high risk for VTE	Lovenox
Treating VTE	Warfarin + either Lovenox or Innohep
Unstable angina OR non-Q-wave MIs	ASA + either Lovenox or Fragmin

Current Labeling for Oral ANTIPLATELET AGENTS				
Indication	**ASA**	**Ticlopidine** (Ticlid®)	**Clopidogrel** (Plavix®)	**ASA/ER DP** (Aggrenox®)
Established PAD	No	No	Yes	No
Recent MI	Yes	No	Yes	No
Recent ischemic stroke	Yes	Yes	Yes	Yes
ASA, aspirin; **ASA/ER DP,** aspirin/extended-release dipyridamole; **PAD,** peripheral arterial disease; **MI,** myocardial infarction				

TICLID

> An antiplatelet agent indicated to reduce the risk of thrombotic stroke (fatal or nonfatal) in patients who have experienced stroke precursors, and in patients who have had a completed thrombotic stroke.

> Because TICLID can cause life threatening hematological adverse reactions including _neutropenia/agranulocytosis and thrombotic thrombocytopeinic purpura (TTP),_ TICLID should be reserved _for patients who are intolerant or allergic to aspirin therapy or who have failed aspirin_ therapy.

PLAVIX

> An adenosine diphosphate (ADP)-receptor antagonist indicated for the reduction of atherosclerotic events (myocardial infarction [MI], stroke, and vascular death) in patients with atherosclerosis documented by recent stroke, recent MI, or established peripheral arterial disease (PAD).
> Does not require routine hematological monitoring.

APLASTIC ANEMIA

1. 2° to a stem cell defect

2. **Pancytopenia**, hypocellular bone marrow

3. **Mortality 80% at 2 years unless allo BMT or ATG (antithymocyte globulin)**

4. Idiopathic is #1 cause; drugs are #2 cause

5. **PNH and infections (Hepatitis C esp.; also Hep B)** ✪ are #3 cause.

6. **Take special care with transfusions!** If transfusions are needed, select nonrelated donors and use leuk-depleted PRBCs and single-donor platelets. Family members should not be transfusion donors since they are more likely to sensitize the patient to minor HLA antigens present in the donor, but absent in the patient.

7. BMT carries a 65% success rate in young patients

8. Treatment options include: immunosuppression with cyclosporine + steroids, BMT, or ATG (anti-thymocyte globulin; if older than 45-50 and no HLA-match).

9. ✪ **Parvovirus B19** can induce transient aplastic anemia in nearly all hemolytic conditions, *including* hereditary spherocytosis, sickle cell disease, thalassemias, red cell enzyme deficiencies, PNH, and autoimmune hemolysis. And unlike B19 patients with erythema infectiosum or arthropathy, those with transient aplastic crisis are viremic and can readily transmit the virus to others.

HEMOCHROMATOSIS (Systemic Disease Of Iron Overload)

1. *Remember*: transferrin sat >60% in men and > 50% in women—best SCREENING test.

2. **CLINICAL:**

   a. **Endocrine**
      i. DM
      ii. Hypogonadism (impotence, libido, amenorrhea)
      iii. Hypopituitarism
   b. **Liver**
      i. Hepatomegaly
      ii. Cirrhosis (can lead to hepatocellular carcinoma)
   c. **Skin**
      i. Bronze ("bronze diabetes")
   d. **Cardiac**
      i. CHF
      ii. Arrhythmias
   e. **Arthropathy**

3. **IRREVERSIBLE COMPLICATIONS** ✪ in hemochromatosis:
   a. *Arthropathy*
   b. *Hypogonadism*
   c. HCC (Hepatocellular carcinoma)
   d. Hepatic cirrhosis

KEY IMMUNE-MEDIATED TRANSFUSION REACTIONS				
	Immediate-Type (ACUTE HEMOLYTIC)	**DELAYED-TYPE**	**FEBRILE**	**URTICARIA**
HEMOLYSIS	Intravascular	Extravascular	Non-hemolytic	None
ANTIBODY	IgM	IgG	N/A	N/A
CAUSE	ABO incompatibility (ABO antibodies to *donor red cells*)	*Amnestic response to other RBC antigens*, so usually in previously transfused patients	Antibodies to *donor leukocytes*	Reaction to *donor plasma proteins*
PRESENTATION	May present with hypotension, tachypnea, tachycardia, fever, chills, hemoglobinemia, hemoglobinuria, chest and/or flank pain	Hemolytic; the alloantibody is detectable 1 to 2 weeks following the transfusion	Fever, chills, rigors are characteristic; Primarily a dx of exclusion	Pruritic rash, edema, headache, and dizziness; The transfusion may be completed after the signs and/or symptoms resolve.
PREVENTION	Proper ABO matching	These reactions occur in previously transfused patients, who've been sensitized to RBC alloantigens and have a negative alloantibody screen due to low antibody levels. As such, prevention is less an issue.	Leukocyte depleted transfusions if suspect; premedication with acetaminophen or other antipyretic	Patients with a history of allergic transfusion reaction should be premedicated with an antihistamine. Cellular components can be washed to remove residual plasma for the extremely sensitized patient.

IMPORTANT PLATELET TRANSFUSION THRESHOLDS:	
PLATELET COUNT $(x\ 10^3\ /\mu L)$	**CLINICAL SCENARIO**
<10	✓ Asymptomatic
<20	✓ Presence of "clinical factors" that might be associated with bleeding in thrombocytopenic patients are present (temperature >38.5°C, infection, concurrent coagulopathy, DIC, or marked splenomegaly) ✓ *Bone marrow aspiration and biopsy* may be performed even in patients with <20,000/μ L *without* platelet supportive therapy, provided that adequate pressure is applied;
<50	✓ *Active bleeding* ✓ Patients requiring *surgery* (eg laparotomy, thoracotomy, hip replacement and craniotomy)
<100	✓ Life-threatening or clinically significant bleeding ✓ Other CNS surgery (including eye surgery)

3 BASIC PROCESSES THAT GIVE THROMBOCYTOPENIA:
> - **Decreased production** (check for *megakaryocytes* on peripheral smear or bone marrow; analogous to checking reticulocyte count in anemia)
> - **Increased destruction** (analogous to hemolysis in anemia)
> - **Splenic sequestration**

> ✓ Once you've ruled out decreased production, consider these as common causes of platelet destruction or consumption → **"SIT *Down*"**: Splenomegaly, ITP, TTP, DIC

ITP (Idiopathic Thrombocytopenic Purpura)
> - **Drugs commonly implicated**→procainamide; quinine; quinidine; heparin; gold; sulfonamides; and rifampin.
> - Remember, thrombocytopenia can be the first sign of disease in patients with SLE and HIV, so these disorders should be ruled out.
> - **TREATMENT ✪**
>   1. *Steroids*—the mainstay of treatment; used first to decrease Ab production. *IV IgG* increases the platelet count faster than steroids and is therefore useful in patients who are actively bleeding and those with dangerously low platelet counts while the steroids are kicking in (usually takes a few weeks)
>   2. If #1 fails or patients relapse after steroid taper → *splenectomy* to remove the predominant site of Ab production and platelet destruction.
>   3. If #2 fails→ *chemotherapy*

APPENDIX

Figure 1. <u>HEMOLYTIC ANEMIA:</u>

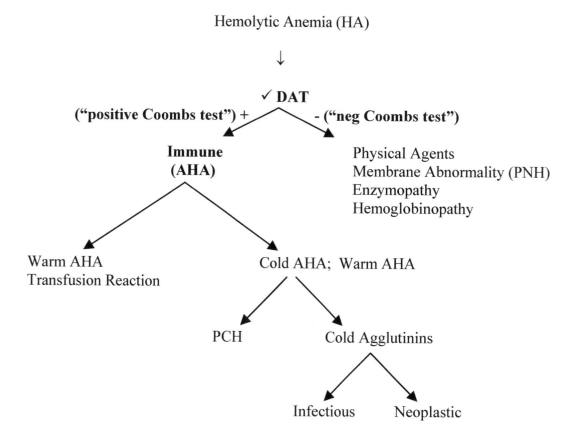

Hemolytic Anemia (HA)

↓

✓ **DAT**

("positive Coombs test") +   - ("neg Coombs test")

Immune (AHA)   Physical Agents
Membrane Abnormality (PNH)
Enzymopathy
Hemoglobinopathy

Warm AHA   Cold AHA; Warm AHA
Transfusion Reaction

PCH   Cold Agglutinins

Infectious   Neoplastic

Figure 2. <u>**OVERVIEW TO THE INTRINSIC & EXTRINSIC CLOTTING CASCADE:**</u>

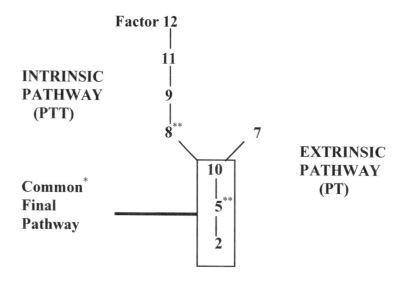

Factor 12

11

**INTRINSIC
PATHWAY
(PTT)**

9

8**   7

**EXTRINSIC
PATHWAY
(PT)**

**Common*
Final
Pathway**

10

5**

2

*Remember: ↑ PT or PTT may also be 2° to deficiencies in factors of the common final pathway.

**Remember too: Protein C(with the help of cofactor Protein S) work to degrade factors 8 and 5; thus deficiencies in these proteins confer a *hyper*coaguable state.

A breakdown of the final steps of the coagulation cascade shows:

- ♦ **Factor 10 + 5 take Prothrombin → Thrombin, which in turn takes Fibrinogen → Fibrin. Then Factor 13 helps to cross-link the fibrin monomers.**

HEPARIN

- ➢ Remember, heparin is a cofactor for AT III, which is the principal inhibitor of Factor 2 (thrombin), and factors 9 thru 11.
- ➢ For this reason think of **antithrombin III deficiency** in patients who have *apparent resistance to heparin.*

LOW-MOLECULAR-WEIGHT HEPARIN

- ➢ Smaller fragments of heparin interact with antithrombin III to give better inhibition of factor Xa and less inhibition of thrombin, which ultimately has several advantages:
    - ✓ *Precludes daily PTT* determination
    - ✓ *Yields a more predictable* response
    - ✓ *Has a better safety* profile (less thrombocytopenia and hemorrhagic complications)
- ➢ Ease of administration
- ➢ And, of course, less time in the hospital

2.   ONCOLOGY

BREAST CA

Who's at risk?
1. Previous h/o breast ca
2. Family history of breast ca
3. early menarche, late first pregnancy, or late menopause—all situations of prolonged estrogen exposure
4. Radiation Exposure at an early age
5. "Benign" breast disease in the form of atypical ductal hyperplasia
6. OCPs and postmenopausal HRT $2°$ to Estrogen

Speaking of HRT…
✪ **Facts you should know about Evista® (RALOXIFENE):**
   ⇒ a SERM (Selective Estrogen Receptor Modulator)
   ⇒ Indicated for prevention of osteoporosis in postmenopausal women;
   ⇒ ↓ risk of breast ca (hormone receptor positive breast ca)
   ⇒ *No* ↑ risk of uterine ca
   ⇒ Does *not* control perimenopausal symptoms, such as hot flashes.

How do you SCREEN? Per ACS guidelines…
1. Monthly self breast exams starting ≥20 yo
2. Clinical breast exam q3y from 20-39 yo
3. Annual clinical breast exam ≥ 40 yo
4. Annual mammogram ≥ 40 yo

Treatment For Breast Cancer *IN SITU*
➢ DCIS (ductal carcinoma in situ) → local excision + radiation versus simple mastectomy.
➢ LCIS (lobular carcinoma in situ) → bilateral breast observation.

PRIMARY TREATMENT OF BREAST CA
▪ Either: a) *MRM* (modified radical mastectomy) + ALND (axillary lymph node dissection) followed by ± XRT (radiation) or b) *lumpectomy* + ALND definitely followed by XRT

ADJUVANT SYSTEMIC THERAPY

▪ *Depends on these 3 factors:*
   i. Pre or Postmenopausal   *and*
   ii. ER + or -   *and*
   iii. Lymph node status (axillary)

If Lymph Nodes + or LN -

	ER +	ER -
PREmenopausal	Chemo *(or Tamox if LN neg)*	Chemo
POSTmenopausal	Tamoxifen	Consider Chemo

✪ CRITICAL GENERAL CONCEPTS IN BREAST CA:

1. The breakdown of breast carcinoma:
   - 80% are infiltrating (or "invasive") ductal
   - 10% are infiltrating lobular
     - ➤ Remember, there is a 50% incidence of *bilaterality* in lobular breast ca
   - The prognosis is similar for infiltrating ductal and infiltrating lobular
   - Medullary and a few others constitute the rest

2. Axillary dissection is needed for *all* patients, whether MRM **or** lumpectomy.

3. If given a breast ca patient with 1 or more *positive <u>Supraclavicular</u> lymph node(s)* on her physical exam, that's automatically <u>Stage 4</u>, because they are **not the natural lymphatic drainage** of the breast, but represent mets.

4. *XRT is not routinely indicated/not necessarily indicated following the lymph node dissection of a MRM* and can unnecessarily result in lymphedema, as opposed to lymph node dissection + lumpectomy, where XRT is always indicated.

5. *Node positive premenopausal* patients get chemo *no matter* what their ER status.

6. *Most patients with node negative disease are cured with primary* treatment alone (i.e. without adjuvant/systemic therapy); adjuvant therapy however offers greater assurance with improved cure rates.

7. In fact, *unless* the patient has *unfavorable tumor features* [high mitotic activity (high S phase), large tumor (> 2.5cm) (another poor feature), undifferentiated/poorly differentiated histology, tumor adherent to skin, chest wall, or pectoralis muscle, matty lymph nodes or + SC nodes, and Her2neu receptor status], **node negative patients with tumors ≤ 1 cm should not receive adjuvant therapy.**

8. In *metastatic ER+* disease, oophorectomy (for premenopausal) or hormonal therapy (for postmenopausal) if there is no visceral involvement.

9. If *metastatic ER -* disease with visceral involvement→CMF or CAF chemo

10. Recall that of all the *prognosticators* in breast ca, positive *lymph nodes* is the most reliable.

11. Remember that *Inflammatory Breast Ca*
   - Requires a biospy to differentiate it from cellulitis or mastitis;
   - It involves rapid progression of skin edema, ridging, and diffuse erythema.
   - Requires aggressive chemotherapy

CERVICAL CA

- Pap smears are critical in screening for this carcinoma.

- *HPV* (Human Papilloma Virus), considered an STD, is the causative agent and, understandably, is rarely, if ever, found in celebate nuns.

- *HSV II* has also been found to be associated with this cancer.

- Screening is recommended with Pap smears as follows
   - *Yearly at onset of sexual activity or starting at age 18*
   - *Every 1-3 years after 3 consecutive smears are negative*

Classification of Preinvasive Cervical Disease			
PAP class	**Dysplasia**	**CIN**	**Bethesda**
I	Normal	Normal	Normal
II	Atypia	Atypia	ASCUS
II or III	Mild dysplasia*	CIN 1	LSIL
III	Moderate dysplasia	CIN 2	HSIL
	Severe dysplasia**	CIN 3	↕
III or IV	CIS	N/A	
V	Cancer	Cancer	
			Cancer

CIN, cervical intraepithelial neoplasia; ASCUS, atypical squamous cells of undetermined significance; LSIL, low-grade squamous intraepithelial lesion; HSIL, high-grade squamous intraepithelial lesion; CIS, carcinoma in situ

* Patients in this category with negative endocervical curettage results should be followed q 4-6 months for up to 2 years with cervical cytologies.
** These patients require cold knife conization and D&C, followed by periodic cervical cytology for 2 years.

- *Women at increased risk for cervical cancer*
   1. $\geq$ 3 sexual partners
   2. Infected with HPV or HIV
   3. History of HSV or other STDs
   4. Cigarette smokers
   5. Previous preinvasive or invasive disease
   6. Lower socioeconomic status
   7. Patients who are poorly compliant with their appointments

COLON CA

Remember...

1. Most tumors start as adenomatous polyps, and the **progression** is from normal mucosa→polyp→cancer over 10 years. Therefore, the risk of a polyp becoming cancerous is related to both size and time. ✪

2. Clinically significant polyps are those measuring > **7mm** (just over ½ cm). ✪

3. After lung, colon ca is the 2nd leading cause of cancer death. ✪

4. After patient's have **Ulcerative Colitis** for 30 years, they have a 1 in 2 chance of developing colon cancer; periodic biopsies should therefore be taken to check for dysplasia, which necessitates colectomy.

5. One's risk of developing colorectal ca is **2-3x ↑ if a first degree relative** has had this carcinoma.

6. **Personal h/o breast, uterine, or ovarian ca doubles your risk.**

7. 100% of patients with **FAP** have become malignant by age 40yo
   a. Screening in affected families: colonoscopy Q year ≥ puberty.
   b. EGD Q 3-5 years after polyps are the first polyps are found.

8. **High fat, low fiber diets** are associated with colorectal ca.

9. In **Peutz-Jeghers syndrome, as opposed to Gardner's syndrome**, the polyps are benign and are not at significant ↑ risk of malignant transformation than regular adenomatous polyps.

10. Recall that polyps are either hyperplastic or adenomatous. Hyperplastic polyps do not have malignant potential. Know that between **tubular** polyps and **villous** polyps, while tubular are much more common, villous polyps are the true "villains" in their malignant potential.

SCREENING—See GI for new ACS criteria on colorectal carcinoma screening/polyp surveillance.

DUKE'S CLASSIFICATION FOR COLORECTAL CA:

Stage	Definition	Treatment
A	Limited to mucosa/submucosa	Surgery
B1	Muscularis mucosa	Surgery
B2	**SEROSA** (into or through)	Surg + Chemo
	(*Remember*, when it comes to the boards, one can never "B2 SERious"...)	
C1	+ regional lymph node mets ≤4	Surg + Chemo
C2	+ regional lymph node mets >4	Surg + Chemo
D	Distant mets	Surg + Chemo

- *CEA* is not for screening! Only use it for follow-up only to check for recurrence.

☞ **5FU (5-fluorouracil) and levamisole** is the Adjuvant Therapy used for Stages ≥ B2

☞ **RECTAL involvement → 5FU and XRT** is the Adjuvant Treatment

✪ CHEMO-RELATED TOXICITIES FOR THE BOARDS

ADRIAMYCIN (Doxorubicin)→dose-related cardiomyopathy and CHF

Bleomycin, **B**CNU (Carmustine), **B**usulfan→ all can give Pulmonary fibrosis. Remember fibrosis is tough, so remember on the boards→"***B tough***!"

CISPLATIN
1. Peripheral neuropathy (similar to Vincristine);
2. Renal tubular damage;
3. Tinnitus & hearing loss.

CYCLOPHOSPHAMIDE
1. Bone: Myelosuppression (see also Melphalan)
2. Bladder: Hemorrhagic cystitis; bladder ca (see also Melphalan)
3. GU: Sterility in males; amenorrhea.

CYCLOSPORINE
1. *Elevations in*: LFTs, K^+, BP (HTN), cholesterol, BUN/creatinine (prerenal picture); hair (hirsutism!)
2. Renal disease*
3. ↓ Mg, tremors, cholestasis

   * Chronic injury results in an irreversible reduction in glomerular filtration rate (GFR), with mild proteinuria and arterial <u>hypertension</u>. <u>Hyperkalemia</u> is a relatively common complication and results in part from tubule resistance to aldosterone. <u>Hypomagnesemia</u> due to urinary magnesium wasting is less common but can cause <u>hypocalcemia</u>.

4. Remember the important <u>drugs which can ↑ cyclosporine (CSA) levels</u>: Might think of stacking (↑) the "<u>DECK</u>": Diltiazem Erythromycin Cimetidine Ketoconazole.

5FU
1. Mucositis
2. Cerebellar ataxia

MELPHALAN
1. Bone: Myelosuppression
2. Bladder: Hemorrhagic cystitis; bladder ca
3. Leukemia

METHOTREXATE
1. Renal toxicity
2. Pulmonary fibrosis (see also Bleomycin)
3. Postnecrotic cirrhosis

MITOMYCIN C → HUS (*Hemolytic Uremic Syndrome*) !

TAMOXIFEN (non-chemo adjuvant tx)
1. Thrombophlebitis
2. ↑ risk of uterine ca
3. ↓ risk of cardiac disease
4. Bone pain, vaginal dryness, hot flashes

TAXOL → Cardiac toxicity

VINCRISTINE → Peripheral neuropathy

✪ POTENTIALLY CURABLE CANCERS FOR THE BOARDS
1. Ewings sarcoma
2. Hodgkin's and NHL
3. Leukemias, acute and chronic
4. Testicular ca

ESOPHAGEAL CA (SCC)

Risk factors:

1. *Alcohol*
2. *Tobacco*
3. Plummer-Vinson syndrome
4. Ingestion of…
    a) Smoked or pickled foods
    b) Lye
6. *Achalasia*
7. Tylosis

HEPATOCELLULAR CA (HCC, "Hepatoma")

1. Any cirrhosis ↑s the risk of HCC, but especially…

    a) HBV, HBC
    b) Alcoholic liver disease
    c) Hemochromatosis

2. Half the time *alpha-fetoprotein* is ↑.
3. Resection is the treatment of choice, as transplantation is complicated by a high rate of recurrence.

✪ LUNG CA

- ***Screening is not warranted*** in lung ca, as opposed to cervical, breast, and colon carcinomas, so "annual chest x-rays" is not appropriate in a preventitive care visit of a low-risk/no-risk non-smoker. In smokers over 50, annual CXR is useful in detecting Stage I disease.

- The main types are **small** cell (also known as oat cell); **squamous** cell; **large** cell; and **adeno** ca. The first 2 are central, and the last two are peripherally located. All four are associated with smoking. Broncho-alveolar lung ca (rare) is not.

  - ✪ Remember, **SMALL** cell and **SQUAMOUS** cell ca lung ca are ***Sentral*** (centrally located).
  - ✪ Remember too, just as **LARGE** cell and **ADENO** ca are peripheral, so either can result in "*peripheral*" findings as seen at the finger tips! (Hypertrophic Osteoarthopathy, HOA)

- Adenocarcinoma: Important points
  - ➢ ***A peripheral non-small cell carcinoma***
  - ➢ **The** most frequently diagnosed lung ca *and* the most common cell-type among non-smokers
  - ➢ Most common cell type in women
  - ➢ also known as ***"scar carcinoma"***.
  - ➢ Weak association with cigarette smoking

- **POTENTIAL COMPLICATIONS** of the four types you must know for the boards:

  - ✪ **SQUAMOUS**→ May Cavitate; ↑ Calcium (ectopic production of **PTH**-like hormone; Sympathetic nerve paralysis ("Horner's syndrome": **m**iosis; **P**tosis; anhydrosis); Pancoast's tumor (with growth into the brachial plexus, C8-T2).

  - ✪ **SMALL CELL**→ "**AACES**":

    ↑**ADH** (SIADH)

    ↑**ACTH** (Cushing's syndrome)

    Carcinoid

    Eaton-Lambert Syndrome
    - Muscle weakness, noted in simple tasks like combing one's hair or rising from a chair
    - Improves with effort/repetitive action

    SVC

☞ Remember the commonly quoted fact in small cell: "The #1 cause of death in survivors of small cell lung ca is ***non-small*** cell lung ca!"

  - **LARGE CELL AND ADENO** *ca*→ HOA (as noted above)

✓ **LARGE CELL only** → **gynecomastia** {that shouldn't be too hard to remember ;) }

✓ **ALL CELL TYPES** are associated with
  ➢ Peripheral neuropathies
  ➢ Subacute cerebellar degeneration
  ➢ Cortical degeneration
  ➢ Polymyositis

STAGING AND TREATMENT

▪ *For treatment purposes, in lung ca the carcinomas are divided into either…*
  1. **Small cell; or**
  2. **Non-small cell**

  … because *staging and managment differ* between small cell and all the others.

✪ Because **Small cell** ca is usually fairly advanced at the time of diagnosis, *Chemo and XRT* are the treatments of choice, **as opposed to Non-small cell,** where *Surgery* is the treatment of choice in the early stages (I-IIIA).

> *Mediastinoscopy/otomy very important in staging; "oscopy" for the right side (no obstruction from the heart, so easier to look around); "otomy" for the left.*

▪ Because of this key difference in mangagement, *staging is viewed slighlty differently* for small cell and non-small cell and goes as follows:

NON-SMALL CELL Lung Ca ✪

Stage	Criteria	Treatment
I	- Hilar nodes	**SURGERY**
II	+ Hilar nodes	**SURGERY**
III A	**IPSILATERAL** involvement of the MED/subcarinal LN or chest wall	**SURGERY**
III **B**	**CONTRALATERAL** mets…	Chemo+XRT ✪
	(*Remember,* "**B**" for "**B**ilateral " & **C**ontralateral → **C**hemo/XRT) …OR supraclavicular mets!	
IV	Distant disease (as always)	Chemo+XRT

SMALL CELL Lung Ca ✪

"Limited Disease"	= Stages I-IIIA*	→	**Chemo** ** **+XRT**
"Extensive Disease"	= Metastases	→	**Chemo only**

* Limited disease, defined as disease confined to the ipsilateral hemithorax and within a single radiotherapy port

** Commonly, *cisplatin and etoposide*.

ADDITIONAL CRITERIA FOR OPERATIVE CANDIDATES (beyond staging):

1. Lung lesion > 2cm from carina

2. Involvement of no major vessels

3. **If preop FEV1 < 2L, MVV <50%, or DLCO <60%, need a quantitative V/Q scan to assess the expected post-op FEV1, which should be > .8L (or 40% of predicted for that patient)**

4. Resting pCO2 >50
   - *Severe COPD and pCO2 >45-50 going into the surgery are considered negative prognosticators.*

HODGKIN'S DISEASE :

1. Central to the diagnosis is the presence of the **Reed-Sternberg cell**, a large cell with a bilobed or multilobulated nucleus with prominent inclusion-like nucleoli, giving the appearance of "owl's eyes."

2. Hodgkin's disease has a bimodal distribution: 20-25 yo and >55 yo.

3. Remember, *staging* in HL is based on *location* of tumor relative to diaphragm, as opposed to staging in NHL, which is based on *histology* /cell type, as specific cell types are classified differently (Low grade; Intermediate grade; High grade; Misc) depending on their aggressiveness. *Treatment*, however, in both HD and NHL is still tied in to tumor location.

4. Remember, the **Cotswolds STAGING system** is an updated or modified Ann Arbor system and is *based on* sites on involvement: *Essentially*, stage **I**: 1 set of nodes on 1 side of the diaphragm; **II**: more than 1 set of LN still on the same side of the diaphragm; **III**: crosses the diaphragm and may include the spleen (III_1 for splenic, celiac, or portal nodes); III_2 for paraaortic, iliac, inguinal, or mesenteric nodes); **IV**: extranodal organ involvement.

   - **Traditionally**, staging *laparotomy* was considered appropriate for all apparent stage I-II disease (essentially, a favorable prognosis buys you surgery) in whom negative results would allow the patient to forgo any unnecessary chemotherapy. That said, staging *laparotomy* is now rarely performed in routine clinical practice, because of the associated morbidity and the apparent lack of survival advantage in patients with favorable prognosis disease, and most patients are *clinically staged, using the same system (below)* through imaging, biopsy, etc.

STAGE	CRITERIA	TREATMENT
I	One LN region, one side of diaphragm	**XRT**
II	Two LN regions, one side of diaphragm	**XRT**
III$_1$	Both sides of diaphragm; specific LN sets	**XRT**
III$_2$	Both sides of diaphragm; specific LN sets	Chemo*
IV	Disseminated disease (bone marrow; liver)	Chemo

* ***Chemo is <u>ABVD</u> (less toxic than MOPP); <u>CHOP</u> is used for NHL.***

☞ Remember, *in Stages II and III,* **<u>add Chemo</u>** *(to XRT)* **<u>for "bulky disease"</u> (the exception).** *Bulky disease* is defined as a mediastinal mass with a maximum width that is ≥ one-third of the internal transverse diameter of the thorax at the level of T5/6 interspace or node or nodal mass **≥ 10 cm** in its largest dimension. Bulky disease is important because it usually warrants the addition of chemotherapy, *even for early stages.* >10 cm maximum dimension of a nodal mass

➢ **In addition, today's approach uses** *prognostic factors* to guide treatment of <u>Stages I and II</u>. Those factors include:

- Large mediastinal adenopathy
- Involvement of ≥4 lymph node regions
- Age over 50 at diagnosis
- A defined combination of B symptoms and elevated erythrocyte sedimentation rate (ESR): B symptoms and an ESR over 30 mm/h or an ESR over 50 mm/h without B symptoms.

☞ Patients with *favorable* prognostic factors are candidates for radiation therapy alone or for modified radiation therapy and chemotherapy. Patients with *unfavorable* prognostic factors should receive chemotherapy and radiation therapy as initial treatment.

---

5. ✪ Histology, nonetheless, is *still* important in prognosis, yes, even in Hodgkin's. For example, "*lymphocyte predominance*" is generally the **best prognosis**, "*nodular sclerosing*" (the **most common** subtype) is common in young patients, classically young women, is frequently mediastinal, and typically responds well to radiation; "*mixed cellularity*" portends an intermediate prognosis and is more common in young to middle-aged men; and "*lymphocyte depletion*" implies the **least favorable prognosis** and is commonly seen in older patients who present with "B" symptoms (as opposed to nodular sclerosis and mixed cellularity, which generally both present with asymptomatic LN enlargement/mass).

---

6. ✪ **<u>Long term complications of chemotherapy</u>** include AML, Solid Tumors, and Diffuse Aggressive Lymphomas; **<u>radiation</u>** leads to an increased incidence of solid tumors, like thyroid, breast, and stomach.

NHL (NON-HODGKIN'S Lymphoma) :

1. Remember, the *staging is based on **HISTOLOGY***
2. **STAGING**: NHL patients fall into one of 3 categories

    i)   **Indolent**
- Small lymphocytic
- Follicular, mixed cleaved
- Follicular, mixed small cleaved and large cell

    ii)   **Aggressive**
- DLCL (Diffuse Large Cell Lymphoma)
- Follicular large cell
- Diffuse small cleaved
- Diffuse mixed small cleaved

    iii)   **Highly aggressive**
- Large cell immunoblastic
- Lymphoblastic
- Small non-cleaved (Burkitt's and non-Burkitt)

  ✓ **INDOLENT** NHL — survival of the untreated disease is measured in **years**
  ✓ **AGGRESSIVE** NHL — survival of the untreated disease is measured in **months**
  ✓ **HIGHLY AGGRESSIVE** NHL — survival of the untreated disease is measured in **weeks**.

3. The **INDOLENT** NHLs are generally associated with reasonably <u>long survival</u>, measured in years, even if left untreated. However, they are usually <u>not curable with conventional treatment</u>. Therefore, *in contrast* to patients with curable aggressive lymphomas, in approaching patients with indolent lymphomas, currently the only major reason for treatment is the alleviation of symptomatic disease.

4. The key **PROGNOSTICATORS** ✪ in NHL are:
   a. LDH (normal vs. elevated)
   b. Age (>60)
   c. ECOG performance status (≥2): A score of 2 or above implies that patient requires rest for ≥ part of the day because of his or her disease, ie *not* "fully ambulatory".
   d. Ann Arbor stage III or IV (this system has some value in NHL too; see below)
   e. Number of extranodal disease sites >1
   f. Tumor burden, which takes into consideration:

- Systemic symptoms
- ≥3 lymph nodes sites >3 cm
- A single lymph node site >7 cm
- Platelets <100,000/μL or absolute neutrophil count <1,000/μL
- Circulating lymphoma cells >5,000/μL
- Marked splenomegaly, compressive symptoms, pleural effusion, or ascites.

5. **TREATMENT**:

GRADE (Histologic)	STAGE	MANAGEMENT
INDOLENT	I, II	XRT
	III, IV	Chemotherapy* + XRT to bulky nodes
AGGRESSIVE	I, II	Chemo + XRT
	III, IV	Chemo as intrathecal methotrexate
HIGHLY AGGRESSIVE	I-IV	As for intermediate III & IV above

* CHOP is the usual regimen; additional agents being used include in various combinations:
  - ✓ Monoclonal antibodies (eg rituximab), interferon, fludarabine and "aggressive combination chemotherapy" regimens, other than CHOP
  - ✓ CHOP + rituxan (anti-CD20 monoclonal Ab) is currently being evaluated into for aggressive lymphomas

6. Between the HLs and NHLs, bone marrow involvement is common only among the low-grade NHLs.

7. Additional points on *highly aggressive* lymphomas:
   - ✓ Often see Neurologic involvement
   - ✓ Allogeneic BMT following remission
   - ✓ ↑↑LDH and U.A. and low phos
   - ✓ 30-40% survival for all comers
   - ✓ "Leukemic" when bone marrow involved

MALIGNANCIES ASSOCIATED WITH AIDS
1. HL and NHL as well as CNS Lymphoma
2. Cervical ca
3. Kaposi's sarcoma
4. Anal carcinoma

MOST COMMON MALIGNANCIES CAUSING SPINAL CORD COMPRESSION
Breast
Lung
Lymphoma
Multiple myeloma.
Prostate

MULTIPLE MYELOMA ✪

- **M-protein is > 3g/dl.** _Remember, though not all patients with myeloma have a monoclonal protein in the serum._ In fact, 20% will only have light chains, which of course, must be measured in a 24-hour urine collection.

- **Plasma cells in the bone marrow > 10%**

- **Urinary light chains (Bence Jones proteins)**

- **Anemia** (normocytic, normochromic)—check for **_Rouleau_** formation on the PBS; ↑ **Ca;** ↑ **creat; osteolytic** (_"punched out"_) bone lesions 2° to **OAF** (osteoclast-activating factor)—invisible on bone scan since no new bone formation occurs. See osteolytic vs. osteoblastic section below.

- **Clinically** in order (most common to least common): bone pain; renal insufficiency; hypercalcemia; weakness, fatigue, and spinal cord compression

- **Know the multiple mechanisms of renal insufficiency or failure in these patients:**
- **"U CLAP"** (you will when you see this): hyperUricemia → uric acid crystallization within the collecting tubules; hyperCalcemia (most common cause); Light chain deposition disease; Amyloidosis; and Plasma cell infiltration

- Often see a decreased anion gap [i.e., $Na^+ - (Cl^- + HCO_3^-)$] because the M component is cationic, resulting in retention of chloride for compensation.

- ↑**Incidence:**
  i. Pneumococcal pneumonia
  ii. Gram-negative infections
  iii. Herpes Zoster

- **_Melphalan and Prednisone_** commonly used in the **_treatment_** of this incurable disease, as it is the least toxic and least expensive regimen Treatment should be **delayed** until **_either_** evidence of progression or imminent complications.

MONOCLONAL GAMMOPATHY ✪ (MGUS is abbrev for "monoclonal gammopathy of undetermined significance")

- The diagnosis of MGUS is made when an _M protein_ (monoclonal protein; M-spike) is _found in the absence of_ multiple myeloma, amyloidosis, Waldenstrom's macroglobulinemia, cryoglobulinemia, or other lymphoproliferative disorder.

- In contrast to multiple myeloma specifically, _there is no_ anemia, no renal failure, no lytic bone lesions, no hypercalcemia, and no urinary Bence Jones proteins.

- Found in up to 10% of individuals > 75yo.

- ▪ **<u>M-protein is < 3g/dl</u>**

- ▪ **<u>Plasma cells in the bone marrow < 10%</u>**

- ▪ While long-term follow-up shows that approximately 25 percent of patients with MGUS eventually transform into myeloma, patients with MGUS pe se require no therapy, and survival, on average is only about 2 years shorter than age-matched controls without MGUS.

OSTEOLYTIC *versus* OSTEOBLASTIC LESIONS

> ✓ **Purely** osteo<u>lyt</u>ic lesions → MM and renal cell ca
> ✓ Osteo<u>blast</u>ic lesions → prostate and breast ca

PANCREATIC CA

- ▪ The primary etiology in " *adenoca of unknown primary*", so when you don't know what the source of the adenoca metastasis is, check either CT or U/S of the pancreas.

- ▪ Remember that even before patient's are told they have pancreatic ca and even before they are symptomatic, there is an ↑ risk of pancreatic ca having an endogenous *depression*, which is felt to be 2° to an unknown paraneoplastic substrate.

- ▪ ↑ incidence of *migratory thrombophlebitis* (so called "Trouseau's Syndrome"✪)

PROSTATE CA

- ▪ *The ACS (American Cancer Society) recommends DRE Q year >40 and PSA Q year > 50. Discontinue when life expectancy< 10 years.*

- ▪ *PSA values: <4 is OK; 4-10 is observation and/or TRUS (Transrectal U/S) ± biopsy; >10 should undergo TRUS + biopsy*

- ▪ *30-40% of men>60 have malignant prostate cells and will die WITH them, not OF them.* Only 8-9% of these individuals will be diagnosed with prostate ca per se. And only a small % of those will die OF prostate ca. Remember, growth into a clinically important ca takes up to 15 years. It's all about the quality and quantity (if any) of years that you're adding by screening and follow-up compared to the side-effects the treatment will cause. These side effects may include: impotence (usually from the XRT or prostatectomy). That's the controversy!

- ▪ **Significance of % Free PSA:**

  - • Useful in eliminating unnecessary prostate biopsies in the diagnostic "gray zone" (PSA 4-10). A *low total % free PSA* (<25%) is associated with ↑ risk of malignancy.

- % free PSA has no role in the initial evaluation of men with an abnormal DRE, as they should all proceed to biopsy.
- For total PSA in the range of 4-10 ng/mL, % free PSA should be measured. If <25% → prostate biopsy. If ≥ 25% → annual total PSA and DRE. Cutoff at this level of 25% eliminates 20% of unnecessary biopsies with resulting sensitivity of 95%.

- The men at ↑**risk** are those African-Americans and those with + Fam Hx.

Risk factor:	*Risk of developing prostate ca:*
A frican-American	2x the relative risk
F ather had it	3x the relative risk
B rother had it	4x the relative risk

Remember "A→F→B" for the order of which is 2, which is 3, and which is 4.

- As with breast ca, this is a hormonally-driven ca, by androgens, no estrogen.

STAGING & TREATMENT

Stage	Criteria	Treatment
A1	*Microscopic*; **<5%** of specimen	Observation
A2	*Microscopic*; **>5%** of specimen	**Prostatectomy versus XRT**
B1	**1** *nodule*, **limited to 1 lobe**	" " "
B2	**Several** *nodules*, **both lobes**	" " "
C	**C**apsular &/or Extra**C**apsular (e.g. the seminal vesicles)	XRT/radioactive seed implant
D1	Pelvic nodes +	(controversial)
D2	Distant mets	Androgen deprivation

➢ Results of *XRT and prostatectomy* are comparable, and XRT is less likely to cause impotence than prostatectomy

➢ Results of *anti-androgen therapy and orchiectomy* are comparable for Stage D2

➢ *Implantable radioactive seeds* are rapidly gaining acceptance, at least as an additional therapeutic alternative to XRT and even prostatectomy.

➤ *Total androgen ablation* is usually achieved using **leuprolide** (Leupron®), actually an LHRH agonist which acts to ultimately inhibit androgen production, plus **flutamide** (Eulexin®), which inhibits androgen binding to its receptor. Remember too that androgens are also produced in the adrenal cortex, and this can be stopped too using **aminoglutethimide**.

MALIGNANT MELANOMA

▪ Similar to breast ca, the *incidence* of malignant melanoma is ↑ing rapidly 2° to earlier dx

▪ Know the *risk factors*…

> ➤ Repeated and/or blistering sun exposure as a child
> ➤ + FH
> ➤ Fair skin
> ➤ Dysplastic nevi—the source of half of melanomas

▪ Of course, *ABCD* keys to diagnosis: Asymmetry; Borders irregular; Color is variable, esp with blues/blacks/tans; Diameter ≥ 6mm

---

✪ *Not to be confused with the above 6mm (!), you should know that the best independent predictor of survival is the thickness of the melanoma on biopsy, and that thickness you hope is ≤.76mm for high chance of survival. See Dermatology for more on this.*

▪ Re: *Moh's surgery* ✪ is both diagnostic and therapeutic and involves essentially shaving off the lesion tier by tier until the margins are clear per the pathologist. Melanoma is not the only indication for Moh's surgery, which can be used in tumors involving cosmetically or aesthetically sensitive zones.

▪ Remember *sentinel lymph node mapping* ✪ is used for melanoma and is increasingly being used for breast ca (to spare the patient unnecessarily extensive lymph node dissections)

SKIN DISEASE AS MANIFESTATION OF MALIGNANCY ✪

1. Acanthosis nigricans (not just DM and obesity!)→GI malignancy, esp gastric; also most conditions associated with insulin resistance. See Dermatology for more on acanthosis nigricans.

2. Actinic keratosis→SCC

3. Café au lait spots→ Von Recklinghausen's disease

4. Dysplastic nevus→Malignant melanoma

5. Epidermal cysts, fibromas, lipomas→Gardner's syndrome

6. Flushing, telangiectasias→Carcinoid tumors

7. Mucosal hyperpigmentation (esp. lips)→ Peutz-Jeghers syndrome

8. Necrolytic erythematous rash (NME: Necrolytic Migratory Erythema)→Glucagonoma

IMPORTANT POINTS ON BRCA1 AND BRCA2:

☞ ↑ Risk of breast and ovarian ca

☞ **BRCA 1 & 2 are <u>tumor suppression genes</u>.** Mutations to these genes "<u>unsuppresses</u>" ca risk and confers an ↑d risk of ca in an autosomal dominant fashion; 5-10% of all cases of breast ca

☞ The cumulative risk (to age 70) of developing **<u>breast ca in females</u>** due to mutations of either BRCA 1 or 2 is 60-80%, vs. cumulative 11% risk in the population at large (up to age 79)

☞ Also, while there is a significant ↑ in relative risk (6% vs. .1% for population at large) of developing **<u>breast ca in males</u>** with BRCA2 mutation, there is no ↑d relative risk in men who have BRCA1.

☞ By age 70, women with BRCA1 mutations also have an **<u>ovarian cancer</u>** risk of up to 40% (20% for BRCA2).

☞ **<u>Genetic testing is indicated</u>** only if the prior probability of abnormalities is ≥ 10%, as revealed by family and clinical history. But in general, testing would be appropriate in each of the following situations:

    1. Patient has ≥ 2 blood relatives—mother, sister, aunt, cousin, or daughter—with premenopausal breast ca or ovarian ca at any age;

    2. Patient has been diagnosed with breast ca, esp premenopause, *and* has a blood relative w/ breast or ovarian cancer;

    3. Patient with ≥ 2 family members with breast cancer diagnosed < 50 yo

    4. Patient has been diagnosed with ovarian ca and has blood relatives who have had ovarian or breast ca;

    5. Patient is related to someone (male or female) who has a BRCA 1 or 2 mutation.

    6. Male patient with breast cancer

    7. Early-onset (<50 yo) breast or ovarian ca in patients of Ashkenazi Jewish ancestry.

☞ Patients found to carry these mutations should be encouraged to commit to an intensive, lifelong program of cancer surveillance.

☞ **Women with a BRCA mutation should have** a:
    ✓ Mammogram every year beginning at age 25 yo
    ✓ Clinical breast exam 1-2 times/y beginning at 25 yo
    ✓ BSE q mo > 18 yo
    ✓ A pelvic exam once or twice a year beginning at 25-35yo
    ✓ Transvaginal U/S with color doppler once or twice a year starting at 25-35 yo
    ✓ Serum CA 125 every year beginning age 25-35 yo.

REVISED CRITERIA FOR THE DX OF HNPCC (Hereditary Nonpolyposis Colorectal Cancer)

    * *≥ 3 relatives with an HNPCC-associated cancer* (colon, endometrium, ovary, small bowel, ureter, renal pelvis)
        * ≥ 1 should be a 1st degree relative of the other 2
        * ≥ 2 successive generations affected
        * ≥ 1 relative diagnosed before age 50

    * *Tumor should be assessed pathologically*
    * *FAP should be excluded*

TESTICULAR CA ✪

Basics first...

1. The #1 ca in males 15-35 yo

2. The biggest risk factor is ***cryptorchidism***, or undescended testes. ***Surgically bringing down the teste does not reduce the risk of ca.*** Klinefelter's is another risk factor.

3. Similar to lung ca or Hodgkins, there are 2 overall categories...
   a. Seminomas
   b. Non-seminomas

4. **SEM**inomas are highly radio**SEN**sitive, and only 10% secrete <u>Beta-HCG</u>; never AFP!!

5. **Non-seminomas** on the other hand do not respond to XRT and secrete <u>both AFP and Beta-HCG</u>. This is clearly summarized in the following table ✪:

	SEMINOMA	NON-SEMINOMA
AFP	<u>**No**</u>	Yes
B-HCG	Yes	Yes

6. ✪ The primary ***treatment*** is radical (inguinal) orchiectomy. Then, if the biopsy shows seminoma, the treatment is **XRT** for Stages 1 and 2. For Stage 1 non-seminoma, surgery followed by observation is usually sufficient. ***For everything else***, it's **platinum-based** chemo!

STAGE	CRITERIA	<u>SEMINOMA</u> vs.	<u>NONSEMINOMA</u>
I	Limited to testes	Surg→**XRT**	Surg→observe
II	→ Peritoneum (low grade: < 6LN+ and LN < 2cm)	**XRT**	Chemo
III	→ Peritoneum (high grade: >6LN+ or LN > 2cm)	Chemo	Chemo
IV	Distant mets	Chemo	Chemo

7. ✪ Remember, ***testicular carcinoma is <u>highly curable, even when metastatic</u>*** (e.g. to the mediastinum).

8. ✪ Finally, remember that if any solitary ***lung mets*** are detected post-chemo, they may be surgically ***removed***.

3. RHEUMATOLOGY

DDX OF MORNING STIFFNESS/PAIN WORSE IN AM
1. **Rheumatoid arthritis**
   - ✓ Difficulty doing up buttons
2. **Ankylosing Spondylitis**
   - ✓ LBP + stiffness radiating to buttocks and thighs
3. **Polymyalgia Rheumatica (PMR)**
   - ✓ Difficulty getting out of bed
4. **Fibromyalgia**

	RHEUMATOID ARTHRITIS	OSTEOARTHRITIS
ETIOLOGY	Autoimmune disease	Degenerative disease
PATTERN of symptoms	Morning stiffness	Worse after effort or as activity progresses; relieved by rest
Predominant HAND joint involvement	PIP, MCP, wrists; symmetric	CMC, PIP, DIP
LAB	+ RF, ↑ESR and C-reactive protein	Normal RF, ESR, CRP
XRAY findings	1. **Periarticular osteopenia** 2. Symmetrical narrowing or the joint space 3. **Marginal bony erosions** 4. Subluxation and gross deformity	1. **Osteophyte** formation 2. **Subchondral sclerosis** (*no* periarticular osteopenia) 3. Joint space narrowing 4. Loose bodies

SEVEN DIAGNOSTIC CRITERIA FOR RHEUMATOID ARTHRITIS*
1. Morning stiffness
2. Arthritis of ≥ 3 joint areas
3. Arthritis of the hand joints
4. Symmetric arthritis
5. Rheumatoid nodules
6. Serum rheumatoid factor
7. Radiographic changes

* In order to have RA, you must have ≥ 4 of the 7 criteria present and #1-4 must be present for at least 6 weeks.

NODES AND NODULES IN RHEUMATIC DISEASE
1. Heberden's nodes→ DIP osteophytes in 1° OA
2. Bouchard's nodes→ PIP osteophytes in 1° OA
3. Rheumatoid nodules
4. Gouty tophi (elbow, ears, heels, PIPs, DIPs)
5. Xanthomata

THERAPEUTIC EMERGENCIES IN RHEUMATIC DISEASE

1. **Atlanto-axial subluxation**
   - Tends to affect RA patients on chronic steroids
   - Treatment→Surgical decompression and fusion for progressive symptomatic disease
2. **Temporal Arteritis**
   - Draw blood for ESR as soon as dx suspected
   - Treat with high dose prednisone (60mg/day) as soon as ESR drawn
   - Biopsy appearances are unaffected by ≤ 48hours of steroid therapy.
3. **Septic Arthritis**
   - Drain joint; gram stain; C&S
   - IV Abx
   - Occasionally, arthroscopic debridement may be necessarily, e.g. if poorly responsive to Abx
4. **Vasculitic Complications**
   - Mononeuritis Multiplex; digital gangrene; bowel infarction
   - High-dose steroids; cytotoxic drugs; surgery
5. **Iridocyclitis**
   - May complicate seronegative spondyloarthropathy (but *not* RA)
6. **Episcleritis**
   - May complicate RA (but not seronegative spondyloarthropathies)

✪ **EXTRA-ARTICULAR MANIFESTATIONS OF R.A. :** **"CLEAN SPUDS"**→
  (*more common in patients with high titres of RF*)

C ardiac
L ymphadenopathy; *Leukocytoclastic vasculitis* (small vessel vasculitis)→*palpable purpura; Low pleural fluid glucose*. Leukocytosis
E *piscleritis* (usually treated topically)
A nemia (normocytic), Amyloidosis
N europathies (e.g. *Mononeuritis Multiplex*)

S jogren's syndrome (*keratoconjunctivitis sicca*, or 2° Sjogren's, is the #1 opthalmic complication)
P ulmonary infiltration→fibrosis; Pleurisy; obstructive lung dz of RA is associated with *keratoconjunctivitis sicca*; Pneumoconiosis→large nodules (*Caplan's syndrome*); Pericarditis
U lcerated legs; Uveitis
D igital vasculitis
S kin nodules (caused by endarteritis, a form of vasculitis)

☞ *Remember*: **Palpable Purpura almost always suggests an antecedent leukocytoclastic vasculitis.**

CHARACTERISTICS OF SYNOVIAL FLUID IN A NORMAL JOINTS:

1. Highly viscous

2. Clear

3. Essentially acellular

4. Glucose concentration similar to that in plasma

✪ SYNOVIAL FLUID ANALYSIS				
FEATURE	**NORMAL**	**NONINFLAMMATORY** (eg osteoarthritis)	**INFLAMMATORY** (eg RA, crystal-induced, spondyloarthropathies, connective tissue dz, HOA)	**SEPTIC**
Clarity	Transparent	Transparent	Transparent	Opaque
Color	Clear	Yellow	Yellow to opalescent	Yellow to Green
Culture	-	-	-	Often +
Glucose	Approximates blood	Approximates blood	>25 mg/dL, but lower than blood	<25 mg/dL
LDH (c/w blood levels)	Low	Low	High	Variable
Viscosity	High	High	Low	Variable
WBCs/mm^3	<200	200-2,000	2000-10,000	>100,000
%PMN	<25	<25	≥50	≥75

* Inflammatory — Inflammatory effusions may be caused by rheumatoid arthritis, acute crystal-induced synovitis, Reiter's syndrome, ankylosing spondylitis, psoriatic arthritis, arthritis associated with inflammatory bowel disease, rheumatic fever, systemic lupus erythematosus (SLE), hypertrophic osteoarthropathy, and scleroderma. Rheumatic fever, SLE, and scleroderma can also cause a noninflammatory effusion.

NOTES ON ASA and NSAIDs→common PRECAUTIONS/INTERACTIONS on boards:

✓ **ASA→** Decreases metabolism of <u>**oral hypoglycemics and therefore ↓s glu values!**</u>

✓ Most **NSAIDs**→diminish the effects of <u>**anti-HTN meds**</u>

✓ While ASA *irreversibly* inhibits cyclooxygenase, NSAIDs *reversibly* inhibit the enzyme.

✪ **IMPORTANT POINTS RE: COX-2 INHIBITORS**

➢ Lower incidence of significant GI toxicity when c/w NSAIDs
➢ No effect on platelet aggregation
➢ Similar renal and hepatic effects c/w NSAIDs
➢ Contraindicated in patients with urticaria, asthma, or other allergic-type reactions to ASA or other NSAIDs
➢ Can be dosed daily for osteoarthritis
➢ Can be dosed without regard to food intake
➢ Celecoxib (Celebrex®) is contraindicated in patients with allergic-type reactions to sulfonamides
➢ Rofecoxib (Vioxx®) can give a dose-dependent ↑ in periperhal edema/HTN/CHF

✪ DMARD Therapy for RA →("GOLD PILE SCAM")		
DMARD	**Potential Toxicities Requiring F/U**	**Monitoring Studies**
Gold IM and PO	Myelosuppression, proteinuria	CBC and urine dipstick for protein
Penicillamine	Myelosuppression, proteinuria	CBC and urine dipstick for protein
Infliximab (Remicade®)*	Flu-like sx, auto-Abs; for patients not responding to methotrexate; given IV	none
Leflunomide (Arava®)	Thrombocytopenia, hepatotoxicity, diarrhea	CBC and AST
Etanercept (Enbrel®) (a TNF α-blocker)	Reactions at site of SQ injection, flu-like sx	none
Sulfasalazine	Myelosuppression	CBC, AST, creatinine
Chlorambucil	Myelosuppression, myeloproliferative disorders, malignancy	CBC
Corticosteroids (PO prednisone, others.)	HTN, ↑glucose, osteoporosis	Baseline BP, chem panel, lipid profile, bone densitometry in high-risk patients; f/u glucose and lipids as indicated
Cyclophosphamide	Myelosuppression, myeloproliferative disorders, malignancy, hemorrhagic cystitis	CBC, urinalysis, and urine cytology
Cyclosporine	Renal insufficiency, anemia, HTN, hirsutism	Creatinine, CBC, K+, LFTs
Azathioprine	Myelosuppression, hepatotoxicity, lymphoproliferative disorders	CBC
Antimalarials (Hydroxycholorquine)	Macular damage	Yearly opthalmologic exams
Methotrexate	Myelosuppression, hepatic fibrosis, cirrhosis, pulmonary infiltrates or fibrosis	CBC, AST, albumin
Minocycline	Photosensitivity, skin discoloration, GI upset, drug-induced hepatitis, dizziness	none

* Remember, infliximab is a chimeric (mouse/human) monoclonal antibody to TNF and must be used in combination with MTX

MORE ABOUT...

Cyclophosphamide (e.g. treatment of **Wegener's**; works by ↓ing B cells, T cells; beware that its metabolite, acrolein, is toxic and can lead to hemorrhagic cystitis, which can be prevented with the use of MESNA; other toxicities include infertility, teratogenicity, and bone marrow suppression); **C**yclosporine; **C**orticosteroids.

Antimalarial drugs (e.g. **hydroxycholorquine**→ **retinopathy** is the major toxicity; clinical response to hydroxycholorquine may not be seen for 2-6 months after initiating); also **A**zathioprine (↓ dose by half if used in simultaneously with *allopurinol*)

Methotrexate (good combination of efficacy and tolerability as seen in **RA**; however, GI toxicity #1 side effect; **CBC, LFTs, PFTs** all should be monitored; beware that **cryptic cirrhosis** may develop **without** ↑LFTs; interstitial lung disease and fibrosis may lead to **↓DLCO on PFTs; however, this can also be 2° to RA itself!**)

DMARDs (Disease-modifying antirheumatoid drugs): 2 KEY POINTS:

1. Do not wait to start patients on DMARDs until after they have failed multiple courses of NSAIDs. Begin therapy with DMARDs as soon as the diagnosis of RA is confirmed.
2. Methotrexate is the DMARD of choice in patients with severe disease. Start therapy with 7.5 mg weekly and raise the dosage at 1- or 2-month intervals until peak efficacy is achieved.

RHEUMATOLOGIC MANIFESTATIONS OF SICKLE CELL DISEASE

1. Gout
2. Sickle crisis→lower extremity arthralgias (knees and ankles most common), myalgias; synovitis
3. 2° hemochromatotic arthropathy (Fe overload 2° to frequent transfusions)
4. **Septic arthritis (or osteomyelitis), esp due to Salmonella, particularly if hyposplenic.**
5. **Aseptic (avascular) necrosis.**

✪ GOUT

1. **Conditions associated** with gout: ("That's a *HARD* 1 ! ")→

   H TN
   A therosclerosis
   R enal stones
   D M

2. While one cannot diagnose gout from noting hyperuricemia alone, it is true that the higher the *serum urate level*, the more likely an individual is to develop gout. In fact, the complications of gout correlate with both the duration and severity of hyperuricemia. Most first attacks of gouty arthritis follow 20 to 40 years of sustained hyperuricemia.

3. The *first metatarsophalangeal joint* is involved in over 50 percent of first attacks and in 90 percent of individuals at some time.

4. _Urate nephropathy_ is a reversible cause of acute renal failure in patients with gout and is due to precipitation of uric acid in, and therefore obstruction of, renal tubules and collecting ducts. Factors that favor uric acid crystal formation include dehydration and acidosis.

5. ✪ The hyperuricemia is either 2° to **OVERPRODUCTION** (> 800mg/24h; 90% of cases; give Allopurinol or colchicine for prophylaxis;) **or UNDEREXCRETION** (<600mg/24h;10% of cases; give Probenicid for prophylaxis) or both. The way to distinguish the two is by ordering a _24hour urine for uric acid levels_. If high, then you have an overproducer. If low, patient is an underexcretor.

6. **COMMON CAUSES OF UNDEREXCRETION** ("That's _HARD_ 2 !") ✪
   ✓ **H**TN
   ✓ Hyp**O**thyroidism
   ✓ Hyp**ER**parathyroidism
   ✓ **A**cidosis (Lactic acidosis, DKA, starvation ketosis)
   ✓ **R**enal insufficiency
   ✓ **D**rugs (esp. thiazide diuretics; alcohol)

7. **COMMON CAUSES OF OVERPRODUCTION** (Here's "_MORE HELP_" for you guys!) ✪
   ✓ **M**yeloproliferative diseases
   ✓ **O**besity
   ✓ **R**habdomyolysis
   ✓ **E**thanol

   ✓ **H**emolytic processes
   ✓ **E**xercise
   ✓ **L**ymphoproliferative diseases
   ✓ **P**. vera; Psoriasis; Purine-rich diet

   Other provocative factors include: stress, trauma, surgery, hospitalization, hyperalimentation, starvation, weight reduction, and infection

8. **COMPLICATIONS OF CHRONIC TOPHACEOUS GOUT**
   ✓ Renal stones
   ✓ Chronic renal insufficiency
   ✓ Proteinuria
   ✓ HTN

9. **NATURAL HISTORY**
   ➢ Some individuals have only a single gouty attack in their lifetime; others can recur.
   ➢ Although the interval between first and second attacks may be over 40 years, 75% of patients experience a second attack within 2 years.
   ➢ The terms "_interval gout_" or "_intercritical gout_" describe the periods between attacks of acute arthritis when the individual has no joint complaints.
   ➢ In severe cases, unless therapeutic intervention occurs, chronic gouty arthritis develops with time.

10. ✪ **NOTES ON TREATMENT:**

   a) **Colchicine** may give severe GI side effects in its PO form only

   b) **Indomethacin** (or other NSAID) should be *avoided in CHF and PUD*

   c) **Probenicid** is a uricosuric (↑s urinary secretion of uric acid) and should not be used if patient either has a h/o kidney stones or has a 24h U.A. level > 1000mg. Simultaneous administration of ASA or Indomethacin should be avoided if possible, as probenicid delays their excretion.

   d) Allopurinol should NOT be given for acute attacks. Instead give either colchicine or indomethacin.

   e) **Allopurinol** is the drug of choice if patient has a 1) overexcretors; 2) recurrent or more frequent attacks; 3) polyarticular disease; or 4) renal calculi/renal insufficiency

   f) Corticosteroids also very useful in mgmt.

   g) **Allopurinol toxicities**: "**FRREE**" (Fever, Rash, Renal, ↑eos, Elevated LFTs) as in "FRREE Gout" (but don't Freakout on the test!)…

   > **F**ever
   >
   > **R**ash—Erythematous, desquamating
   >
   > **R**enal insufficiency
   >
   > **E**os ↑
   >
   > **E**levated LFTs

11. Uric acid crystals are <u>negatively birifringent, as opposed to Pseudogout, which is Positively birifringent</u> under polarized light microscopy. Remember 5-10% of patients will have both gout and pseudogout.

12. **<u>For the exam, serum hyperuricemia is neither necessary nor sufficient to make the diagnosis of gout</u>**. A synovial fluid aspirate is necessary for definitive diagnosis. Always remember, for definitive diagnosis, to send the synovial fluid for crystal analysis, gram stain, C&S. Nevertheless, the aspirations will not always reveal crystals either, so the absence of crystals does not necessarily rule out gout.

13. **<u>Alcohol/diet/diuretics</u>** are the most common cause of acute gout in the outpatient population

14. Gout is very uncommon among premenopausal women.

PSEUDOGOUT [CALCIUM PYROPHOSPHATE DISEASE (CPPD)]

1. *Associated conditions include*: hyperparathyroidism, hemochromatosis-hemosiderosis, hypothyroidism, gout, ↓Mg, ↓ Phos, Wilson's disease, aging, and amyloidosis.
2. Can mimic and coexist with gout.
3. *Similar to gout, surgery, trauma, and alcohol may precipitate* (so to speak!)
4. Treatment options are similar to gout, except for allopurinol, of course.

CRYSTAL ANALYSIS: GOUT VERSUS PSEUDOGOUT		
Feature	**Gout**	**Pseudogout**
Crystal	Monosodium urate	Calcium pyrophosphate
Color under polarized light	Yellow	Blue
Shape of crystal	Needle	Rhomboid
Birifringence/ rotation under polarized light direction	Negative (counterclockwise)	**P**ositive (clockwise)

STILL'S DISEASE

1. Systemic onset juvenile R.A.

2. **Triad** of Still's however, is the **F**ever, the **A**rthritis, and the **R**ash (*FAR*): Think "Board scores are *STILL FAR* away"

3. High spiking fevers; arthralgias/arthritis; seronegativity (-RF; -ANA); ↑WBC; macular rash; serositis; lymphadenopathy; hepato/splenomegaly

DIAGNOSIS OF FELTY'S SYNDROME

1. *Neutropenia caused by hypersplenism and antineutrophil antibodies in a patient with rheumatoid arthritis*

2. *Triad* of ✪…Neutropenia; Seropositive RA ; Splenomegaly/hypersplenism

3. Frequent concomitants
   a) Serious infections
   b) Leg ulcers
   c) Mononeuritis Multiplex
   d) Anemia, thrombocytopenia
   e) LN, Hepatomegaly
   f) Sjogren's syndrome
   g) Weight loss

4. Laboratory clues
    a. _Antineutrophil antibodies_
    b. ↓WBC and ↓ platelets (2° to splenic sequestration)
    c. ↓serum Complement
    d. + ANA, high titre RF (IgM)

5. Response to splenectomy (Recurrent life-threatening infection or life-threatening
              hemolytic anemia are indications for splenectomy)
    a. Arthritis not affected
    b. ↓WBC frequently improves, though only temporarily

✪ STILL'S VS. FELTY'S: A SELECTIVE COMPARISON:

STILL'S DISEASE	FELTY'S SYNDROME
↑WBC	↓WBC
Fever	No fever necessary
Seronegative RA	Seropositive RA
Splenomegaly	Splenomegaly

✪ DDX OF ORAL + GENITAL ULCERATION

1. Behcet's syndrome → Painful
2. E. multiforme   →   Painful
3. HSV →   Painful
4. Pemphigus →   Painful
5. Crohn's disease→   Pain_less_
6. Reiter's syndrome → Pain_less_
7. Syphilis →   Pain_less_

DIFFERENTIATING REITER'S VS. BEHCET'S:

FEATURE	Reiter's	Behcet's
M:F	10:1	2:1
Ulcers	Painless	Painful
Predominant ocular disease	Conjunctivitis	Uveitis
Long-term ocular disability	rare	also rare
Long-term joint disability	frequent (50%)	rare
Spondylitis/sacroiliitis	frequent	rare
HLA association	B27	B12, B5 (esp ocular disease and colitis)
Important in pathogenesis	Infection is	Racial factors are
Treatment	NSAIDs	Immunosuppressives

CLINICAL SPECTRUM OF BEHCET'S SYNDROME

1. Ocular disease—occurs in 80%; more common in HLA B5 and Japanese men; eg *uveitis*
2. *Genital ulcers*
3. *Oral ulcers* (98%)
4. *E. nodosum* (F>M; assoc'd with non-deforming arthritis); occur in 80%
5. Thrombophlebitis (30%)
6. CNS disease (30%)
   a) Aseptic meningitis
   b) TIA-like episodes
   c) Cranial nerve palsies
7. Colitis (30%)
   a) *Associated with HLA-B5*
   b) May lead to perforation
   c) Clinically overlaps with IBD
8. Spondylits, sacroiliitis
   ✓ *When present, linked to HLA-B27*

DIAGNOSTIC CRITERIA FOR PMR (Polymyalgia Rheumatica)

1. Age > 50
2. ESR > 40 mm/h
3. Neck/bilateral shoulder/pelvic girdle AM **stiffness**
   a) Symptomatic episodes >1h in duration
   b) Clinical history >1 month duration
4. Response to *low-dose (≤15 mg/day) steroids*
5. *Minor criteria include*:
   a) Weight loss; fever; night sweats
   b) Symmetrical proximal muscle tenderness
   c) ↑alk phos/GGT
   d) Normocytic anemia
   e) Synovitis
   f) Normal CPK, EMG, muscle biopsy

EXCLUSION OF COEXISTING TEMPORAL ARTERITIS (Giant Cell Arteritis) ✪

1. *Presentation (classical) of Temporal Arteritis*→ H/A; *scalp tenderness; jaw claudication*; sudden visual loss.
2. 50% of TA patients have symptoms of PMR
3. 10-20% of patients with *clinically pure* PMR (i.e. only symptoms of PMR) will be found to have TA on biopsy.
4. 50% of *all* PMR patients (± TA symptoms) will be found to have giant-cell arteritis on TA biopsy.
5. *Remember, PMR patients complain more of stiffness than pain.* ✪
6. False-negative biopsies may occur 2° to presence of 'skip lesions' (if a 2cm biopsy is taken the false-neg rate is < 5%; therefore a 3-5cm segment biopsy is recommended)
7. Height of initial ESR cannot be used to predict disease severity or likelihood of complications.

✪ **IMPORTANT SIDE EFFECTS OF CHRONIC USE OF STEROIDS—for the exam…**
1. <u>**Proximal myopathy**</u>
2. <u>**Avascular Necrosis (e.g. hip)**</u>
3. <u>**2° Osteoporosis**</u>
4. Cataracts
5. Glucose Intolerance
6. Poor sleep; psychiatric changes
7. Striae
8. Weight gain

RELAPSING POLYCHONDRITIS

1. Associated with autoimmune disease in 30%
2. Leads to <u>**fever, arthralgias, episcleritis, swollen floppy ears**</u>
3. Nasal septum collapse (<u>**the other 'saddle nose'**</u> deformity, i.e. not just Wegener's)
4. <u>**Laryngeal disease→hoarseness; respiratory obstruction**</u> ✪
5. Tracheobroncial degeneration→recurrent infections, respiratory arrest
6. AI/ MVP/Aneurysm in ~ 10%

SPONDYLOARTHROPATHIES

☞ "Spondyloarthropathy" means *disease of the axial skeleton.*

A. <u>**DDx of Spondylitis**</u>
1. Ankylosing spondylitis
2. Other seronegative arthritides→psoriatic, Reiter's, juvenile RA
3. IBD; 'reactive' spondyloarthritis
4. Infection
   a) Septic arthritis
   b) TB
   c) Brucellosis
B. <u>**Characteristics**</u> ✪:
1. SI joint involvement
2. Peripheral arthritis (usu asymmetric and oligarticular)
3. Seronegativity (absence of RF or other autoantibodies)
4. Association with HLA-B27
5. Relatively early age of onset (<40)
6. Enthesopathy

C. <u>**HLA-B27 Rheumatic Diseases**</u> ✪:
1. Ankylosing Spondylitits (>90% are HLA-B27+)
2. Reiter's Syndrome or reactive arthritis (>80%)
3. Enteropathic Spondylitis (75%)
4. Psoriatic Spondylitis (50%)

D.   An **offspring of a person with HLA-B27** has a 50% chance of inheriting the antigen.

E.   Among **HLA-B27 persons in the <u>general population</u>**, only 2-10% will develop disease.

F.   **ANKYLOSING SPONDYLITIS**

   1. **LBP**
      a) Onset between 15-40yo
      b) Insidious
      c) <u>**Early AM back stiffness**</u>
      d) Improves with exercise

   2. **Radiographic findings**
      a) Erosions
      b) Syndesmophytes
      c) <u>**'Bamboo spine'**</u>

   3. <u>**Enthesopathic** involvement</u>
      a) Plantar fasciitis
      b) Achilles tendinitis
      c) Costochondritis

   4. <u>**Iritis**</u> (an important clue in spondyloarthropathies)

   5. **Among the differentials of ank. spond. is <u>DISH</u>** ✪ ('Diffuse Idiopathic Skeletal Hyperostosis', *a form of 1° osteoarthritis*)

      a) Patients with DISH are often obese and 60% have diabetes;
      b) **Sensation of 'stiffness' at the spine, yet relatively well-preserved spinal motion;**

      c) **Criteria for DISH...**
         ✓ <u>**'Flowing' ossification along the anterolateral aspects of ≥4 contiguous vertebral bodies with preservation of disk height**</u>
         ✓ No apophyseal joint involvement
         ✓ Absence of SI joint involvement
         ✓ Extraspinal ossification

      d) <u>**Marked calcification and ossification of paraspinous ligaments**</u> occur in DISH. <u>**Ligamentous calcification and ossification in the anterior spinal ligaments give the appearance of "flowing wax"**</u> on the anterior vertebral bodies. However, **a radiolucency may be seen between the newly deposited bone and the vertebral body, differentiating DISH from the marginal osteophytes in spondylosis.**

      e) Intervertebral disk spaces are preserved, and sacroiliac and apophyseal joints appear normal, **helping to differentiate DISH from spondylosis and from ankylosing spondylitis**, respectively.

      f) The radiographic changes are generally much more severe than might be predicted from the mild symptoms.

6. **Spinal fracture is the #1 cause of death and disability** in Ank Spond 2°
   to relatively minor trauma to a rigid spine.

7. *Don't be fooled*→ **HLA-B27 is *neither necessary not sufficient* for the dx**.

G. REACTIVE ARTHRITIS

1. An acute nonpurulent arthritis induced by a host response to an infectious agent
   elsewhere in the body.

2. Examples of reactive arthritis <u>include</u> rheumatic fever and <u>Reiter's</u> syndrome.

3. Follows *infections of GI and GU systems*. The *organisms that trigger* it are:

   a) Salmonella, Shigella flexneri
   b) Yersinia enterocolytica
   c) Campylobacter jejuni
   d) Ureaplasma Urealyticum, Chlamydia (non-gonococcal urethritides)

4. *Sacroiliitis and HLA-B27 commonly associated.*

5. Clinical features of Reiter's may ensue.

H. REITER'S SYNDROME

1. *A subset of reactive arthritis following venereal infections or dysentery that may
   include many of the following (and need not include all):*

   a. *Conjunctivitis,*
   b. *Urethritis (or cervicitis in females),*
   c. *Arthritis,* and
   d. *Characteristic mucocutaneous lesions:*

      i. Painless ulcers of the oral mucosa
      ii. **Circinate Balanitis** (rash on glans penis)/oral ulcers/keratoderma
      iii. **Keratoderma Blenorrhagicum** (indistinguishable clinically and
          histologically from psoriasis)

2. *C. trachomatis* has been recovered from the urethra of up to 70 percent of men with
   untreated nondiarrheal Reiter's syndrome and associated urethritis

3. Most commonly affects males in their 20s and 30s.

4. The term is now largely of historical interest only, and reactive arthritis is now
   commonly used instead.

I. ARTHRITIS ASSOCIATED WITH IBD

1. A non-deforming asymmetric arthritis, principally affecting knees, ankles, and PIPs,
   occurs in approximately 15%.

2. E. nodosum, uveitis, oral ulcers and pyoderma *occur in association with peripheral
   arthritis* in IBD.

3. This **PERIPHERAL** arthritis tends to occur ≥ 6 months after the onset of bowel disease. Its **severity reflects/parallels that of the bowel disease** ✪. Colectomy rids it.

4. **Spondylitis/Sacroiliitis** (considered more **CENTRAL** arthritis) occur in ~ 5%, may predate the onset of bowel symptoms, and are **associated with HLA-B27**. They are **independent of bowel disease activity** ✪, and so unaffected by colectomy.

5. Among patients with IBD + Ank Spond, ~75% are HLA-B27 +.

6. However, patients with IBD alone do not have an ↑d frequency of HLA-B27, nor do they have higher risk for developing spondylitis.

J.   **PSORIATIC ARTHRITIS**
      ☞ *Of patients with psoriasis, only 7% develop the arthritis.*

CLINICAL PATTERNS:

1. *Oligoarticular, asymmetric type* (70%)→see **'sausage digits' (dactylitis),** which represents flexor tendon sheath effusions (dactylitis may also be seen in Reiter's, Crohn's, and other diseases)

2. *DIP joint type* (15%)→usually seen in assn with psoriatic **nail disease** (i.e. pitting and onycholysis); **pitting of the nails is strongly associated with joint disease**

3. *Pseudorheumatoid type*
   a) Seronegative
   b) M=F
   c) Severity of arthritis correlates with severity of **skin disease**

4. *Ankylosing Spondylitis type*
   ✓ **HLA-B27 positive in >90%** only (less common than in 1° Ank Spond or Reiter's)

5. *Arthritis Mutilans*
   a) **Sacroiliitis** often assoc'd
   b) **'Telescoping digits'** (radiographically 'pencil-in-cup' appearance)

LYME DISEASE

1. Caused by the spirochete bacteria ***Borrelia Burgdorferi***, which is carried by the ***Ixodes dammini*** tick (the vector)
2. It is seen primarily in **summer and fall.**

3. ✪ **Very early Lyme disease (4-6 weeks post-exposure) may show negative serology, so the patient's history, flu-like symptomatology, and ECM rash become critical in deciding whether or not to treat.**

4. **Stages:**

    Stage I
- a) 3-32 days after the tick bite
- b) Flu-like illness
- c) **ECM (Erythema Chronicum Migrans**; 60%)

    Stage II
- a) Weeks to months following bite
- b) 10-15% develop neurologic abnormalities (e.g. **Bell's palsy**) and/or carditis);
- c) **Arthritis develops in 30-50%**

    Stage III
- a) Can become chronic
- b) **Arthritis develops in 50%**
- c) Synovium resembles that of rheumatoid arthritis;
- d) Unique feature of lyme arthritis is **obliterative endarteritis** of synovium
- e) Those with chronic joint disease have ↑ frequency of **HLA-DR4**

5. Carditis and facial palsy are commonly reversible; prognosis is usually favorable

6. *Lyme test should be used only for confirmation if suspect the disease, and not for screening*, because of false positives and false negatives. False positives may be seen with infectious *mono, RA, SLE, and other spirochetal* disease. If suspect a false positive and/or the patient has one of these diagnoses→√ Western blot

7. **Complications by system…**

- a) Skin lesions (ECM)
- b) Neurological –Cranial nerve palsies; peripheral neuropathies; meningitis
- c) Cardiac—AV block; myopericarditis
- d) *Arthritis—recurrent, asymmetric; often affects the knee.*

8. **Treatment:**

- a) Early (ECM)→Doxy or Amox or Biaxin x 2-3 wk; or Cefuroxime x 3 wk
- b) Carditis→Ceftriaxone/Cefotaxime/PenG x 2-3 weeks IV
- c) Facial nerve paralysis→Doxy or Amox x 3-4 weeks
- d) Meningitis→Ceftriaxone IV x 3weeks
- e) Arthritis→Doxy or Amox—duration unknown
- f) Pregnant women→No doxycycline!

✪ HYPERTROPHIC PULMONARY OSTEOARTHROPATHY (HOA)

1. Presentation also similar to RA
2. **Periosteal new bone formation** occurs at the end of long bones, giving **tenderness and soft-tissue swelling.**
3. This renders a so-called **spongy sensation** on palpation of the fingernail beds.
4. If lower extremities involved, **lowering the legs characteristically improves the pain**.
5. Usually 2° to **lung carcinoma or bacterial endocarditis**

CAUSES OF CLUBBING: " 7 C'S "→

C ardiac: SBE; cyanotic congential heart disease
C hest: cystic fibrosis; empyema; bronchiectasis; lung ca; TB (if extesive fibrosis); abscess
C rohn's disease; celiac disease; cirrhosis
C irculatory: AV fistula in upper extremities
C arcinoma: gastric, etc.
C ongenital clubbing
C ervical rib (unilateral)
     Plus : thyrotoxicosis

AVASCULAR NECROSIS OF BONE

1. Associated conditions include
   a) Alcohol
   b) **Chronic steroid use** ✪
   c) SLE and other connective tissue diseases
   d) Hemoglobinopathies, e.g. **sickle cell disease**
2. **Hip involvement** (at least on the exam)
3. **MRI** is best diagnostic tool on the exam! ✪

INFLAMMATORY MYOPATHIES—KEY CONCEPTS ✪

1. Muscle biopsy is mandatory in each of these.
2. **Polymyositis and Dermatomyositis** → **proximal muscle weakness** (e.g. rising from chair, brushing hair, or walking up the stairs); similar to steroids in this respect. *You might also think "proximal" esophagus since first third is skeletal muscle →dysphagia presentation*
3. Speaking of which, steroids are the treatment of PM and DM, until the CPK normalizes.
4. Dermatomyositis → *heliotrope rash; Gottren's papules; poikiloderma; photosensitivity*
5. **Inclusion Body Myositis**; unique in the following respects ✪…
   a) Responds poorly to steroids
   b) Proximal *and distal* muscle involvement

✪ COMPLEMENT LEVELS IN RENAL VS. SYSTEMIC DISEASE

	↓ Serum C′	Normal Serum C′
PRIMARY renal dz	Poststrep GN **MPGN** (membranoproliferative) *Lie down in PM*	Berger's Dz (IgA) Alport's Syndrome **RPGN** (p- or c-ANCA+) *"BAR"*
SYSTEMIC disease	**SLE** Infective Endocard Mixed essential cryo *"SLIM down"*	Goodpasture's Dz **HUS** **O**ccult Abscess **S**ystemic Vasculitis (Wegener's; PAN; HSP) **T**TP *"GHOST"*

SYSTEMIC LUPUS ERYTHEMATOSIS (SLE) ✪

A. **SLE Renal Disease**
- Mesangial changes alone→ No aggressive treatment needed
- Active diffuse, proliferative GN→ High-dose steroids ±
  immunosuppressives
- Focal proliferative GN and membranous GN→treatment controversial/prognosis
  favorable; renal biopsy often helpful in directing therapy

> ➢ So, **proliferation/inflammation/necrosis/crescent** formation→all
> requireTx

B. **↓Total C' correlates with active disease.**
C. **↓CH50 complement levels in SLE→usually mean renal or skin disease**.
D. Anti ds DNA levels also fluctuate with disease activity in general.
E. Neonatal SLE implies congenital heart block associated with *maternal* anti-SS-A
   (anti-Ro) antibody
F. SLE patients may show a **false-positive VDRL 2° to cross-reaction of an antiphospholipid Ab to VDRL**.
G. Most (80%) of SLE patients with a false + VDRL have circulating lupus 'anticoagulant' (really a '*pro*-coagulant', since predisposes to thrombotic disease)
H. Management:
   1. **Mild** disease→NSAIDs, hydroxychloroquine
   2. **Flares and moderate-to-severe disease**→ PO or IV steroids; steroid-sparing
      agents (eg methotrexate, azathioprine, and cyclophosphamide)
   3. **Severe** lupus **nephritis**→intravenous pulse cyclophosphamide

ANTI-NUCLEAR ANTIBODY FLUORESCENT PATTERNS ✪ :

FLUORESCENT PATTERN	ANTIGEN	RHEUMATIC DISEASE
Homogeneous/diffuse	DNP*	SLE (chronic)
Rim, peripheral	DNA	SLE (acute)
Nucleolar	RNA	Scleroderma
Speckled	ENA**	MCTD, SLE, Polymyositis

    *   DNP=Deoxyribonucleoprotein
   **   ENA=Entractable nuclear antigens

RHEUMATOLOGIC AUTOANTIBODIES ✪:

➢ **Anti-dsDNA→SLE** (70% sensitivity; highly specific); **Anti-ssDNA**→SLE (100% sensitivity, low specificity)

➢ **Anti-Sm (Smith)**→SLE (30% sensitivity but highly specific *if* you see it)

➢ **Anti-RNP** (Ribonuclear protein)→**MCTD** (Mixed Connective Tissue Disease)

➢ Anti-**SS**-A ('anti-Ro') and -B ('anti-La')→**S**jogren's **S**yndrome (also SLE)

➢ **Antihistone→Drug-induced SLE (hydralazine and procainamide)**

➢ Anti-**Scl**-70→**Scl**eroderma (progressive systemic)

➢ Anti**C**entromere (anti-topoisomerase)→**C**REST

✪ Remember, **numerous drugs can cause a + ANA without ever resulting in the clinical syndrome of drug-induced lupus**. Hydralazine and procainamide are important and common exceptions. If a patient is clinically stable on one, say, procainamide for an arrythmia, and his ANA is 1:640, you need not discontinue the medicine based on the ANA alone, unless symptomatic for drug-induced lupus (fever, arthralgias, pleurisy).

✪ **Anti-Jo-1** (Ab vs histidyl-tRNA synthetase)→**Polymyositis > Dermatomyositis esp with lung involvement, eg PM- and DM-related Interstitial Pulmonary Fibrosis.** Anti-Jo-1 antibody is associated with PM and DM only 25% of the time. **Remember too, ~ 10% of patients >40 with PM and 30% with DM have an associated malignancy.**

CREST Syndrome:

C alcinosis cutis

R aynaud's phenomenon

E sophageal dysmotility

S clerodactyly

T elangietasias

SCLERODERMA (Systemic Sclerosis)

S tiffness and aching. Skin feels thick and inelastic

C alcinosis, sclerodactyly and telangiectasia (CREST variant)

L oss of weight

E levated pulmonary pressure (**pulmonary HTN 2° to interstitial pulmonary fibrosis →
   cor pulmonale**.) A significant **↓ DLCO** can be present on PFTs despite normal CXR.

R aynaud's syndrome

O esophagus (dysphagia)

D yspnea (50%)

E SR ↑

R ecurrent ulcers: **R**aynaud's; **R**enal HTN (**TREAT SCLERODERMA HTN WITH AN ACE I**)

M outh: skin contracts. Muscle weakness

A rthritis, acrosclerosis

S jogren's syndrome

RAYNAUD'S PHENOMENON
1. Abnormality in microvasculature
2. F>M
3. Usually not associated with connective tissue disease, unless ANA+
4. Definitive dx by skin capillary microscopy→shows torturous, dilated capillary loops
5. Treatment:
   a) Wearing gloves
   b) Biofeedback
   c) Nitrates
   d) Calcium Channel Blockers
   e) D/C smoking (similar to Buerger's Disease—see later)
   f) Beta-blockers are contraindicated, as will ↑ the spasm

6. Differentiating 1° vs. 2° Raynaud's phenomenon...

1° RAYNAUD'S	2° RAYNAUD'S
Females	Males and Females
All digits	**Single digit**, usually
Frequent attacks	Infrequent attacks
Can be precipitated by emotional stress	Not precipitated by emotional stress
Digital ulceration rare	**Common**
Livedo Reticularis common	Uncommon

Antiestrogenic and Estrogenic Activities of Raloxifene and Tamoxifen:

Tissue	Raloxifene	Tamoxifen
Bone	E	E
Breast	AE	AE
CNS	AE	AE
Endometrium	AE	E
Liver	E	E
Vagina	AE	AE

Abbreviations:
> E=Estrogenic effect
> AE=Antiestrogenic effect

OSTEOPOROSIS

1. ↓ in bone mass usually in postmenopausal women 2° to ↓ estrogen levels

2. ***Important 2° causes*** ✪ that must be ruled out include...

   a) *Endocrine {↑steroids; ↑T4; ↑PTH 2° ↑resorption; ↑sugars (DM)}*
   b) Malignancy
   c) Immobilization
   d) Prolonged use of steroids or *heparin*
   e) *Alcoholism*; malabsorption
   f) Hypogonadism (↓LH and FSH)
   g) Smoking; Alcohol; Obesity

3. Calcium homeostasis is unaffected; ***serum Ca is normal***.

4. ***Bone densitometry*** is the gold standard for diagnosis.

5. ***Treatment***: Calcium; Vit D; Weight-bearing exercises; Estrogen asap after menopause—add Progesterone if uterus is intact; if contraindicated or high risk of complications, may **try Raloxifene (Evista®)→does not improve the hotflashes, but will lower the LDL**; ALSO cut out any tobacco/excess alcohol/extra weight.

6. Remember, a ***thin, white, postmenopausal smoker has 4 risk factors*** for developing osteoporosis. Risk factors, in general, may be considered modifiable vs nonmodifiable as seen below...

RISK FACTORS FOR OSTEOPOROSIS IN WOMEN	
(National Osteoporosis Foundation)	
NONMODIFIABLE	**MODIFIABLE**
Personal h/o fracture as an adult	Cigarette smoking
History of fracture in a 1st-degree relative	Low body weight (< 127lb)
Caucasian race	Estrogen deficiency
Advanced age	Prolonged premenopausal amenorrhea (> 1y)
Early menopause	Low calcium intake (< 400 mg/d life-long)
Dementia	Alcoholism (> 3 drinks/d)
Poor health/frailty	Poor health/frailty
	Recurrent falls
	Inadequate physical activity

7. NATIONAL OSTEOPOROSIS FOUNDATION GUIDELINES

- *Calcium intake*: 1200 mg/d

- *Vitamin D*: 400-800 IU/d for high-risk patients

- Regular *weight-bearing exercise*

- Avoid smoking; moderate alcohol consumption

- Treat all vertebral and hip fracture cases for osteoporosis

- *Begin prophylactic treatment when*

  - T-score below –2.0
  - T-score below –1.5 with risk factors

- *HRT is first-line therapy* !

BONE MINERAL DENSITY TESTING	
W.H.O. Diagnostic Criteria For Adult Women	
CATEGORY	**CRITERIA**
Normal	BMD within 1 Standard Deviation of the young adult reference mean
Low bone mass (*osteopenia*)*	BMD >1 **SD** below the young adult mean
*Osteoporosis**	BMD ≥2.5 **SD** below the young adult mean
Severe (established) osteoporosis*	BMD ≥2.5 **SD** below the young adult *mean in the presence of an osteoporotic fracture*.

   * Candidates for HRT/alendronate/calcitonin

OSTEOMALACIA ✪

1. Considered in the differential of osteoporosis
2. *Failure of __Mineralization__* of the bone due to …
   a) ↓ Vit D
   b) Vit D resistance
   c) ↓ phosphate
   d) Abnormal bony matrix
3. *↓Ca, ↓Phos, ↑alk phos*
4. *__Pseudofractures__* (noted radiographically as "__Looser's zones__"), which are thin radiolucent zones representing focal accumulations of nonmineralized osteoid
5. Obviously one can have both osteoporosis and osteomalacia.
6. AKA "rickets" in children
7. *__Renal osteodystrophy (2° hyperparathyroidism)__*
   a) Related to phosphate retention, ↓ vit D, and acidosis—all part of CRF
   b) Syndrome consists of…
      i) Osteitis fibrosa
      ii) Osteomalacia
      iii) Hyperparathyroidism
8. Similar to osteoporosis, Vit D and Calcium are important in treatment.

PAGET'S DISEASE ✪

1. *__Bone is structurally weakened 2° to disorganized bone remodeling__*
2. *__Normal serum Ca__* (similar to osteoporosis), except with immobilization
3. *↑alk phos (similar to osteomalacia) and it correlates with disease activity*.
4. Unknown cause
5. Affects axial>appendicular skeleton, with particular preference for:
   a) Spine, sacrum, pelvis
   b) Femur
   c) Tibia
   d) Skull (lytic lesions here called osteoporosis circumscripta)
6. Skeletal pain ;deformities; fractures
7. High Output cardiac failure
8. ↑ Urinary hydroxyproline and ↑ 24 hour urine *N-telopeptide* are very useful markers
9. Nuclear bone scans see "hot" spots of Paget's dz, and are far better than plain films in dx
10. *__Potential for malignant transformation__*, esp tumors of the humerus and femur)
11. Calcitonin and bisphosphonates (e.g. etidronate) commonly used in management.

✪ LABORATORY COMPARISON OF COMMON METABOLIC BONE DISEASES:			
Bone Disorder	**Serum calcium**	**Serum phosphorus**	**Alkaline phosphatase**
Osteoporosis	NL	NL	NL
Osteomalacia	↓	↓	↑
Hyperparathyroidism	↑	↓	↑
Renal failure/ osteodystrophy	↓	↑	↑
Paget's Disease	NL	NL	↑↑

OSGOOD-SCHLATTER DISEASE

- *Osteochondritis of the tibial tuberosity* (where the quadriceps tendon inserts)
- Usually *unilateral*
- This *epiphysitis* is seen exclusively in *young men > women under the age of 19* whose growth centers are still active.
- Can be seen following trauma or exercise
- Xrays can show *irregular ossification and calcified thickening* at the tendonous insertion
- Treatment is *rest/NSAIDs*; usually *remits spontaneously*; steroids if persists

POPLITEAL CYST

- *An extension of inflamed synovium into the popliteal space*; also known as a '*Baker's cyst*'
- A *ruptured Baker's cyst* may resemble acute DVT, and has therefore also been referred to as '*pseudophlebitis*'
- Ultrasound is typically the initial imaging modality of choice
- **DDx** is primarily DVT; popliteal artery aneurysm; LNs; and tumor.

FIBROMYALGIA

- A diagnosis of exclusion
- F>>M
- Pain must be present for ≥ 3mo
- Multiple tender, painful points
- Patients are poorly able to localize their pain, which is ↑ in Ams
- Patients frequently do not feel rested on awakening
- Nervousness is a frequent concomitant.

VASCULITIDES ✪

PALPABLE PURPURA
- Pathognomonic of *vasculitis*
- *Palpable since* blood and fluid escape from affected vessels into the extravascular space
- *Do not blanch* since they are extravascular

PAN (Polyarteritis Nodosa)

A. COMMON MANIFESTATIONS
1. Commonly involved organs include: *intestine, kidneys, skin, peripheral nerves, and joints; the lungs are usually spared*.
2. Abdominal pain/ischemic bowel→*abdominal aneurysms*
3. Focal necrotizing GN→*HTN & impaired renal function*
4. *Palpable purpura and livido reticularis*
5. *Mononeuritis multiplex* (similar to RA)
6. Asymmetric polyneuropathy
7. Mesenteric (or other) angiogram may show"beading"

8. **Other Signs & symptoms**
   - *Constitutional*: fatigue, weight loss, myalgia, fever
   - Hematochezia or melena
   - *Testicular pain*
   - Arthralgia
   - Multiple mononeuropathies

---

9. **PAN**→ **p-AN**CA (as opposed to **We**gener's = **c-AN**CA →"**We cAN**").
However, in vasculitides, cannot rely on the ANCA for dx; need biopsy!

---

10. Treatment → high-dose prednisone; or cyclophosphamide + prednisone

B. **Less Frequent Manifestations**
   1. MI, CHF
   2. CVA, Sz
   3. Retinal hemorrhage
   4. Interstitial pneumonitis

HYPERSENSITIVITY VASCULITIDES (HV) ✪—term encompasses 3 disorders:

➢ Mixed essential cryoglobulinemia
➢ Henoch-Schonlein purpura
➢ Serum sickness

☞ **Leukocytoclastic vasculitis** with palpable purpura is the major clinical sign of HV. The term *leukocytoclastic* refers to the neutrophils that have infiltrated the perivascular space during the acute stages of (predominantly cutaneous) vasculitides on (usually skin) biopsy, but it can also be seen in a variety of other conditions, like acute bacterial endocarditis, EBV, HIV, chronic active hepatitis, UC, and PBC. *Palpable purpura* is essentially the physical manifestation of leukocytoclastic vasculitis, when seen in HV.

CRYOGLOBULINEMIA

➢ Remember, cryoglobulins are *antibodies that precipitate when cooled*; when they do, they yield a *leukocytoclastic vasculitis*.
➢ Exacerbations of disease activity can, therefore, *follow cold exposure*
➢ Should be considered a type of vasculitis since the cryoglobulins precipitate in the dermal vessels.

A. **Type I** (MONOCLONAL)
   1. Single, *monoclonal* cryoglobulinemic antibody
   2. Associated with **MULTIPLE MYELOMA, WALDENSTROM'S**, lymphoma, and leukemias
   3. Symptoms, if any, are usually related to **hyperviscosity**, e.g.:

      a. H/As

      b. Blurry vision

      c. Epistaxis

      d. Raynaud's phenomenon

      e. Ischemic ulcers; skin necrosis

B. Types II & III (MIXED) ✪

1. _Polyclonal or "mixed"_ cryoglobulinemic antibodies (usually IgG and anti-IgG)

2. Commonly associated with **autoimmune disorders and chronic infections (must know HEPATITIS C)**

3. The typical presentation for essential mixed dz is glomerulonephritis, arthralgias, hepatosplenomegaly, and lymphadenopathy in addition to skin involvement (**palpable purpura; urticaria; skin ulcers**)

4. Over the long run, nephritis/**progressive renal disease** is a common complication

5. Labs for essential mixed cryoglobulinemia include: hypocomplementemia, ↑ LFTs, and cryoglobulin titer

6. _Plasmapheresis_ temporarily lowers the level of globulins, removes the immune complexes, and improves symptoms. However, long-term management should include, if possible, _control of the underlying disease_ that produces the abnormal globulins or immune complexes.

DON'T CONFUSE COLD AGGLUTININS & CRYOGLOBULINS : Know'em _cold_ ! ;)

	COLD AGGLUTININS	**CRYOGLOBULINS**
Etiology	Antibodies (Ig **M**) vs. RBCs	Immunoglobulins that precipitate in the cold—may be monoclonal (type I) or polyclonal (types II and III)
Associated conditions[1]	Measles, mumps Mono Mycoplasma	Lymphoma Multiple myeloma Waldenstrom's

[1] In mycoplasma pneumoniae, mononucleosis, and other viral diseases, the titer of antibody is usually too low to cause clinical symptoms, but its presence is of diagnostic value; only occasionally is hemolysis present.

HENOCH-SCHONLEIN PURPURA ("HSP")

> *Palpable purpura (most commonly distributed over the buttocks and lower extremities), arthralgias, gastrointestinal signs and symptoms, and glomerulonephritis.*

> It is a small vessel vasculitis.

> While usually seen in children, may also be seen in adults.

> **Ig A** is the culprit antibody in this immune-complex disease, and in fact, IgA levels are elevated in about one-half of patients.

> *Not unlike Berger's (Ig A nephropathy!) and poststreptococcal GN, HSP **also** often follows a URI.*

> The prognosis of Henoch-Schonlein purpura is excellent, with either complete spontaneous resolution of disease or improvement with steroids.

SERUM SICKNESS

> An immune response most commonly triggered by a drugs such as penicillins, sulfonamides, phenytoin, ASA, and even heparin

> A classic arthrus or Type III hypersensitivity reaction with immune complex disease.

> Presentation typically includes fever, lymphadenopathy, urticaria, and arthralgias occurring 7-10 days after initial exposure to the agent or 2-4 days after subsequent exposure

CHURG-STRAUSS SYNDROME

1. **Asthma + peripheral eosinophilia**

2. 3 STAGES (need not occur in this order):

   a. Usually a prodrome of **upper respiratory** disease in the form of…
      i. Allergic rhinitis, or
      ii. Asthma
      iii. Nasal polyposis

   b. **↑Blood and tissue eos** (eg pulmonary infiltrates re PIE)

   c. **Coronary vasculitis**

3. **HTN**

4. **p-ANCA** (similar to PAN; in fact, there is a lot of clinical overlap between Churg-Strauss and PAN); think *pulmonary* involvement more for Churg-Strauss versus *renal and GI* more for PAN

BUERGER'S DISEASE

1. Seen in *young adult smokers*, usually less than 30 yo; M>F
2. Present with *instep claudication and digital infarction*
3. Pathology is intraluminal thrombus-containing microabscesses to small and mid-size arteries and veins; aka thromboangiitis obliterans
4. Unlike atherosclerotic disease, the upper extremities are usually involved.
5. *Quitting smoking stops the disease* progression

CHOLESTEROL EMBOLI

1. Be able to identify *procedures involving large arteries (e.g. catheterizations and vascular surgery*) as the commonly presented risk factor, occurring as 'showers' of cholesterol-containing microemboli that become dislodged from atheromatous plaques. Incidentally, cholesterol emboli may also occur following anticoagulant therapy or appear spontaneously due to disintegration of atheromatous plaques.

2. Signs to look for include: *livedo reticularis*, *gangrene of toes with distal pulses that are characteristically **intact***, ischemic ulcerations, and *orangeish cholesterol retinal plaques*.

3. Peripheral *eosinophilia* is common, as is *acute renal failure*, which in this syndrome, is *irreversible*

WEGENER'S GRANULOMATOSIS

1. **ACR Criteria for Wegener's Granulomatosis (≥ 2 of the following):**
   a. Nasal or oral inflammation: Development of painful or painless oral ulcers or purulent or bloody nasal discharge
   b. Abnormal CXR: Film shows nodules, fixed infiltrates, or cavities
   c. Urinary sediment: Microhematuria (> 5 RBCs/HPF) or RBC casts seen
   d. Granulomatous inflammation on biopsy: Histologic changes that show granulomatous inflammation within the wall of an artery or in the perivascular or extravascular area (artery or arteriole)

2. **Pulmonary-renal syndrome (others include** Goodpasture's; Churg-Strauss; SLE; cryoglobulinemic vasculitis; leukocytoclastic vasculitis, i.e. small vessel vasculitis)

3. Pulmonary manifestations include hemorrhage and thick-walled, centrally-**cavitating nodules**

4. Renal manifestation is **Focal Segmental** GN

5. **ELKS** summarizes the organs affected:

> **E** NT (eg sinusitis, bloody nasal discharge)
> **L** ung
> **K** idney
> **S** kin

6. Treatment → oral cyclophosphamide and prednisone

4. GASTROENTEROLOGY

PARACENTESIS:

	Transudates	**Exudates** (*everything "EXceeds"**)
	CHF/cirrhosis/nephrosis	TB (infEXtion)
	Portal HTN	Fungal (infEXtion)
	↓Albumin	SBP (infEXtion)
	Meig's Syndrome	Cancers (e.g. hepatoma; mesothelioma; mets; ovarian) ("My EX"!)

	Transudates	**Exudates***
Ascites protein	<3 g	>3g
Ascites LDH	<200	>200
Ascites/serum LDH	<0.6	>0.6
Ascites/serum protein	<0.5	>0.5

ALBUMIN GRADIENT

> ☞ The 'albumin gradient' is actually the difference between the serum and the ascites albumin, or Serum-Ascites Albumin Gradient (SAAG).
>
> ✪ If this **gradient ≥1.1 g/dl** → indicates **portal HTN** (97% accuracy), which β-blockers, like *propranolol* can treat to ↓ the risk of variceal bleeding.
>
> ✪ SAAG < 1.1 means abnormal capillary permeability. The broader ddx includes:
>
> | **Low SAAG** (< 1.1 g/dL) | **High SAAG** (≥ 1.1 g/dL) |
> |---|---|
> | Nephrotic syndrome | *Cirrhosis*; alcoholic hepatitis |
> | Pancreatitis | CHF |
> | Peritoneal TB | Massive liver mets |
> | Peritoneal carcinomatosis | |
> | Serositis | |

✪ SBP (SPONTANEOUS BACTERIAL PERITONITIS)

1. Is exactly that, and nearly always involves a *single organism* (key culprits include→ enterobacteriaceae 63%, strep pneumo 15%, and enterococci 6-10%)
2. Fever/abdominal pain and tenderness/ascites
3. ✪ Check the cell count of the ascitic fluid: **PMNs→ usually > 250/mm³ (*or* WBC > 500)**; often culture negative, so don't necessarily rely on the culture, and **when you do culture→innoculate bottles at bedside! Instead, if see ↑PMNs and suspect clinically, → start patient on a 3rd generation cephalosporin.**
4. 10-20% of cirrhotic patients develop SBP
5. Treatment is 3rd generation cephalosporin for ≥ 5days; other options include Timentin™, Augmentin™

HEPATORENAL SYNDROME ✪

1. *ARF with normal tubular function/normal urinalysis in a patient with cirrhosis*
2. The onset of renal failure is typically insidious, but *can be precipitated by* an acute insult such as gastrointestinal bleeding, infection, or aggressive diuresis, all of which are common scenarios in cirrhosis.
3. *Urine sodium is < 10 meq/L* (off diuretics) and urine osm > plasma osm.
4. Can be distinguished from hypovolemia (prerenal indices can look similar) by the patient's *failure to respond to a fluid challenge*.
5. Carries a *high mortality*
6. Treatment is largely *supportive*. Patients with hepatorenal syndrome who progress to renal failure can be treated with *dialysis*. Survival on dialysis is generally limited by the severity of the hepatic failure. The best hope for reversal of the renal failure is an *improvement in hepatic function* due to partial resolution of the primary disease or to successful *hepatic transplantation*. *Combination therapy with midodrine* (a selective alpha-1 adrenergic agonist) *and octreotide* (a somatostatin analog) has shown some success. The rationale for such therapy is that, since midodrine is a systemic vasoconstrictor and octreotide is an inhibitor of endogenous vasodilator release, combined therapy would improve renal and systemic hemodynamics.

SUDDEN ↑ IN ASCITES IN PREVIOUSLY STABLE CIRRHOSIS ✪

1. SBP (esp if fever/chills/abdominal pain)
2. Hepatic vein thrombosis (Budd-Chiari syndrome)
3. Hepatoma (hepatocellular carcinoma); √ alpha fetoprotein; re: Hep B and C carry ↑ risk of cirrhosis→hepatoma; Hep A does not.
4. Acute deterioration in hepatocellular function; e.g....
    a) Sepsis
    b) Hemorrhage
    c) Alcohol binge
5. Hepatorenal syndrome

RISK OF REBLEEDING IN PUD BASED ON HOW THE BLEED APPEARS AT ENDOSCOPY

1. *Clot visualized* overlying site of bleed→ 10-40% risk of rebleed→Observation
2. *No overlying clot* seen; *only flat spot* →0-10% risk of rebleed →Observation
3. *Culprit vessel visualized* on exam →50-70% risk of rebleed →Requires treatment via endoscopy (e.g. laser photocoagulation, sclerotherapy, etc)

BLEEDING TENDENCY IN ALCOHOLIC CIRRHOSIS

1. *↓Synthesis of coagulation factors (↑PT)*: remember, since the half life of factor VII is only 6 hours, the PT is a sensitive index of hepatic function; albumin is the other important index of hepatic function. Sometimes, it is difficult to determine if a patient's ↑ PT is 2° to liver disease or ↓ vit K, so remember this trick: If factor 5 is ↓, it's liver disease; if Factor 5 is normal, vitamin K deficiency.
2. *Platelet function defect (↑bleeding time)*
    a) Cirrhosis-induced von Willebrand-type defect
    b) Separate alcohol-induced platelet function defect

3. ***Thrombocytopenia***
    a) Hypersplenism*
    b) Marrow suppression
4. ***Local factors***
    a) Varices
    b) PUD
    c) Gastritis
    d) Mallory-Weiss tears
        ➢ Mucosal laceration at EG junction
        ➢ 75% of patients have a history of retching and vomiting before bleeding.
    * *Note:* **Splenomegaly and hypersplenism** should not be used interchangeably. Splenomegaly (SM) is simply a palpable spleen tip, whereas hypersplenism implies hyperfiltration of erythrocytes, leukocytes, or platelets. All patients with hypersplenism have SM, but the reverse is not true.

ESOPHAGEAL VARICES ✪

1. Beta-blockers, like propranolol are the *primary prevention* of choice.
    a. Non-selective beta blockers (eg, propranolol and nadolol) block the adrenergic dilatory tone in mesenteric arterioles resulting in unopposed alpha adrenergic mediated vasoconstriction and therefore a decrease in portal inflow. At the present time, these are <u>the only drugs recommended for prophylaxis against a first variceal hemorrhage</u>.
    b. Beta blockers *decrease initial variceal hemorrhage* by 45 percent *and bleeding-related deaths* by 50 percent.
    c. **TIPS** is <u>not</u> used for *primary* prophylaxis due to expense and higher morbidity and mortality and high incidence of shunt stenosis, and recurrent portal hypertension. Accepted indications for TIPS include:
        i. *Active* hemorrhage despite emergent endoscopic treatment
        ii. *Recurrent variceal* hemorrhage despite emergent endoscopic treatment
2. Although selective beta blockers also reduce portal venous pressure, the effect is not dramatic and their use remains to be validated in large scale clinical trials.
3. *Band ligation* is the endoscopic treatment of choice for the *long-term management* of variceal hemorrhage

BOERHAAVE'S SYNDROME

1. *<u>Severe retching and vomiting followed by excruciating retrosternal chest and upper abdominal pain. Odynophagia, tachypnea, dyspnea, cyanosis, fever, and shock</u>* develop rapidly thereafter.
2. Esophageal perforation which commonly occurs after *dilatation of esophageal strictures;* medical procedures cause over one-half of all perforations
3. Similar to Mallory-Weiss, it often follows violent retching, as after an alcoholic binge; a history of *alcoholism or heavy drinking is present in 40 percent*.
4. The diagnosis of esophageal perforation should be confirmed by *water-soluble contrast esophagram (Gastrograffin®)* which reveals the location and extent of extravasation of *contrast material.*
5. *Treatment* is primary surgical repair of the ruptured esophagus, mediastinal debridement, and pleural drainage. Continuous NG suction, IV broad-spectrum antibiotics, and TPN.

HEPATOMEGALY + HEART FAILURE—not just CHF !
1. Alcoholic cardiomyopathy with fatty liver
2. Amyloidosis
3. Carcinoid syndrome
4. Constrictive pericarditis
5. Hemochromatosis
6. Right ventricular failure ± tricuspid incompetence
7. Left heart failure (!) which is the #1 cause of right heart failure.

HEPATIC ASCITES—*Causes by Location*:
➢ **Presinusoidal** → eg Portal vein thrombosis
➢ **Sinusoidal** (most common) → Cirrhosis is the typical culprit
➢ **Postsinusoidal** → Budd-Chiari syndrome (hepatic vein obstruction); veno-occlusive disease
(= *hepatic venule obstruction; think of this when see ascites in the setting of BMT, chemo, and oral contraceptive use*)

DDX OF FLAPPING TREMOR…
1. Hepatic encephalopathy
2. Wilson's disease
3. Uremia
4. CO_2 narcosis

IRRITABLE BOWEL SYNDROME (IBS) ✪
1. ↑ # of bowel movements *correlated with* ↑*stress*;
2. Abdominal pain *relieved by defecation*. *Pain in IBS does not awaken the patient from sleep.*
3. *Pencil-thin stools*
4. Chronic or recurrent *constipation* and/or abdominal *distension*; *dyspepsia*
5. Feeling of incomplete evacuation
6. *Management*
   ➢ Fiber to help prevent constipation
   ➢ Loperamide for diarrhea
   ➢ Antispasmodics [eg dicyclomine (Bentyl) and hyoscyamine (Levsin)] to reduce abdominal pain by decreasing intestinal contractions
   ➢ TCAs, SSRIs:
      ✓ Antidepressants have analgesic properties independent of their mood improving effects and may therefore be beneficial in patients with neuropathic pain.

↑ ALK PHOS—FACTORS FAVORING HEPATIC ORIGIN
1. ↑GGT
2. ↑5'-nucleotidase

GENERALLY, LFTs REFLECT 2 PATTERNS OF LIVER INJURY:
1. Cholestatic → Alk phos, GGTP
2. Hepatocellular → AST, ALT, and LDH

LABORATORY INDICATORS OF ALCOHOLIC LIVER DISEASE:
1. ↑GGTP
2. ↑MCV; macrocytosis
3. AST/ALT > 2:1 (remember, 'S' for Superior)
4. Blood alcohol (if suspect daily drinking)
5. AFP (if hepatoma suspected)

GILBERT'S DISEASE
1. **#1 cause of isolated ↑ indirect bili, which is, in turn, the #1 cause of hyperbilirubinemia.**
2. Usually caused by **fasting states** and resolves after patient has eaten.

REFEEDING SYNDROME
> This term refers to the metabolic disarray (ie ↓ phos, ↓K, and ↓ Mg) that can be seen with cardiopulmonary and neurologic complications in *severely malnourished patients being refed enterally or parenterally*.

UNDERSTANDING BILIRUBIN AND JAUNDICE

	Normal U.Urobilinogen	↑U. Urobilinogen
↑ Conjugated Bili (Direct)	Common Bile Duct Obstruction	Acute **H**epatitis
↑ UNconjugated Bili (Indirect)	**Gilbert's** Disease **Crig**ler-Najjar ("Under Gilbert's crib")	**H**emolysis

IMPORTANT CAUSES OF CHRONIC HEPATITIS: → "*ABCDEF*": ✪

A utoimmune Hepatitis (✓anti-smooth muscle Ab; anti-LKM; soluble liver Ag); Alpha-1-antitrypsin deficiency

B iliary cirrhosis (✓ anti-mitochondrial Ab); hepatitis **B**

C opper excess (*Wilson's* disease → ✓serum/urine/liver copper ↑; ceruloplasmin usually ↓) Hepatitis **C;** Cholangitis, sclerosing

D rugs

E thanol

F e overload (*Hemochromatosis*→ ✓ transferrin saturation)

✪ CIRRHOSIS—IMPORTANT CAUSES & OVERVIEW		
Etiology	**DIAGNOSIS**	**KEY TREATMENTS**
Alcoholic Liver Disease	GGT, MCV, AST/ALT	Abstinence
Hepatitis B	serology	Interferon α-2b Lamivudine (3TC)
Hepatitis C	serology	Interferon alfacon-1 Interferon α-2b + ribavirin
Hemochromatosis	Transferrin sat; ferritin; hepatic Fe index; HFE gene	Phlebotomy
Autoimmune hepatitis	ASMA (anti-smooth muscle antibody); anti-LKM; soluble liver Ag; ANA	Prednisone, azathioprine
Primary Biliary Cirrhosis	AMA (anti-mitochondrial antibody)	Ursodiol
Wilson's disease	Serum and urine copper, Ceruloplasmin	D-penicillamine; zinc
Alpha-1-antitrypsin deficiency	Alpha-1-antitrypsin level (<11 μmol/L or 80 mg/dL)	Enzyme replacement ("augmentation" as IV infusions); liver transplant (for end-stage hepatic disease)

HEPATITIS B SEROLOGY SIMPLIFIED ✪ ...

1. + Hep BsAg (**surface antigen**)→ means <u>active infection</u>; persistence beyond 6 months indicates chronic infection

2. + anti-HepBs (**surface antibody**) →means <u>recovery and immunity</u>

3. + Hep BeAg ('**e' antigen**) → a marker for infectivity for acute and chronic infections

4. + anti-HepBe means ('**e' antibody**) →usually means patient is <u>no longer infectious</u> (since it indicates a nonreplicative state *versus* 'e'Ag and HBV DNA which indicate a replicative state). For example, HBsAg carrier mothers who are HBeAg-positive almost invariably (□90 percent) transmit hepatitis B infection to their offspring, while HBsAg carrier mothers with anti-HBe rarely (10 to 15 percent) infect their offspring.

5. HepBcAg (**core antigen**) is not routinely detected in peripheral blood

6. + IgM anti-HBc (**core antibody**) →means <u>acute infection</u> with Hep B. It is also significant because, in some cases of acute Hep B, it may be the only marker to appear (and therefore the only way to make the diagnosis) between the early and recovery phases, that is, during the so-called "*window period*", which is seen after surface Ag and 'e' Ag disappear *but before* antibodies to 1) Hep B core (IgG); 2) surface Ag; and 3) 'e' Ag appear.

7. Persistence of anti-HBc (**core antibody**) means <u>chronic infection</u>, especially chronic active hepatitis (CAH—not to be confused with the other CAH, congenital adrenal hyperplasia!—see Endocrine lecture); in the presence of anti-HBs, it is an important tool in <u>distinguishing natural immunity from vaccination</u>

8. Hep BsAg (**surface antigen**) can be ordered first. If negative, order surface and core antibodies. <u>If the surface Ag or core Ab are + for more than 6 months</u> (serologically, chronic hepatitis—re: ↑ transaminases ≥ 6 mo is more commonly used to define "chronic hepatitis"), <u>request 'e' Ag and Ab to evaluate for infectivity.</u>

9. <u>If a chronic surface Ag carrier presents with unexplained exacerbation, request *delta agent antibody*. The delta agent is important in the conversion of chronic persistent →chronic active hepatitis, and is strongly associated with IV drug abuse.</u> Remember, CAH can be treated with alpha-interferon.

10. If see **<u>sudden ↑ in ascites</u>** in a patient with history of Hep B or C → **✓ alpha fetoprotein (hepatoma) and R/O SBP (spontaneous bacterial peritonitis)**

11. If patient with **chronic Hep B** presents with **<u>new or sudden abdominal pain</u>** that cannot be accounted for by liver disease per se, R/O **PAN** (polyarteritis nodosa).

12. If a non-immune individual is exposed to Hep B, s/he may be protected by giving HBIG (**passive** Hep B immunoglobulin); but s/he will still require **active** immunization with a routine series of 3 shots can be given if patient is going to be continously exposed to the virus.

13. If patient not found to have Hep B (or **Hep C, which can simply be checked with Hep C antibody, although dx must be confirmed via a <u>RIBA</u>** for Hep C), then additional testing may be done for other causes of usually ↑ transaminases

    ☞ **<u>Natural history of Hep C</u>**: 50% of patients with HepC go onto become chronically infected, and 50% of *those* develop CAH; 20% develop cirrhosis; Re: Hep C is the #1 cause of post-transfusion hepatitis.

    ☞ Remember to **R/O Hep C in patients with** isolated ↑ **ALT.**

    ☞ **<u>HepA</u>** can go onto develop fulminant hepatitis (very rare), but never get chronic infection or cirrhosis.

A DIAGNOSTIC APPROACH TO PATIENTS WITH SUSPECTED HBV ✪

✓ HBsAg, or **surface Ag**: if +, then HBV present, so ✓ **<u>IgM core antibody</u>** to see if it's acute or chronic.
   ☞ If **<u>IgM core antibody</u>** is +, then patient has *acute* infection; observe these
   ☞ If **<u>IgM core antibody</u>** is -, then patient likely has *chronic* infection; re✓ surface antigen in 6 months to confirm:
      a. <u>If surface Ag still there at 6 months</u>, pt definitely has *chronic* infection
         ☞ If **'e' antibody** is +, BUT eAg/HBV DNA/& ALT are all normal → then the pt is an HBV *carrier*; observe these.

☞ If **'e'** <u>**antigen**</u> is + and HBV DNA is + → then pt has *active infection*→ **consider for treatment** (biopsy, etc).
　　b. If surface Ag negative at 6 months, then the infection has *resolved*.

✪ ASSOCIATIONS/COMPLICATIONS OF HEPATITIS <u>B</u> TO KNOW:

1. **Aplastic anemia**

2. *Glomerulonephritis*

3. *Hepatocellular carcinoma* (hepatoma)

4. *Polyarteritis nodosa (PAN)*

5. *Mixed cryoglobulinemia (Hep C > B)*

6. *Arthralgias/arthritis*

✪ DIAGNOSTIC TESTS FOR HEPATITIS C:

Category	ALT	EIA	RIBA	HCV RNA (RT-PCR)
False positive EIA	N	+	-	-
Resolved infection or	N	+	+	-
HCV Carrier	N	+	+	+
Chronic Hep C intermittent viremia	↑	+	+	+

✪ IMPORANT BASIC POINTS ON TESTING FOR HCV:

☞ **First** ✓ the **ELISA** (Enzyme Immunosorbent Assay) antibody is done.

☞ *Generally speaking,* all positive EIA results must be <u>confirmed</u> with a supplemental assay such as the RIBA or qualitative RT-PCR. Only 30 to 40 percent of EIA-positive patients with a normal serum ALT (eg blood donors) will be RIBA positive.

☞ The real value of the <u>RIBA</u> is to decrease false positive ELISA tests that may still be seen in individuals with *no apparent risk factors* for HCV, i.e. low-risk populations, such as *prospective blood donors* with a positive anti-HCV screen; the 40 to 50 percent false positive rate in this setting warrants supplemental testing.

☞ On the other hand, in *high-risk individuals*, the positive predictive value of the <u>ELISA</u> test is >95% and in the presence of ↑ALT levels virtually establishes the diagnosis. If confirmatory tests are performed, molecular assays (such as RT-PCR) for HCV RNA are more appropriate than RIBA

☞ Remember if the patient has a + <u>ELISA</u> and a + confirmatory <u>RIBA</u> for Hep C, but the <u>PCR</u> is negative, this indicates the patient had *prior exposure* to Hep C infection.

☞ Re also: Because some HCV-infected patients may be only intermittently HCV RNA +, a single negative test cannot be used to R/O chronic infection, and repeat testing at 3-6 mo intervals by PCR is indicated to check for **chronic infection with intermittent viremia**.

☞ Re: EIA-2 detects anti-HCV generally by 10 weeks of exposure, while qualitative RT-PCR detects presence of virus as early as 1-2 weeks post-exposure.

☞ **HCV GENOTYPE**: <u>There are 6 genotypes. *Genotype 1 is the most common in the US and is associated with lower response rates to current therapy*.</u> HCV genotyping is therefore useful for guiding the duration of therapy and predicting the likelihood of response.

CURRENT TREATMENT GUIDELINES IN HEP C	
(from the National Concensus Development Conference Panel Statement: Management of Hep C)	
Patient Characteristics	**Recommendations**
Persistent HCV viremia; persistently ↑ ALT; & liver biopsy showing portal or bridging fibrosis or moderate inflammation or necrosis	Consider Rx with interferon and ribavirin
Persistently normal ALT	Observe
↑ ALT, minimal abnormalities in biopsy	Observe, serial ALTs, consider biopsy q3-5y
Compensated cirrhosis	Observe, consider treatment
Decompensated cirrhosis	Consider liver transplant

NATURAL HISTORY OF CHRONIC HEP C:

Chronic Hepatitis ——— **Cirrhosis** ——— **Hepatocellular Ca** ——— **Death**

20-30years   5-10years   variable

- Acute infection goes onto chronic infection >85% of the time
- Chronic infection leads to cirrhosis in 20-40% of cases

✪ THE 'RULE OF 20s' WITH HEP C:

➢ *20%* of patients with acute Hep C have **symptoms**
➢ 15-*20%* of patients with acute Hep C *clear the virus*
➢ In *20%* to 40% of patients with chronic Hep C, *cirrhosis* develops over *20* years
➢ Cirrhosis leads to *liver failure* in *20%* of these patients, and to *HCC* in another *20%*
➢ *20%* of patients without cirrhosis who receive *interferon* will obtain a *sustained response*.

PREVENTING HEP C TRANSMISSION—GUIDELINES FROM THE NIH

1. Adherence to universal precautions to protect medical personnel and patients against HCV should be sufficient.
2. Advise patients with HCV infection not to donate blood, organs, tissues, or semen
3. Strongly encourage safer sexual practices, including the use of latex condoms, in patients with multiple sexual partners.
4. *The risk of transmission is low (<3%) in monogamous long-term relationships; therefore, no changes in sexual practices are recommended to these individuals*
5. *HCV Ab testing is recommended for the sex partners of infected patients.*
6. Advise patients not to share razors and toothbrushes. Covering an open wound is recommended. However, it is *not* recommended to avoid close contact with family members or to avoid sharing meals or utensils.
7. *Pregnancy is not contraindicated in women with HCV infection. The risk of transmission to the fetus is low (3-6%)*
8. *There is no evidence of transmission during breastfeeding; thus, breast-feeding is considered safe and should be encouraged.*

✪ EXTRAHEPATIC MANIFESTATIONS OF CHRONIC HCV INFECTION

1. *Porphyria cutanea tarda*
2. *Mixed Cryoglobulinemia (Hep C > B)*
3. *Leukocytoclastic vasculitis*
4. *Membranoproliferative GN*
5. Thyroiditis
6. Sjogren's Syndrome
7. Lichen Planus
8. B-Cell Lymphoma; plasmacytoma

Typical Transaminase Ranges for Various Diseases:

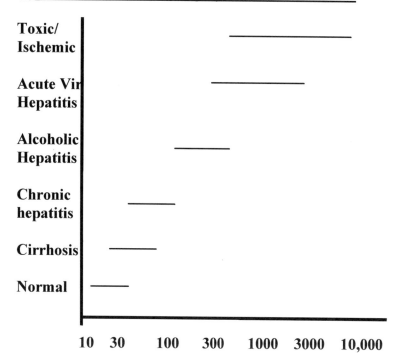

IMPORTANT POINTS ON HEPATITIS D

- HDV is an RNA virus that is unable to replicate on its own and requires HBV

- HDV can occur as a "_superinfection_" in patients with underlying _chronic_ HBV or as a "coinfection" during acute HBV infection.

- ☞ The major significance of HDV is its ability to ↑ the severity of HBV infection. For example, fulminant hepatitis is more likely in patients who have acute HBV + HDV _coinfection_. And patients with chronic HBV who become _superinfected_ with HDV may have an acute worsening of liver disease and a more rapid progression to cirrhosis.

HEPATITIS E

- Enterically transmitted
- Resembles Hep A
- ☞ If a **woman in her 3rd trimester** acquires Hep E→ high risk of going onto fulminant hepatitis.

HEPATITIS G ✪

- _Asymptomatic_ carrier
- A _chronic_ hepatitis, or "_cryptogenic_" non-A/B/C/D/E cirrhosis
- Present in nearly _2% of eligible blood donors and 1.5% of donors with ALT > 45_
- Among new cases of non-A, non-B hepatitis in the U.S., _nearly 20% are positive for Hep G, 80% of whom are also infected with Hep C._
- _Among patients with Hep C, 10-20% have evidence of Hep G in their serum_

AUTOIMMUNE HEPATITIS ✪

- ☞ _**Young women, primarily; average 10-20 yo**_
- ↑↑serum gamma globulins
- + ANA
- ☞ + **anti-Smooth muscle Ab;** _have been associated with_ **anti-LKM (liver-kidney-microsomal antibodies)** _and_ **soluble liver antigen.**
- ☞ Treatment is _**steroids**_ ± azathioprine

ALCOHOLIC HEPATITIS

- A histological diagnosis (e.g. _**Mallory bodies**_, etc)
- Clinical: N/V; anorexia; abdominal pain; ↓ weight
- #1 sign is hepatomegaly
- ↑AST (_**AST/ALT >2/1**_)
- Poor prognosticators: spider nevi; ↑ PT; bili>20; renal failure; ascites; encephalopathy.

PRIMARY BILIARY CIRRHOSIS (PBC) ✪

1. Idiopathic disease of ***middle-aged women***
2. Affects the SMALL bile ducts
3. ↑*alk phos* and ↑ IgM; + ***AMA (anti-mitchondrial antibody)***
4. ***Pruritis***, steatorrhea (2° to progressive cholestasis)
5. Treatment: ursodeoxycholic acid (***UDCA***); colchicine.

PRIMARY SCLEROSING CHOLANGITIS ✪

1. LARGER bile ducts (extra and intrahepatic) suffer an obliterative inflammatory **fibrosis**
2. Also felt to be autoimmune
3. *Clinical presentation* generally includes: fatigue, RUQ pain, jaundice, pruritus, and weight loss. (not to be confused, of course, with ascending cholangitis, which can give *fever* + RUQ pain + jaundice = Charcot's triad; chills, hypotension/shock; etc.)
4. Dx→Cholangiography (MRCP, ERCP): thickened ducts with multifocal stricturing or "beading" of extrahepatic and intrahepatic bile ducts.
5. **Ulcerative Colitis associated** in 70% of cases (may come **before, during, or after** the PSC). One important clue in patients with preexisting UC is **asymptomatic elevations in alk phos**. Moreover, *for all patients initially diagnosed with sclerosing cholangitis, one should rule out an incipient UC.*
6. ↑ **risk of** **cholangiocarcinoma** (i.e. bile duct ca; remember too that UC per se also has an ↑ risk of cholangiocarcinoma, i.e. *irrespective* of PSC)
7. Treatment is primarily supportive, although many patients require liver transplant.

INDICATIONS FOR LIVER TRANSPLANTATION —Liver transplantation is indicated for acute or chronic liver failure *from any cause*. The most frequent indications for liver transplantation include:

- Chronic liver failure from cholestatic disorders (eg, primary biliary cirrhosis [PBC], sclerosing cholangitis [PSC], and extrahepatic biliary atresia); chronic hepatitis (eg, hepatitis B, hepatitis C, and autoimmune hepatitis); alcoholic liver disease; metabolic diseases (eg, Wilson's disease, hereditary hemochromatosis, alpha-1-antitrypsin deficiency, nonalcoholic steatohepatitis); and cirrhosis of unknown cause (cryptogenic cirrhosis)
- Acute liver failure (fulminant hepatic failure of any cause)
- Hepatocellular carcinoma [HCC]

ORAL CONTRACEPTIVE USE AND LIVER DISEASE ✪

1. **Adenomas** ± intraperitoneal **rupture** (also seen in pregnancy)
2. **Cholelithiasis; cholestasis**
3. **Focal nodular hyperplasia**
4. **Hepatic vein thrombosis**
5. **Peliosis Hepatis** (*blood-filled cysts in the liver*)

PELIOSIS HEPATIS, ASSOCIATIONS WITH...

1. OCPs

2. Pregnancy

3. Anabolic steroids (also ↑ risk of angiosarcoma)

4. Bartonella henselae *(re: cause of cat-scratch disease and bacillary angiomatosis)*

MORE USEFUL MNEMONICS..

LIVER DYSFUNCTION IN IBD→ *"CCCHHH"*

C holelithiasis in Crohn's disease (re: "stones in Crohn's)
C holangiocarcinoma
C holangitis (either pericholangitis—usually minimally symptomatic ↑alk phos—or *sclerosing cholangitis*)

H epatitis (CAH)→cirrhosis; granulomatous)
H epatic infiltration (fat, amyloid)
H epatic vein thrombosis *(see next section)*

HEPATIC VEIN THROMBOSIS MAY COMPLICATE THESE ✪: *"HOPING"* you remember this !

H epatoma

O CPs—as noted above

P Vera; P NH

I BD-as noted above

N ephroGenic carcinoma (renal cell ca)

FATTY LIVER MAY BE CAUSED BY ✪: *"PIC-A-DOT"*; *or remember you have to store all your excesses somewhere! ...*

P regnancy (↑β-HCG)
I BD (↑ inflammation)
C ushing's syndrome (↑cortisol)
A lcohol (↑Etoh)
D M (↑ glucose)
O besity (↑ fat)
T hyrotoxicosis (↑thyroxine)

ACALCULOUS CHOLECYSTITIS

- Severe inflammation of the GB in the absence of gallstones.
- *Associated with a high incidence of complications* (e.g., necrosis, gangrene, and GB perforation), *so early recognition is important* !
- *Risk factors include*: serious trauma or burns, **postop**, prolonged parenteral hyperalimentation (**TPN**), GB adenocarcinoma, **diabetes** mellitus, torsion of the GB, and bacterial and parasitic infection

THE MIRIZZI SYNDROME

- Refers to *common hepatic duct obstruction caused by an extrinsic compression from an impacted stone in the cystic duct.*
- Part of the differential diagnosis of *obstructive jaundice.*
- Most patients present with the clinical triad of *jaundice, fever, and right upper quadrant pain* (also = Charcot's triad for ascending cholangitis).
- The major laboratory findings are elevations in the serum concentrations of *alkaline phosphatase and bilirubin* in over 90 percent of patients.
- Imaging studies — Ultrasonography and CT scanning are commonly employed in patients with obstructive jaundice. Ultrasonography in this setting generally reveals gallstones and a contracted gallbladder. Additional features suggestive of Mirizzi syndrome include:
  - Dilatation of the biliary system above the level of the gallbladder neck.
  - The presence of a stone impacted in the gallbladder neck.
  - An abrupt change to a normal width of the common duct below the level of the stone.
- Associated with a high frequency of gallbladder cancer.
- Surgery is the mainstay of therapy, permitting removal of the causal factors: the inflamed gallbladder; cystic duct; and impacted stone.

NONOPERATIVE THERAPIES FOR SYMPTOMATIC GALLSTONES:

AGENT	RESULTS	NOTES
Oral bile acid dissolution: (eg ursodiol=Actigall)	30-90 % successful dissolution; no mortality	50% recurrence rate; dissolves noncalcified cholesterol stones; optimal for *free-floating stones <5mm*;
Contact solvents: methyl *tert*-butyl ether/*n*-propyl acetate	50-90%	70% recurrence rate; duodenitis, hemolysis, nephrotoxicity, mild sedation
Lithotripsy	70-90%	70% recurrence rate; selection criteria→*no more than 1 radiolucent stone <20mm* in diameter, patent cystic duct, functioning gallbladder in a patient with symptomatic stones without complications

GIANT GASTRIC RUGAE
1. **Malignancy** (e.g. lymphoma, leiomyoma)
2. **Gastrinomas**

DIAGNOSIS OF LACTOSE INTOLERANCE
1. History of *loose bm's/flatulence/cramps* after milk products
2. Successful *therapeutic trial of milk-free diet*
3. Positive *hydrogen breath test* following oral lactose.

INVESTIGATING SUSPECTED LAXATIVE ABUSE
1. ↓ Serum K+
2. + KOH test
3. + Urinary Phenolphthalein
4. **Melanosis coli** on endoscopy; barium enema shows a **loss of haustra** (beware, both of these findings can also be seen in Carcinoid syndrome)

✪ **BLOODY DIARRHEA or FECAL LEUKOCYTES: BACTERIAL CAUSES**

"*YE³S², Can Cause!*"

1. Yersinia
2. Entameba histolytica
3. Enteroinvasive E. Coli
4. E. Coli 0157H7
5. Salmonella
6. Shigella
7. Campylobacter jejuni
8. C. diff colitis (5% of cases present this way)

✪ **HEMOCHROMATOSIS**

1. A disorder of Fe metabolism and Fe overload, with subsequent Fe deposition in multiple organs (heart, pancreas, gonads, joints, skin)

2. Laboratory:
   ➢ *Serum **TRANSFERRIN SATURATION**, preferably in the fasting state, is the best initial **SCREENING** test for hemochromatosis.*
   ➢ While iron-binding saturations of **>90% are typical**, hemochromatosis **should be suspected at levels > 60% in men and 50% in women**
   ➢ Serum ferritin > 1000
   ➢ ↑ serum Fe, reduced TIBC
   ➢ Liver biopsy→grade 3 or 4 Fe stains

3. **PHLEBOTOMIZE** to keep Hgb<10, male ferritin <350, female ferritin< 200. This approach prevents the development of liver disease, cardiac disease, or skin bronzing. A typical phlebotomy regimen would be qw or biw for 2—3 years,

then every 3-4 months for life. Chelation with deferoxamine and watching one's dietary intake of iron, except for avoiding MVI containing Fe, pale in comparison to phlebotomy and actually do not play a significant role.

4. *Arthropathy* and *hypogonadism* and *cirrhosis* are the irreversible complications; the insulin requirement in established diabetics is rarely eliminated, although control may improve.

5. Re: ↑ risk of hepatoma in patients with cirrhosis.

WILSON'S DISEASE ✪

1. Autosomal dominant disease, where, **secondary to decreased biliary copper excretion** *in the liver*, **it is deposited in a variety of tissues** (as opposed to hemochromatosis, which is 2° to ↑Fe *absorption*→mechanism unknown)—both, however, give a transaminitis.

2. Definitely must know what's ↑ and what's ↓:
   a) Copper in the serum, urine, and liver are **ALL INCREASED**
   b) **DECREASED serum ceruloplasmin** (carrier protein for Cu) <200. In 5%, though, >200.

3. **Kaiser-Fleischer rings** (a brownish pigmented ring at the edge of the cornea)
4. *Neurologic signs*→ eg flapping tremor; chorea; rigidity; dysarthria; parkinsonism; abnl gait
5. **HEMOLYTIC ANEMIA (Coombs' negative)**

6. TREATMENT:
   a. **Lifelong oral chelation with PENICILLAMINE** ↑s urinary Cu excretion;
      i. Penicillamine greatly increases the urinary excretion of copper to above 1200 μg/day (normal 30 μg/day).
      ii. The initial goal is urinary copper excretion of 2000 μg/day. The rate of copper excretion falls as copper stores become depleted.
      iii. Values usually fall to below 500 μg/day at four to six months. *At this time, the dose of penicillamine can be lowered or the patient can be switched to oral zinc (↓absorption) for maintenance.*
      iv. Penicillamine inactivates pyridoxine. Thus, small doses of pyridoxine, 25 mg per day, should be given to patients treated with penicillamine to prevent pyridoxal phosphate deficiency
   b. **ORAL ZINC**
      i. Oral zinc acetate (50 mg PO three times a day) has been used successfully *to prevent the reaccumulation of copper in patients who have already responded to penicillamine, and in patients who responded poorly to penicillamine*, particularly those who have neuropsychiatric disease.
      ii. Zinc works to inhibit copper absorption and even promotes copper excretion in stool.

7. The **prognosis** in patients with Wilson's disease is excellent in all but those with advanced disease and those who present with rapidly progressive liver failure and hemolysis. The neurologic, psychiatric, and hepatic abnormalities gradually improve with treatment, and liver function test results usually return to normal.

⊗ **DRUG-INDUCED HEPATIC DISEASE:**

OFFENDING AGENTS	HEPATOTOXICITY
Halothane; INH; ketoconazole	Viral Hepatitis
ASA; valproate	Reye's syndrome
TCN; AZT; valproic acid	Steatosis
Long-term MTX; amiodarone; ↑VitA; vinyl chloride	Crytogenic cirrhosis
Chlorpromazine (Thorazine®)	Primary Biliary Cirrhosis
Methyldopa; INH; nitrofurantoin; dantrolene	Chronic Active Hepatitis (CAH)
Synthetic estrogens	Budd-Chiari Syndrome
Allopurinol	Granulomatous (hypersensitivity) hepatitis
Amiodarone	Can mimic alcoholic liver dz
Acetaminophen (SGOT>4000)—may occur at relatively low doses in alcoholics	Acute Hepatitis
Cocaine	Massive ischemic necrosis
Androgenic steroids; OCPs	Peliosis Hepatis
Vinyl chloride; thoratrast; anabolic steroids	Angiosarcoma
Amoxicillen-clavulinate; oral contraceptive pills	Cholestatic Hepatitis

GUT ENDOCRINE TUMORS (PANCREATIC ISLET CELL TUMORS)

GLUCAGONOMA ✪

1. Primary *α-cell* _pancreatic tumor→glucagon excess._
2. Clinically, remember these patients on your **"WARD's"**; *that's* →**W**eight loss, **A**nemia, **R**ash (NME, or necrolytic migratory erythema), and **D**iabetes mellitus/**D**iarrhea
3. The diarrhea is non-steatorrheal.
4. _**Necrolytic Migratory Erythema**_ is a transient bullous or crusting rash, most commonly involving perineum or central face, and leaves residual pigmentation.
5. Additional clinical findings: ↓cholesterol; stomatitis, glossitis, thromboembolism.
6. Spontaneous, asymptomatic remissions common.
7. Tx: Somatostatin for the diarrhea, anticoagulants for any thromboses, insulin if required.

INSULINOMA

1. Symptoms do develop early, so that tumors are usually small (most are < 2cm in diameter) and solitary at the time of diagnosis.
2. As with gastrinomas, insulinomas are frequently (10%) associated with MEN I
3. **Diagnosis** of insulinoma is made by demonstrating fasting hypoglycemia in the presence of normal or elevated plasma insulin levels. Think of insulinoma as part of the differential of hypoglycemia and the exercise therein! It is important to rule out exogenous insulin administration as well as surreptitious sulfonylureas. _Exogenous insulin suppresses endogenous insulin secretion, and therefore the C-peptide (which only comes from endogenous production of proinsulin)._ ✓ out this chart:

✪ LABORATORY EVALUATION OF HYPOGLYCEMIA

Diagnosis	Glucose	Insulin	C-PEPTIDE	Proinsulin
Sulfonylurea abuse	↓	↑	↑ *	↔
Surreptitious insulin	↓	↑↑	↓**	↓
Insulinoma	↓	↑	↑	↑

* **HIGH C-peptide** implies *endogenous* insulin secretion, which can result from:
  a) Insulinoma; *or*
  b) Sulfonylurea abuse—this can be confirmed by simply *checking urinary sulfonylurea levels.*
    - *Consequently, in hyperinsulinemic patients, the exclusion of sulfonylurea abuse points to insulinoma.* Remember, sulfonylureas promote insulin secretion by the β cells.
** **LOW C-peptide**, on the other hand, implies *exogenous* source, such as surreptious insulin

ZOLLINGER-ELLISON SYNDROME

1. **Remember**, as with essentially all of the GI endocrine tumors (pancreatic islet cell tumors), this is an "**APUD**" tumor (recall the embryological origins of most GI endocrine tumors): *that's → **Abdominal Pain, Ulcers, Diarrhea"**.* 50% of cases present with diarrhea or steatorrhea. *Diarrhea* results from large amounts of HCL secreted and may precede the ulcer symptoms. *Steatorrhea* results from inactivation of pancreatic lipase and precipitation of bile salts.

2. *Gastrinoma* → ectopic G cell tumor with hypersecretion of gastrin and usually found in the *pancreatic head* (60%) or duodenum (30%)

    ➢ 2/3rds of them are malignant
    ➢ ¼- ½ of the gastrinomas are associated with MEN I (*pituitary* hyperplasia or adenoma; *pancreatic islet cell* hyperplasia or adenoma *or carcinoma; parathyroid* hyperplasia or adenoma)
    ➢ 90-95% develop *ulceration*; 75% involve the *duodenal bulb* (a single duodenal ulceration is the most common radiographic finding in ZES)
    ➢ Suspect gastrinoma if you see: *recurrent* duodenal ulcers; PUD that is *poorly responsive* to the usual treatment; ulcers in patients with stigmata of *MEN I*; *post-bulbar or multiple* ulcers; and prominent gastric folds noted on barium

3. Serum *fasting gastrin level (>1200* pg/ml + low pH) is the most sensitive and specific test (although hypergastrinemia is noted in several other disorders, including: pernicious anemia and chronic atrophic gastritis)

4. *Secretin test*→ normal gastrin (↓) response in patients with simple duodenal ulcer (secretin normally inhibits gastrin); *paradoxical ↑ in gastrin response with ZES*.

5. Intraoperative localization can be difficult. Selective arteriograms see 1/3 of them, as do CT scans.

6. H2-receptor blockers, proton pump inhibitors, somatostatin, and surgery are important in management. 20-25% of gastrinomas are surgically respectable. **If** the resection is curative→ the patient can expect a normal life expectancy; **if not**→ the average life expectancy is only 2 years.

SOMATOSTATINOMA

1. *The delta cells of the* <u>*pancreas*</u> *→overproduction of somatostatin.*
2. **Remember, "<u>S</u>^{3}"; that's → Steatorrhea, Stones (cholelithiasis), and Sugar (diabetes)**
3. *Stimulates gastric emptying, but inhibits almost everything else* (gastric acid/pepsin secretion; pancreatic and biliary secretions; celiac blood flow; release of GH, TSH, insulin, glucagon, gastrin, and secretin)
4. Octreotide is actually successfully used in VIPoma diarrhea control; gastrinoma; insulinoma; glucagonoma; used also in GI hemorrhage and pancreatitis.

VIPoma (vip=vasoactive intestinal peptide)

1. Similar to somatostatin, VIP is also elaborated by the pancreatic delta cells
2. Primary tumor usually pancreatic, producing ↑VIP, resulting in…
3. *Profuse, watery diarrhea* (**secretory** diarrhea—frequently nocturnal or fasting; >3L/d in most patients), dehydration/hypotension/flushing; ↓K+
4. *Non-anion gap acidosis 2° to bicarb wasting*
5. Other clinical…
   a) Colicky abdominal pain (so-called "**pancreatic** cholera")
   b) Achlorhydria
   c) Hypercalcemia in 2/3rds of patients
   d) Hyperglycemia in half of patients resulting from hypokalemia- and VIP- induced glycogenolysis in the liver.
6. Treatment: Somatostatin drug of choice for symptom control

CARCINOID SYNDROME—CLINICAL PRESENTATION—<u>*ABCDEF*</u>:

1. **A** sthma (wheezing)
2. **B** ig belly! (ascites)
3. **C** or Pulmonale
4. **D** iarrhea
5. **E** ndocardial fibrosis
6. **F** lushing; facial edema

REMEMBER…
   ➢ Order a <u>*urinary 5-HIAA*</u> levels (a serotonin metabolite) for diagnosis
   ➢ Vital signs: ↑Temp, ↓BP (2° to vasodilatation), ↑Pulse
   ➢ Re: 90% of the tumors are in the *terminal ileum*

> ## *If the gut is normal, look for tumor in the bronchus or gonads*

> As for *management*, surgical resection can cure small carcinoids, but cure is not possible *if mets are present*, at which point *somatostatin analogues, like octreotide®, are effective for flushing, diarrhea, and carcinoid crisis* . Remember, secondaries in or beyond the liver produce the symptoms (for "syndrome", there must be hepatic metastasis present)

> Of note, in referral centers, this is the #1 cause of watery diarrhea:
> - Proctoscopy reveals *melanosis coli and absent haustra* (similar proctoscopy to laxative abuse)

STRESS ULCERS ✪

1. Cushing's and Curling's ulcers

2. **Curling's ulcers** follow *burns* (might think: "Curling iron")

3. **Cushing's ulcers** are seen in 50-75 % of *head injuries* (might remember: the injury could have been prevented had they been wearing their helmet, or "cushion")

4. Bleeding occurs in 10-20% from 3-7 days following the stress (trauma, stress, illness, burns, etc) if no prophylactic regimen is instituted (Sucralfate; H_2 blockers)

✪ THE BERNSTEIN TEST (Acid Perfusion test) in the Diagnosis of GERD

The Bernstein test consists of infusions of solutions of 0.1 N HCl and normal saline into the esophagus. It is *valuable in diagnosing reflux that is not obvious on endoscopy*. The test is positive if infusion of acid, but not of saline, *reproduces the symptoms* of heartburn in patients with reflux esophagitis. Infusion of acid in normal subjects usually produces no symptoms.

KEY INDICATIONS FOR ESOPHAGEAL pH RECORDING*

1. To document abnormal esophageal acid exposure in an endoscopy-negative *patient being considered for surgical antireflux repair*

2. To evaluate patients *after antireflux surgery who are suspected to have ongoing* abnormal reflux

3. To evaluate patients with either *normal or equivocal endoscopic findings and reflux symptoms that are refractory to proton pump inhibitor*

4. Esophageal pH recording is not indicated to detect or verify reflux esophagitis (this is an endoscopic diagnosis).

    * pH study done after withholding antisecretory drug regimen for ≥one week

MEDS FREQUENTLY ASSOCIATED WITH ESOPHAGITIS ✪
"QUINcy PAID 'N Cash"

1. **Q** uinidine
2. **P** otassium chloride
3. **A** lendronate/**A**spirin
4. **I** ron sulfate
5. **D** oxycycline/Tetracycline
6. **N** SAIDs
7. **C** vitamin

BARRETT'S ESOPHAGUS ✪

1. Columnar-lined esophageal metaplasia; complication of chronic reflux;

2. Associated with a 30-fold ↑ risk of esophageal **adenoca**

3. Remember, while much ado is made about Barrett's→adenocarcinoma, 98% of esophageal ca is actually squamous cell carcinoma. **Squamous** cell carcinomas are more common in blacks than whites, while adenocarcinomas are more common in whites than blacks, and in fact, Barrett's **rarely develops in blacks.**

4. **Squamous** cell carcinomas and adenocarcinomas of the esophagus cannot be distinguished radiographically or endoscopically

5. While Barrett's is an important risk factor for adenocarcinoma, *risk factors to know for* **SQUAMOUS CELL CARCINOMA** *include*: **alcohol, tobacco**, lye stricture, pickled or smoked foods, achalasia, Plummer-Vinson syndrome, and tylosis.

6. While indeed 30% of patients presenting with carcinoma in Barrett's have no prior history of reflux, Barrett's esophagus is found in 10% of biopsies for esophagitis and 40% of patients with chronic peptic strictures. Therefore, endoscopic surveillance important: if multiple foci of high-grade dysplasia develop, resection may be indicated.

RECOMMENDATIONS BY LEVEL OF DYSPLASIA ON ENDOSCOPY

No dysplasia:
Repeat endoscopy q2y
PPI (proton pump inhibitor) therapy for symptoms

Low-grade dysplasia: Intensive PPI therapy
Repeat endoscopy @ 8wk. If dysplasia found, repeat endoscopy every 6 mo until 2 consecutive exams show no dysplasia, then q year

High-grade dysplasia: Confirm dx with another pathologist
Intensive PPI therapy
Esophagectomy or endoscopic ablation therapy

PLUMMER-VINSON SYNDROME

1. Hypopharyngeal *webs* (esophageal stricture)
2. *Fe deficiency anemia*
3. Classically *middle-aged women*
4. *15% chance of developing oropharyngeal or esophageal carcinoma*

DYSPHAGIA

1. Intermittent dysphagia is caused by rings/webs/motility disorders.

2. 2 causes: **mechanical (obstruction) vs. functional (motility)**

3. Diagnosis by **history** can usually be had by getting this information on the dysphagia

   a) Is it to solids or both solids and liquids?
   b) Progressive or intermittent?
   c) Is there associated heartburn?

4. **Schatski's ring** is *a ring at the level of the LES that can present with episodic dysphagia to solid food at diameters less than 1.3cm*

5. **Zenker's diverticulum** (Aka "crycopharyngeal diverticulum")

   a) Clinical: *halitosis, regurgitation, dysphagia, chronic cough, recurrent pneumonia.*

   b) Treatment is surgical excision of the diverticulum

✪ UNDERSTANDING DYSPHAGIA BY PRESENTATION:

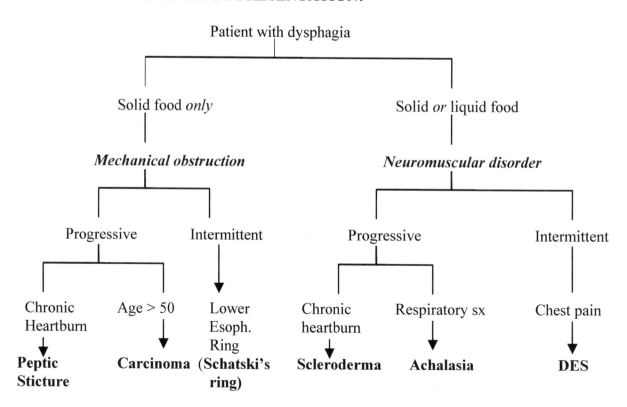

SCLERODERMA ✪

1. GERD; **peptic strictures** very common
2. Progressive dysphagia to solids & liquids
3. Look for these on the UGI:
   - ✓ **Common E-G tube**
   - ✓ **Pseudoobstruction**
   - ✓ **Wide-mouthed jejunal diverticula**
4. Motility studies show
   - ✓ **LOW resting LES pressures**
   - ✓ **Aperistalsis** in the body of the esophagus; LES incompetence→ severe reflux.

ACHALASIA ✪

- ➢ Achalasia a Greek term that means "does not relax".
- ➢ Mechanism is the *__incomplete relaxation of the LES__*
- ➢ Manifests clinically as solid and liquid dysphagia
- ➢ Regurgitation of material retained in the flaccid esophagus may be troublesome, especially during recumbency at night, and may result in aspiration.
- ➢ Patients with achalasia are also *at substantially increased risk for developing squamous cell esophageal cancer.*
- ➢ *Endoscopic evaluation* is generally recommended for most patients with achalasia primarily *to exclude malignancies at the esophagogastric junction that can mimic primary achalasia* clinically, radiographically, and manometrically (so called "pseudoachalasia").

- ➢ **IMAGING ✪**
  - ▪ **Radiography**
    1. **"Bird's beak" sign** on UGI → dilated esophagus with tapered lower end that is due to a beak-like narrowing caused by the persistently contracted lower esophageal sphincter (LES)
    2. Absent of the normal gastric A/F (air/fluid) level caused by the failure of LES relaxation that prevents air from entering the stomach
  - ▪ **Manometry**: 3 characteristic features:
    1. **HIGH resting LES pressure**
    2. **Incomplete LES relaxation**
    3. **Aperistalsis** is seen in the smooth muscle portion of the body of the esophagus. Tertiary contractions may be seen replacing peristaltic activity at all levels.
- ➢ **TREATMENT** options include: 1) Botulin toxin injection (Botox®); 2) bougienage; 3) pneumatic dilatation; 4) surgical myotomy; and 5) medical therapy with nitrates or calcium channel blockers.

MANAGEMENT OF DES (Diffuse Esophageal Spasm) (AKA 'nutcracker' esophagus)

1. Avoid stress and cold or hot liquids, all of which exacerbate the episodes of chest pain.
2. Be sure you've ruled out CAD/gallstones/PUD
3. Nifedipine
4. Nitrates

VERTICAL TRANSMISSION OF HEPATITIS IN PREGNANCY

1. HBV most likely to be transmitted if acquired in the 3rd trimester
2. Neonates at risk should be immediately started on both active and passive immunization; 90% of infected neonates become chronic carriers.
3. Approximately 50% of vertically-infected children ultimately die of cirrhosis or hepatoma

HEPATIC ADENOMAS IN OCP USE (OR PREGNANCY)...

☞ May present with **acute RUQ pain and hemodynamic compromise 2° to bleeding/ rupture**.

GLUTEN-SENSITIVE ENTEROPATHY ✪ (aka <u>CELIAC SPRUE</u>, or "sprue", as opposed to "tropical sprue")

1. AutoAbs may be seen: + *<u>Anti-endomysial Ab</u>*; + *<u>Anti-gliadin Ab</u>*; + *<u>Anti-reticulin Ab</u>*
2. Persistent non-specific GI upset
3. Celiac disease, classically, has been said to be a cause of *<u>iron deficiency anemia</u>* that *<u>doesn't respond to oral iron</u>*.
4. Steatorrhea
5. Growth retardation
6. *<u>Osteomalacia</u>*(2° to ↓ vit D)
7. *<u>Dermatitis Herpetiformis</u>*—classic rash of celiac disease
8. Proctalgia fugax
9. *Remember, the most definitive diagnosis is had by noting symptomatic resolution on a <u>gluten-free diet</u>* :
    AVOID → Barley Rye Oats Wheat (these should raise your "<u>BROW</u>")
    MAY HAVE→ rice, corn, soybean
10. Howell-Jolly bodies on peripheral blood smear may be seen
11. ↓ RBC folate seen in 70%

INFECTIONS OF THE ESOPHAGUS

1. Candida, HSV, and CMV are the most important causes of odynophagia
2. CMV: severe inflammation with *very large ulcers*
3. HSV: barium and EGD show small, discrete ulcers; biopsy shows *intranuclear inclusions* (*Cowdry bodies*)

COMPLICATIONS OF GASTRECTOMY-*6 D'S*: (Remember botulism has 6 D's too! --see section on "Toxigenic Diarrheas")

D umping
D iarrhea
D izziness
D ysphagia
D eficiencies (vitamins, Fe)
D istension after eating

BLIND-(or "Stagnant"-) LOOP SYNDROME —"_SALAD_":

S teatorrhea
A nemia
L oss of weight
A bdominal pains
D eficiencies of vitamins

- _**Mechanism of BLIND-LOOP SYNDROME**_→Bacterial overgrowth occurs in the **afferent loop** and causes malabsorption (as bile salts are deconjugated) and **megaloblastic anemia** as bacteria consume B12; ↓**B12** may also be 2° to loss of Intrinsic Factor that occurs with gastrectomy. Treatment is to convert the Bilroth II→Bilroth I or Roux-en-Y. This **syndrome should not be confused for "afferent loop syndrome"**, which is another complication of Bilroth II that occurs earlier than blind loop syndrome and results, not from bacterial overgrowth complications, but from partial obstruction of the afferent loop.

BRIEF SYNOPSIS OF THE TREATMENTS FOR MALABSORPTION DISORDERS:	
Diagnosis	**Treatment**
Abetalipoproteinemia	Low-fat diet; fat-soluble vitamins
Bacterial overgrowth	Antibiotics
Crohn's disease	5-ASA, steroids
Intestinal infection with: Giardia lamblia Isospora belli Strongyloides stercoralis	 Metronidazole TMP/SMX Thiabendazole
Lactase deficiency (Lactose intolerance)	Lactase supplementation
Lymphangiectasia	Address the causative disease
Pancreatic insufficiency	Pancreatic enzyme supplements
Short-gut syndrome	Medium-chain triglycerides, low-oxalate diet, parenteral nutrition as appropriate

Sprue
  Celiac
  Tropical
	
	Gluten-free diet
	B12, folate, TCN

Whipple's disease	Initial IV tx then PO x 1year with Bactrim-ds bid or Cefixime 400 qd(see "Whipple's" below)

INITIAL SCREENING TESTS FOR SUSPECTED MALABSORPTION
    STOOL Tests
        1. 72h quantitative fecal fat
        2. O&P
    BLOOD Tests
        1. Alkaline phosphatase
        2. Blood levels of vitamin B12, folate, vitamin D and K, Calcium, carotene
        3. CBC
        4. Serum protein
        5. Thyroid function

✪ DIAGNOSTIC APPROACH TO MALABSORPTION:

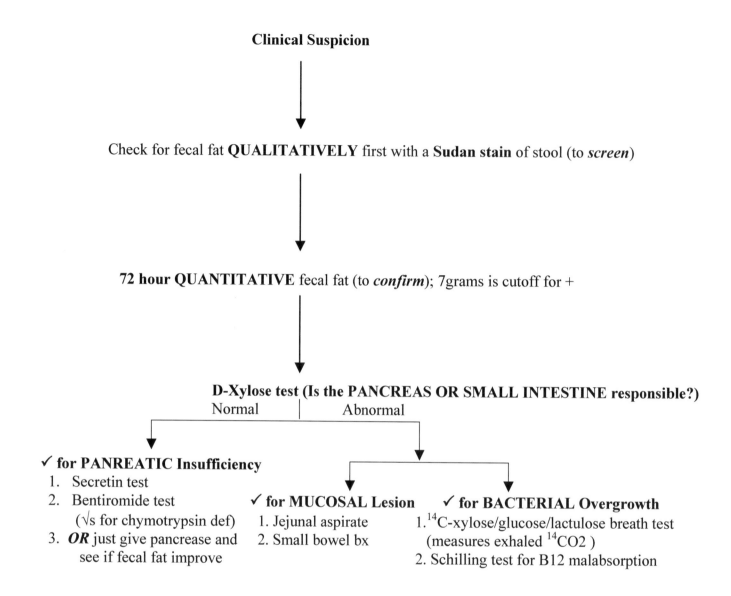

Clinical Suspicion

↓

Check for fecal fat **QUALITATIVELY** first with a **Sudan stain** of stool (to *screen*)

↓

72 hour QUANTITATIVE fecal fat (to *confirm*); 7grams is cutoff for +

↓

D-Xylose test (Is the PANCREAS OR SMALL INTESTINE responsible?)

Normal | Abnormal

✓ for PANREATIC Insufficiency
1. Secretin test
2. Bentiromide test
   (√s for chymotrypsin def)
3. **OR** just give pancrease and
   see if fecal fat improve

✓ for MUCOSAL Lesion
1. Jejunal aspirate
2. Small bowel bx

✓ for BACTERIAL Overgrowth
1. ^{14}C-xylose/glucose/lactulose breath test
   (measures exhaled $^{14}CO2$)
2. Schilling test for B12 malabsorption

IMPORTANT NOTES:

- **D-Xylose test**— A good screening test for carbohydrate malabsorption due to small intestinal disorders (eg celiac sprue). A 5-hour urine xylose excretion < 4.5g following ingestion of 25g of d-xylose is +.
- **Secretin test**—Under fluoroscopic guidance, pancreatic secretions are collected in the second part of the duodenum before and after an IV dose of secretin; diagnostic of pancreatic exocrine insufficiency if there is a ↓ in pancreatic fluid output and bicarbonate secretion after secretin; highly sensitive & specific, but invasive and requires excellent patient cooperation. *This ≠ the secretin test in Zollinger-Ellison Syndrome!* (see that section)
- **Bentiromide test**—Normally, after oral administration, bentiromide is metabolized in the small intestine by chymotrypsin with the liberation of PABA, which is rapidly absorbed and excreted in the urine. Lower urinary levels of PABA are seen in pancreatic malabsorption.
- **^{14}C-xylose breath test**—Elevated levels indicate bacterial overgrowth. *This ≠ the D-Xylose test.*
- **Hydrogen breath test**—Tests for lactose intolerance (although trial of avoidance should be done first).

EXTRAINTESTINAL SIGNS OF MALABSORPTION (Mayo IMBR):

EXTRA-GI SYMPTOM	RESULT OF
Muscle wasting, edema	↓Protein absorption
Paresthesias, tetany	↓Vit D and Ca absorption
Bone pain	↓Ca absorption
Muscle cramps; weakness	↓ K+
Easy bruising, petechiae	↓ Vit K absorption
Hyperkeratosis, night blindness	↓ Vit A absorption
Pallor	↓ Vit B12, folate, or Fe absorption
Glossitis, stomatitis, cheilosis	↓ Vit B12, folate, or Fe absorption
Acrodermatitis	↓ Zinc absorption

BILE ACID MALAPSORPTION ✪

1. Diarrhea following ileal disease or resection
2. If the disease/resection is <100 cm→ treatment is **cholestyramine**
3. If the disease/resection is > 100cm→ treatment is **medium chain triglycerides** with a low fat diet

ILEAL RESECTION AND RENAL STONES ✪

- ✓ **Hyperoxaluria** → **calcium oxalate** stone formation.
- ✓ **Treatment** of enteric hyperoxaluria is directed toward *diminishing intestinal oxalate absorption.* The initial regimen consists of a low oxalate diet, high fluid intake, potassium citrate to correct metabolic acidosis if present, and oral calcium carbonate (1 to 4 g/day) to bind oxalate in the intestinal lumen. Although some of the calcium is absorbed, there is a proportionately greater fall in oxalate excretion.

MECKEL'S DIVERTICULUM—*RULE OF 2'S*:

- ✓ 2:1 Male: Female ratio
- ✓ 2 complications: hemorrhage and perforation
- ✓ 2 types of ectopic tissue: gastric and pancreatic
- ✓ Confused with 2 other problems: ulcers and appendix
- ✓ 2% incidence on autopsies (i.e. affects 2% of population)
- ✓ Usually occurs within 2 feet of the ileocecal valve
- ✓ Usually presents within the first 2 years of life
- ✓ Usually about 2 inches in length

CLINICAL FEATURES OF **ACUTE** PANCREATITIS—"*AMYLASE*"

A cute pain; **A** lcohol is the #1 cause (acute on chronic) and gallstones are #2.

M id-abdominal staining (Grey Turner's and Cullen's signs)—loin and periumbilical respectively

Y ellow (ascites)

L ipase ↑; **L** eft-sided pleural effusion

A mylase ↑ (usu. > 1000)

S entinel loop (**S** mall bowel ileus overlying the pancreatic area)

E mesis and nausea

CLINICAL FEATURES OF **CHRONIC** PANCREATITIS—"*C MAIDS*"

(think "Old maid(s)" for chronic)

C alcification, pancreatic; **C** hronic (!)

M alabsorption

A bdominal pain (Alcohol is the #1 cause, similar to AP)

I cterus

D iabetes

S teatorrhea

✪ **POOR PROGNOSTICATORS IN ACUTE PANCREATITIS (RANSON'S CRITERIA)**

At Time of Admission or Diagnosis:
1. Age>55yo
2. WBC>16
3. Glucose (serum)>200
4. LDH>350
5. SGOT (ALT) > 250 IU/L

During Initial 48 hours: "*Ranson's BASeline BUNdle Sure CAn Help Out*"

B ase deficit > 4 mEq/L	4
B UN increase of > 5 mg/dl	5
S equestration of fluid > 6 L	6
C alcium < 8 mg/dl	8
H ct decrease > 10%	10
O xygen < 60 mm Hg	60

CONDITIONS ASSOCIATED WITH ACUTE PANCREATITIS
1. *Hypertriglyceridemia (Types 1,4,5)* ✪
2. *Hypercalcemia*. If see, R/O: ✪
   - ✓ Multiple myeloma
   - ✓ Hyperparathyroidism
   - ✓ Metastatic Ca.
3. Pancreas divisum--failure of ventral and dorsal pancreas to fuse during organogenesis;
4. *Post-ERCP*

✪ **KEY DRUGS that can cause PANCREATITIS:** *"PD FAST VET"* (as in "Pretty Fast corVETte"):

P entamidine
D di (didanosine**)**

F urosemide
A zathioprine
S ulfa
T hiazides

V alproic acid
E strogen
T etracycline

COMPLICATIONS OF ACUTE PANCREATITIS

1. *Phlegmon*—a mass of inflamed pancreatic tissue

2. *Pseudocysts* ✪—<u>**fluid collections—resolve spontaneously most of the time within weeks**</u>

3. *Hypocalcemia* (2° to accumulation/precipatation of calcium salts)

4. *Pancreatic abscess* ✪—<u>**usually occurs 2-4 weeks after the acute episode: see fever; persistent abdominal pain; persistent ↑ amylase. These MUST be drained!**</u>

5. *ARDS*; and left-sided pleural effusion

PANCREATIC PSEUDOCYSTS
➤ Seen in approx 15% of cases of acute pancreatitis
➤ 85% are located in the body and tail of the pancreas
➤ They represent collections of tissue, fluid, debris, pancreatic enzymes, and blood which develop over a period of 1 to 4 weeks after the onset of acute pancreatitis.
➤ In contrast to true cysts, pseudocysts do not have an epithelial lining; rather, the walls consist of necrotic tissue, granulation tissue, and fibrous tissue.
➤ Usually resolve spontaneously; however, <u>pseudocysts that are greater than 5 cm in diameter and that persist for longer than 6 weeks</u> should be considered for drainage due to an increased risk of complications.

PANCREATIC CA
1. The 5 year survival rate is < 2%, since most patients present late in the course of their disease. If patients are diagnosed early enough (tumor<2cm; no nodes; no mets)→Whipple procedure.
2. <u>Courvoisier's sign</u>=painless jaundice with a palpable gallbladder→pancreatic ca
3. <u>Trousseau's sign</u>=recurrent migratory thrombophlebitis→associated with pancreatic ca.
4. <u>"Double-duct" sign</u>=obstruction and therefore visible dilatation of both bile and pancreatic ducts, and is secondary to pancreatic ca; a classic presentation.

WHIPPLE'S DISEASE ✪

1. *Diarrhea (malabsorptive)*

2. *Fever*

3. *Lymphadenopathy*

4. *Migratory arthralgias*

5. Neurologic symptoms

6. Causative organism (found in these macrophages) is Tropheryma Whippllii, a gram + bacillus

7. Treatment: *Initial IV*: Ceftriaxone 2.0g bid + Streptomycin 1.0g qd; *then PO Rx for 1 year with either* TMP/SMX-DS bid or Cefixime 400mg PO qd.

MEDICAL CONDITIONS THAT ↑ RISK FOR GASTRIC CANCER: *"SAM's PUB!"* ✪

➢ **S**urgery (prior gastric)
➢ **A**lcohol (!); Atrophic gastritis (below) (*H. pylori* → chronic atrophic gastritis→gastric ca)
➢ **M**enetrier's disease (extreme hypertrophy of the gastric rugal folds)

➢ **P**ernicious anemia
➢ **U**lcers **(gastric)**
➢ **B**lood type A

Of course, the long-term ingestion of foods containing high concentrations of nitrates in dried, smoked, and salted foods is also associated with a higher risk.

CHRONIC ATROPHIC GASTRITIS ('Nonerosive Gastritis'): TYPES A & B ✪

TYPE A		TYPE B
1. *Associated with* **pernicious Anemia** & gastric carcinoids	⟷	*Associated with* **H. Pylori** (& PUD) (H. Pylori **B**acteria is actually responsible!)
2. *Body/fundus* of stomach	⟷	*Antrum* of stomach
3. Serum gastrin ↑	⟷	*Normal* serum gastrin

- *Both* types are associated with *adenocarcinoma*.
- *Both* are usually *asymptomatic*.
- In patients with type B gastritis, eradication of *H. pylori* is generally not recommended in the absence of documented peptic ulcer or MALT lymphoma.

H. PYLORI AND PUD

- H. Pylori is responsible for <u>chronic (type B) antral gastritis</u> and accounts for 80% and 90% of <u>gastric and duodenal PUD</u> respectively.

- Eradication of H. Pylori, using various combinations of bismuth, proton pump inhibitor, H2-receptor antagonists and antibiotics ↓ the rate of recurrence of both gastric and duodenal ulcers.

- H. Pylori can be tested in the gastroenterologist's office using a <u>CLO test</u> on the endoscopy specimen→agar changes color when presented with the urease-splitting organism.

- ☞ H. Pylori is also implicated in the etiology of <u>gastric ca</u>.

- ☞ Re: duodenal ulcers are 4x more common than gastric ulcers in this country. Recall that gastric ulcers, if > 2.5cm or suspicious in radiologic appearance, require endoscopy with biopsy, as gastric ulcers have an ↑ risk of malignant transformation.

POINTS ON H. PYLORI TESTING

- **The Urease Breath Test**. The UBT employs ^{13}C and ^{14}C-labeled urea to detect **active** H. Pylori infection. ***The test works as follows****:* if the bacteria are present in the stomach, the urease they produce will hydrolyze labeled urea ingested by the patient, resulting in the release of labeled CO_2, which is measured as the patient breaths into a collection device.

- ☞ The ^{13}C and ^{14}C UBTs **can also be used to confirm eradication after treatment** (stool testing is another noninvasive method shown to compare will with the breath test). However, ***proper*** ***timing is important****:* testing must be done ≥ 2 weeks after cessation of maintenance antisecretory therapy and ≥ 4 weeks after completion of antibiotic therapy (4 weeks post treatment for stool antigen detection). Remember, **antibody testing with ELISA** is less useful in the evaluation of posttreatment response because high levels of antibodies to H. pylori remain for variable and extended periods. However, for an individual more than a year out from therapy, seroconversion is a reliable indicator of successful eradication.

DIARRHEAS

<u>OSMOTIC DIARRHEA</u>	<u>SECRETORY DIARRHEA</u>
1. Diarrhea stops with fasting	Diarrhea persists despite NPO
2. Stool has + **anion gap**	No anion gap
3. Volume<1L/day	Volume >1L/day

- In acute diarrhea, no evaluation is necessary unless there are bloody stools and fever, or infection is suspected. In these cases, classically at least, antimotility drugs should *not* be administered.

RIGHT-SIDED DIARRHEA

1. Large stool volume
2. *No* urgency/tenesmus/mucus/blood
3. Anemia, insidious

LEFT-SIDED DIARRHEA

1. Small amounts of stool
2. *May* note: urgency, tenesmus, mucus, or blood
3. Constipation/obstipation; usually presents sooner

- **Chronic diarrhea** lasts *longer than 4 weeks* by definition. The #1 cause is IBS. Must r/o Lactose intolerance (lactase deficiency). Be able to ddx <u>organic</u> (e.g. food poisoning) vs. <u>functional</u> (e.g. IBS) diarrheas. Essentially, in **IBS**, there is no weight loss; no blood in stool; so-called "pencil" (thin) stools; chronicity (> 6 mo); small stool quantity; diarrhea occurs primarily in AMs and rarely wakens the patient; significant association of bowel symptoms with level of stress. These are all in contrast to organic diarrheas.

✪ Key Features of <u>TOXIGENIC</u> Bacterial Diarrheas—*<u>WATERY</u>; <u>NO</u> fecal leukocytes...*

Staph aureus	Rapid onset(2-4h) after custard-filled pastries and delicatessen meats.
Clostridium botulinum (botulism)	Neurotoxin interferes with presynaptic ACh release, causing the other 6D's→Dilated fixed pupils; Diplopia; Dysarthria; Dysphagia; Dry tongue; Descending paralysis.
Clostridium perfringes	"Church picnic"/buffet diarrhea; precooked foods; later in onset than Staph aureus
E. Coli, enterotoxigenic	Traveler's diarrhea; Cipro prophylactically; if develops, may take Cipro bid for 3 days, although usually self-limiting.
Vibrio cholerae	The only toxigenic bacterial diarrhea where Abx clearly ↓ disease duration (TCN)
B. Cereus	Fried rice in oriental restaurants

✪ Key Features of some <u>INVASIVE</u> Bacterial Diarrheas—*Fever; BLOODY stools; and + fecal leukocytes...*

Salmonella	**No antibiotics, unless** + blood culture; also do **not** see bloody diarrhea with Salmonella (the exception); eggs/poultry/fecal-oral route
Vibrio parahemolyticus	Undercooked shellfish
Yersinia enterocolytica	DDx includes AP and Crohn's disease; dairy products
E. Coli 0157H7 (enterhemorrhagic E. Coli)	**No** fever here; tainted beef/milk→HUS; Also, **no antibiotics** → treatment of E. Coli 0157H7 infection is supportive, with monitoring for the development of HUS.
Vibrio vulnificus (noncholera)	Skin/muscle inflammation/infection after exposure to seawater or cleaning fish; & septicemia/necrotizingvasculitis/gangrene/ shock after ingesting raw oysters.
Others: Shigella; Campylobacter (below)	

CAMPYLOBACTER JEJUNI ENTERITIS

1. Remember the association with **_Guillain-Barre Syndrome_** ✪ (<u>ascending</u> paralysis—as opposed to the descending paralysis of botulism, above)
2. More common cause of enteritis than Salmonella or Shigella.
3. Bloody diarrhea/toxic megacolon/HLA B27+ reactive arthritis are all potential complications and may therefore resemble Ulcerative Colitis.
4. Treatment is Erythromycin.

SYSTEMIC MASTOCYTOSIS ✪

1. 2° to proliferation of mast cells in numerous organs
2. ↑histamine released; 50% of patients have GI symptoms, such as PUD and diarrhea
3. _Urticaria pigmentosa_
4. _"Bath pruritis" (similar to P. Vera)_
5. ✓ _urinary histamine levels_
   ☞ The measurement of histamine in a 24 hour urine collection has been used in the diagnosis of systemic mastocytosis, particularly prior to the availability of tryptase measurements. However, an increased histamine level in urine obtained during a symptomatic episode, such as flushing or syncope, _does not distinguish between anaphylaxis and systemic mastocytosis_. In such cases, an evaluation of the ratio of total (A + B) tryptases to B tryptases can differentiate (<10 in anaphylaxis; >20 in SM)
6. SM is strongly suspected in patients with _baseline levels of total tryptases of greater than 20_ ng/mL _and with a ratio of greater than 20 between total tryptase and beta tryptase_ (yes, that's 20-20!)

AMYLOIDOSIS _("AMY gives her P's TLC")_ ✪

1. **M**acroglossia (**T**ongue)
2. **H**epatomegaly (**L**iver)
3. **C**ardiomegaly (**C**ardiac)
4. **P**roteinuria
5. **P**eripheral neuropathy
6. **P**alpable **P**urpura
7. **P**inch (post-traumatic) purpura
8. **P**eriorbital ecchymoses **P**ost-**P**roctoscopy
9. GI symptoms, such as motility disorders and malabsorption, are 2° to amyloid infiltration into muscle and nerve.
10. Skin-**P**opping in type B ("AA"), not type A ("AL") phenotype
11. Fat and rectal biopsies very useful in diagnosis.
12. _Management_:
    a **Primary** amyloidosis → Melphalan and prednisone (_Remember_→ Melphalan and prednisone are also the treatment for Multiple myeloma)
    b **Secondary** amyloidosis → Treatment of the primary disease
    c **Light chain disease** → No effective treatment; poor prognosis

CLASSIFICATION OF AMYLOIDOSIS		
SUBTYPE	**ASSOCIATED CONDITIONS**	**PROTEIN SEEN**
Systemic Primary	B-cell or plasma cell **neoplasms** (multiple myeloma!)	**AL** (remember L for "Light" chains)
Secondary	**Chronic illnesses**, eg TB, RA, or osteomyelitis	**AA**
Familial	Familial	Prealbumin fibrils
β 2-microglobulin	**Long-term hemodialysis** usually with cuprophane membranes	**β2-microglobulin** as amyloid fibrils in the musculoskeletal system
Localized	N/A	N/A

β2-MICROGLOBULIN VARIANT OF AMYLOIDOSIS

1. Seen in *long-term dialysis* patients
2. *Carpal tunnel* syndrome
3. *Arthropathy*
4. *Cystic bone* lesions
5. Pathologic *fractures*

PSEUDO-OBSTRUCTION

1. Acute intestinal pseudoobstruction is often referred to as *Ogilvie's syndrome*.
2. Clinical findings of mechanical obstruction but without occlusion of the lumen; usu. the colon
3. *Abnormal esophageal motility* in most patients
4. *Steatorrhea (caused by bacterial overgrowth)*
5. *2° causes include* → amyloidosis, Parkinson's disease, myxedema, hypoparathyroidism, L-Dopa, TCA's, clonidine, phenothiazines, and narcotics.

ULCERATIVE COLITIS AND CROHN'S DISEASE ✪

1. UC involves the **colorectal intestine**
   - While Crohn's may involve **any** part of the intestinal tract (other than the rectum—"rectal sparing"), and is associated with **perianal** disease (e.g.strictures/fistulas/abscesses→Flagyl)

2. Generally, UC is associated more with frequent **bloody** stools, while Crohn's disease is associated more with crampy, abdominal **pain**, fewer BMs, and less bleeding. ("Crohn's moans; Ulcers bleed")

3. UC may have **pseudopolyps and crypt abscesses.** <u>**Toxic megacolon**</u> is a complication of particular concern in **UC**, and opiates may precipitate (just as anti-motility drugs can in patients with hematochezia and fever, e.g. many of the invasive bacterial diarrheas)

    a Medical **treatment for toxic megacolon** includes NPO, nasogastric suction, serial abdominal exams as well as aggressive use of steroids, antibiotics, fluid-electrolyte replacement, and blood transfusion.

    b **Surgery is appropriate** if resolution does not occur within 24-48 hours

4. **Colonoscopy is contraindicated in acute UC due to the ↑ risk of perforation.**

5. Among the extraintestinal manifestations: *__the severity of joint and skin disease mirrors the severity of colitis__* ✪. On the other hand, ankylosing spondylitis and sacroiliitis do not mirror the colitis.

6. Remember, **C** rohn's→ Calcium oxalate stones **(C→C)**
   U C   → Uric acid stones   **(U→U)**

7. General Overview of <u>**Medical Management in Crohn's**</u> ✪

    ➤ Start with an *__oral 5-ASA product__ (e.g. mesalamine) __or sulfazalazine__*
    ➤ If no or poor response, can consider *__antibiotics__* (usual: metronidazole ± cipro, or clarithromycin)
    ➤ If still no response, *__oral steroids__* can be considered. (5-ASA agents and antibiotics and prednisone are commonly used together in various combinations.
    ➤ For *refractory disease*, i.e. patients who remain symptomatic despite adequate doses of steroids (steroid-resistant), 5-ASA agents, and antibiotics, or for patients who flare once their prednisone is decreased or stopped (steroid-dependent), *__immunomodulators, ie azathioprine, 6-mercaptopurine, or methotrexate__*, should be considered. Remember, unlike UC, where colectomy is curative, surgery is accompanied by a high recurrence rate.
    ➤ Immediate *hospitalization* is required for patients who present with severe symptoms or appear toxic. Therapy should consist of bowel rest, parenteral nutrition, and parenteral corticosteroids.

8. <u>**Medical Thrapy in UC**</u> (by location) ✪

    ➤ *Mesalamine*:   1) RowASA suppository/enema for relief of *__proctitis__*
                        2) PentASA for relief of *__small bowel__* inflammatory disease; work by releasing ASA into small bowel
                        3) ASAcol best choice for *__terminal ileum__* disease.

    ➤ *Olsalazine and Sulfasalazine*: For *__colonic__* disease, releasing ASA into the colon.

    ✓ *Note, sulfasalazine is important in __maintaining__ remission in __UC__ only; mesalamine for maintenance in Crohn's.*
    ✓ For **Crohn's, metronidazole** is commonly used for *__perianal__* disease; one can go from sulfasalazine to metronidazole, but not vise versa.

KEY POINTS IN THE MEDICAL MANAGEMENT OF ULCERATIVE COLITIS

- ➤ *Mild to moderate disease* → *Mesalamine or sulfasalazine* for active disease or maintenance.
  - ○ Topical rectal mesalamine are particularly helpful in patients with urgency, pain, and tenesmus
  - ○ Add a daily hydrocortisone enema for those who do not respond to rectal mesalamine after 2-3 weeks of treatment
- ➤ *Mod to severe disease* → *Systemic steroids* (PO/parenteral) to induce remission. Consider colectomy or immunosuppressive therapy for patients who do not respond to systemic steroids.
  - ○ Avoid giving steroids to maintain disease; *azathioprine or 6-mercaptopurine can be used to wean from steroids*
- ➤ *Annual surveillance* colonoscopy with biopsy → for patient with *pancolitis and left-sided colitis as they are at ↑ risk for colorectal carcinoma. Consider colectomy for* patients with long-standing UC, esp if the disease is refractory or requires immunosuppressive therapy.

RISK OF COLORECTAL CANCER IN UC ✪

1. Depends upon the duration and extent of disease. In addition, patients with UC complicating **primary sclerosing cholangitis** (PSC) may be at increased risk for CRC compared to those without PSC.

2. In **patients with pancolitis**, the risk begins to increase 8 to 10 years following the onset of symptoms. The approximate cumulative incidence of CRC is 5 to 10 percent after 20 years and 12 to 20 percent after 30 years of disease.

3. The presence of "**backwash ileitis**" (in which mucosal inflammation involves the terminal ileum) may be an independent risk factor for CRC.

4. **Left-sided** colitis and ulcerative **proctitis** have a very favorable prognosis and probably cause no increase in mortality rate; similarly, the long-term prognosis for extensive colitis has improved greatly.

INDICATIONS FOR COLECTOMY IN ULCERATIVE COLITIS ✪

1. *Acute complications* (eg toxic megacolon that does not respond to medical mgmt in 24-48h; colonic perforation; severe hemorrhage; or intractable pararectal or extraintestinal complications)
2. *High grade dysplasia and carcinomas* (colonic or cholangiocarcinoma)
3. Fulminant colitis

RESPONSE OF COMPLICATIONS OF ULCERATIVE COLITIS TO COLECTOMY ✪:

1. *Positive* Response
   a. **P**eripheral arthropathy (don't confuse with hemochromatosis, where treatment *does not* improve the arthropathy)
   b. **P**yoderma gangrenosum (and the other noteworthy dermatologic manifestation, erythema nodosum)
   c. **P**ara-rectal disease

2. *Unresponsive*
   a. **S** pondilitis, Ankylosing (remember, 'S' for stays the **S**ame)
   b. **S** clerosing cholangitis (remember, 'S' for stays the **S**ame)

PROCTOCOLECTOMY & POUCHITIS

> For the surgical treatment of *ulcerative colitis and familial adenomatous polyposis* (FAP), proctocolectomy with ileal pouch-anal anastomosis (IPAA) is the favored alternative to proctocolectomy with permanent ileostomy since it preserves intestinal continuity and sphincter function and removes the entire colorectal mucosa. This procedure consists of total abdominal colectomy, stripping of the rectal mucosa with preservation of the anal sphincter, and the construction of an ileal pouch that is anastomosed to the anus.

> *The most frequently observed long-term complication of IPAA is acute and/or chronic inflammation of the ileal reservoir, called pouchitis.*

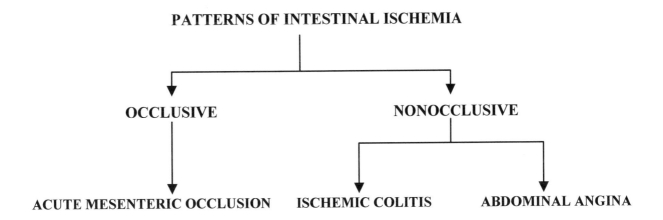

✪ ACUTE MESENTERIC ISCHEMIA

1. <u>Usually 2° to *Afib or h/o heart disease*→ *emboli* to the SMA (superior mesenteric artery)→ ischemia→gangrene</u>; comorbid abdominal vascular *thrombosis* is a less frequent presentation.

2. Radiography may show gas in the portal vein; "***thumbprinting***" (2° thick, edematous bowel wall); A/F levels may be seen

3. ***Severe abdominal pain*** ("out of proportion to the exam") ± shock

4. ↑Anion Gap 2° to lactic acidosis; ↑WBC

5. High mortality

6. **Immediate surgical resection** of the diseased bowel is the treatment.

✪ ISCHEMIC COLITIS

➢ Ischemic colitis, on the other hand, is almost always a *nonocclusive* disease.

➢ This is *more of a subacute* disease, producing *less pain and bleeding* and often occurring over several days or weeks.

➢ Mucosal ischemia is a result of *transient low blood flow or poor perfusion through* atherosclerotic splanchnic vasculature as well as "*watershed*" area of the intestine

➢ *Angiography is not usually indicated* because almost all cases are nonocclusive.

➢ *Surgery is not required* except for obstruction secondary to postischemic stricture.

➢ May see *thumbprinting* here too.

✪ ABDOMINAL ANGINA

➢ As in angina pectoris, the pain *of chronic mesenteric insufficiency* occurs under conditions of *increased demand for splanchnic blood flow.*

➢ *Midabdominal pain that occurs 15-30 minutes after eating* due to insufficient postprandial mucosal blood flow, typically *lasting several hours*

➢ Abdominal angiogram usually demonstrates *complete or near complete occlusion of at least two of the three major splanchnic arteries*, usually the celiac and superior mesenteric arteries.

AMEBIC COLITIS

1. *Bloody diarrhea with fever, tenesmus, and abdominal cramps.*
2. Proctoscopy shows *discrete ulcers.*
3. Concentric narrowing of the cecum 90% of the time.
4. Treatment is *metronidazole.*

PEARL: *If you're presented with a case of Strep Bovis endocarditis, √ the colon for diverticulosis or colon ca !* ✪

OVERVIEW OF COLONIC POLYP PATHOLOGY ✪

1. **HYPERPLASTIC**—these are benign
2. **ADENOMATOUS**
   a) *Villous*—**the real "villains"**, i.e. *carry a greater risk of malignant transformation* (3 times that of tubular)
   b) *Tubular*—much smaller risk of transformation
   c) *Tubulovillous*—halfway in between the two in risk of transformation.

✪ REVISED ACS Guidelines For SCREENING And Surveillance For COLORECTAL POLYPS/CA

Risk Category	Recommendation[1]	Age to Begin	Interval
Average Risk			
Patients ≥ 50 yo not in any of the categories below	One of the following: 1. FOBT plus FS[2]; or 2. TCE[3]	Age 50	1. FOBT every year and FS q5y 2. Colo q10y or DCBE q5-10y
Moderate Risk			
Single small (<1cm) adenomatous polyps	Colonoscopy	At the time of initial polyp diagnosis	TCE within 3y after initial polypectomy; if normal, as per average recommendations (above)
Large (≥1 cm) or multiple adenomatous polyps of any size	Colonoscopy	At the time of initial polyp diagnosis	TCE within 3y after initial polypectomy; if normal, TCE q5y
Personal h/o curative-intent resection of colorectal ca	TCE[4]	Within 1y after resection	If normal, TCE in 3y; If still normal, TCE q5y
Colorectal ca or adenomatous polyps in 1st degree relative <60 or in ≥2 1st degree relatives of any age	TCE	Age 40, or 10y before the youngest case in the family, whichever is earlier	Q5y
Colorectal ca in other relatives (not included above)	As per average-risk recommendations (above); may consider screening before 50yo		
High Risk			
Family h/o adenomatous polyps	Early surveillance with endoscopy, counseling to consider genetic testing, and referral to a specialty center	Puberty	If genetic test is +, or polyposis is confirmed, consider colectomy; otherwise, endoscopy q1-2y
Family h/o HNPCC	Colonoscopy and counseling to consider genetic testing	Age 21	If genetic test is +, or if patient has not had genetic testing, colonoscopy q2y until age 40, and then q year
IBD	Colonoscopies with biopsies for dysplasia	8 years after the start of pancolitis; 12-15 y after the start of L-sided colitis	Q1-2 y

DCBE=double-contrast BE; FOBT = fecal occult blood test; FS = flex sig; TCE = total colon examination
1. Digital rectal exam should be done at the time of each flex sig, colonoscopy, or DCBE.
2. Annual FOBT has been shown to reduce mortality from colorectal ca, so it is preferable to no screening.
3. TCE includes either DCBE or TCE.
4. This assumes that a perioperative TCE was done.

> ✪ The likelihood that any polypoid lesion in the large bowel contains invasive cancer is **RELATED TO THE SIZE** of the polyp, being **negligible (<2 percent) in lesions smaller than 1.5 cm**, **intermediate (2 to 10 percent) in lesions 1.5 to 2.5 cm in size**, and **substantial (10 percent) in lesions larger than 2.5 cm**.

SYNDROMES OF MULTIPLE INTESTINAL POLYPS Commonly Addressed On The Exam...

1. Familial adenomatous polyposis

2. Gardner's syndrome

3. Peutz-Jeghers syndrome

FAMILIAL ADENOMATOUS POLYPOSIS (FAP)

➤ Autosomal dominant disease caused by mutations in the adenomatous polyposis coli (APC) gene

➤ Approximately *one-third of patients with FAP have no family history* of the disease and probably represent new germ-line APC mutations.

➤ The diagnosis of FAP is based upon the presence of more than 100 adenomatous colorectal polyps.

➤ Polyps *also* occur commonly in the *upper gastrointestinal tract* of patients with FAP (30 to 100 percent in various series)

➤ The risk of colon adenocarcinoma in classic FAP approaches 100 percent by age 45, so total *colectomy should generally be performed as soon as possible following the diagnosis*.

GARDNER'S DISEASE

➤ Adenomatous polyposis syndrome associated with an ↑ risk of colon ca

➤ **Keep an eye out for**: *skeletal osteomas; fibromas; lipomas; epidermoid cysts; neurofibromas; desmoid tumors; retroperitoneal fibrosis*.

➤ As with FAP, the colonic polyps are generally evident in affected individuals by age 25, and if the polyposis is not treated surgically, colorectal cancer will develop in almost all patients before age 40.

✪ PEUTZ-JEGHERS Syndrome

➤ A polyposis syndrome characterized by the presence of numerous *pigmented spots on the lips and the buccal mucosa*, and multiple gastrointestinal hamartomatous polyps.

➤ The hamartomas are primarily of the small intestine. *The malignant potential is PRESENT, BUT QUITE LOW (<3%)*

➤ The risk of gastric, small intestinal, and colorectal cancer is thought to occur via *adenomatous change within the hamartomas*. Adenomatous changes have been found in 3 to 6 percent of hamartomas removed from patients with PJS.

5. INFECTIOUS DISEASE & HIV

VIRAL DISEASES

THE WEST NILE-LIKE VIRUS

➤ A mosquito-borne virus which can cause encephalitis or meningitis
➤ It is spread to humans by the bite of a mosquito that becomes infected when feeding on infected birds.
➤ The virus cannot spread directly from person to person and there is no evidence that a person can get the virus from handling an infected bird.
➤ The incubation period in humans is 5-15 days
➤ Most infections are mild. Symptoms include fever, H/A, and myalgias, often with a skin rash, and lymphadenopathy.
➤ More severe infections may be marked by H/A, high fever, neck stiffness, stupor, disorientation, coma, tremors, convulsions, muscle weakness, paralysis, and rarely, death
➤ Therapy is supportive, as there is no directed therapy.

✪ EBV and INFECTIOUS MONO

1. Look for '**atypical lymphocytes**' on exam
2. Symptoms: fever, fatigue
3. Signs: **splenomegaly**; + LN; exudative pharyngitis
4. Official clinical 'triad' is → 1) Fever; 2) pharyngitis; and 3) cervical lymphadenopathy
   a) Lab: ↑**LFT's** (in 80-90%); + **Monospot** (in 90%).
   b) *However*, remember, that 15 % of patients will be negative Monospot and still have the disease. So, when the Monospot is neg but you still suspect EBV, ✓ EBV-specific antibodies, especially Ig M to viral capsid antigens ("VCA"; *Extremely useful in heterophile-negative cases; the best test for confirming acute* disease), and antibodies to early antigens ("EA"; these appear within 2-3 weeks of symptom onset).

      ➤ EBNA Antibody (<u>IgG</u>) appears late and indicates *prior infection*; persists lifelong. VCA (viral capsid antibody; <u>IgG</u>)—Positive indicates *past or present* infection

5. **If Ampicillen is given, a rash usually always develops.**
6. Remember, EBV is also associated with Hodgkin's/B-cell/Burkitt's lymphomas; nasopharyngeal ca.; and oral hairy leukoplakia

---

Remember, **EBV and CMV** mononucleosis syndromes can look similar clinically. To rule out EBV, ✓ VCA IgM. To rule out CMV, ✓ CMV IgM. Note that 'atypical lymphocytes' may be seen in either EBV, CMV, or Toxo, all of which give mono-like syndromes.

CMV

1. Causes a **heterophile-negative** (negative Monospot) mononucleosis syndrome
2. Otherwise it is a fairly benign virus in immunocompetent individuals.
3. CMV is **transmitted via granulocytes**, which harbor the virus. Thus, in immunosuppressed individuals, blood products often require a "Leukotrap" or WBC filter to prevent CMV transmission.
4. In *AIDS and transplant patients, CMV may cause...*

> a) ✪ <u>Retinitis</u> (so-called '**ketchup-and-mustard**' or '**pizza pie**' fundoscopic appearance); patient with AIDS complains of <u>floaters</u>; treatment with **Gancyclovir (re: bone marrow suppression)** or **Foscarnet (re: nephrotoxicity)** or Cidovidir.

   b) Encephalitis
   c) Pneumonia (more in transplant patients—mortality 50% in these patients)
   d) Esophagitis
   e) GI ulcers
   f) Adrenalitis

VZV (VARICELLA ZOSTER VIRUS)

1. Causes Varicella (chicken pox) and Zoster (shingles)
2. *"Dewdrops on a rose petal"*, the phrase that applies to the rash in chickenpox where papules evolve into vesicles.
3. Vesicular lesions follow a dermatomal distribution in Zoster
4. *May disseminate, particularly in immunocompromised patients, to give pneumonitis or encephalitis.*
5. **Ramsay Hunt syndrome**→ A collection of findings that includes pain + vesicles on the external auditory meatus + loss of taste on the anterior two thirds of the tongue + ipsilateral facial palsy with involvement of the geniculate ganglion
6. Most common complication→Post-herpetic neuralgia

> Patients who have never had chicken pox can get chicken pox by exposure to someone with shingles (*but can't get zoster* since to contract zoster you have to have had chicken pox, as zoster is a manifestation of reactivation of a previous infection). Seen diagrammatically:
>
> Zoster ⟷ Chicken pox, but *never* Zoster ⟶ Zoster
>   (can go either way)

HSV-1 and HSV-2

1. Among **genital** HSV infections, HSV-2 is responsible for 75%; HSV-1 for 25%
2. As for **oral** lesions, the distribution is usually the other way around
3. **HSV-1** is usually responsible for **disseminated** HSV infection
4. Encephalitis shows a predilection for the **temporal lobes**
5. **Herpetic whitlow** is a painful finger infection, usu contracted thru needle sticks.
6. Remember, Dermatitis Herpetiformis is a bullous skin complication related to Celiac Disease (gluten-sensitive enteropathy) and has nothing to do with herpes per se.

PARVOVIRUS B19 ✪

1. Can have a *variety of presentations* that include: **1) polyarthropathy; 2) anemias; 3) aplastic crisis**; and 4) erythema infectiosum (children; aka 'fifth disease', 'slapped-cheek syndrome')

2. Many of the severe manifestations of B19 viremia relate to the propensity of the virus to *infect and lyse erythroid precursor cells in the bone marrow. Giant pronormoblasts* are often seen on bone marrow exam; marrow is hypoplastic in patients manifesting with aplastic crisis.

3. Found in patients with **pure red blood cell aplasia**

4. Can cause **chronic infection with anemia** in *immunocompromised* patients. In the *normal host*, the immune response controls the infection in 10 days to two weeks, red cell production returns, and there is no clinically apparent anemia. In *immunocompromised* patients, lysis of red cell precursor cells continues, leading to prolonged cessation of red cell production and a severe, chronic anemia.

5. Parvovirus B19 infection is the cause in most instances of **transient aplastic crisis** developing suddenly in patients with chronic hemolytic disease. *Nearly all hemolytic conditions can be affected by B19 infection*, including sickle cell disease, erythrocyte enzyme deficiencies, hereditary spherocytosis, thalassemias, paroxysmal nocturnal hemoglobinuria, and autoimmune hemolysis.

6. **Polyarthropathy**
   - ✓ In adults (F>>M)
   - ✓ Usually symmetric and most commonly involve the hands, wrists, knees, and feet.
   - ✓ Joint symptoms may or may not be accompanied by rash or other symptoms
   - ✓ Usually resolves within a few weeks.
   - ✓ The arthritis associated with acute B19 infection does not cause joint destruction.

7. **Treatment** is individualized based on the clinical manifestation, eg NSAIDs are appropriate for the arthritis and arthralgias; transfusions (and O2 prn) for transient aplastic crisis; *IV IgG + transfusions for chronic infection with anemia.*

HPV—CLINICAL ASSOCIATIONS ✪ *–see Dermatology for more re: specific subtypes*

1. *Plantar* warts

2. *Flat* warts

3. *Skin* squamous cell carcinoma in transplant patients

4. *Genital* warts (condyloma acuminata)

5. *Oral leukoplakia*

6. Squamous cell carcinoma of the *cervix or genitalia*

PRECURSORS TO INVASIVE CERVICAL CARCINOMA

Low-grade Lesions
- ° Cellular changes associated with **HPV** infection
- ° Mild dysplasia (CIN I)

High-grade Lesions
- ° Moderate dysplasia (CIN 2)
- ° Severe dysplasia (CIN 3)
- ° Carcinoma-in-situ

INFLUENZA

1. Type A most common
2. Those ≥65yo have by far the highest mortality
3. Strep and Staph can secondarily infect
4. **Amantadine** is only effective vs. Type A and can shorten the course of disease in influenza only if given **within 48 hours** of symptom onset (Amantadine as *TREATMENT*)
5. Amantadine + Vaccine confers ± 95% protection (Amantadine as *PROPHYLAXIS*)
6. Amantadine toxicity = restlessness, insomnia, dizziness, renal
7. The flu vaccine **may in fact be given along with Pneumovax**
8. The following **risk groups** should receive annual vaccine

    a. ≥65
    b. > or < 65 with chronic medical problems, such as cardiopulmonary disorders and DM
    c. Nursing home residents and residents of other long-term care facilities, as well as their staff
    d. Health care personnel
    e. House-hold members of high-risk groups
    f. Healthy pregnant women who will be in their 2nd or 3rd trimesters during the flu season.
    g. HIV and immunocompromised
    h. Anyone who wishes to reduce the likelihood of becoming ill with influenza

9. The **neuraminidase inhibitors, Relenza® (zanamivir) and Tamiflu® (oseltamivir)** are indicated for uncomplicated acute illness due to influenza in patients who have been symptomatic **for ≤ 2 days**.

    a. They are effective vs. both influenza types A and B.
    b. Neuraminidase is a viral glycoprotein whose function is to break the bond holding new virus particles to infected cells. Once these bonds are broken, new viruses are free to infect other cells.
    c. These inhibitors of neuraminidase, *therefore*, are thought to reduce the spread of the virus. Relenza® is the inhaler. Tamiflu® is the capsule.

RABIES

1. A virus that spreads along peripheral nerves → CNS
2. Cats, dogs, skunks, foxes, raccoons, bats harbor the virus
3. Consider rabies in cases of myelitis or encephalitis of unclear etiology
4. Diagnostics:
   a) Serum and CSF may be tested for rabies Ab
   b) DFA (Direct Fluorescent Ab) testing of biopsy taken from back of neck may be used to detect rabies Ag
   c) Negri bodies seen on hippocampal biopsy specimen are definitive
5. **HRIG** (Human Rabies Immune Globulin) **+ vaccine** are useful, **but only if begun before the onset of symptoms.**

   ✪ N.B. Half of the **HRIG** dose should be injected directly into the **wound** and the rest in the *gluteal* area.
   ✪ In adults the **Vaccine** should only be given at the *deltoid* area: re **days 0,3,7,14,28**

RABIES POST-EXPOSURE PROPHYLAXIS ✪ —*Cleansing wound with soap & water shown to be protective in 90% of experimental animals.*

ANIMAL	EVALUATION/ DISPOSITION OF ANIMAL	RECOMMENDATION FOR PROPHYLAXIS
Dogs, cats	Healthy and available for 10d observation →	Don't start unless animal develops sx, then start HRIG (IgG) + vaccine
	Rabid/suspected rabid →	Immediate vaccination
	Unknown (escaped) →	Consult public health officials
Skunks, raccoons, bats, foxes, most carnivores	Regard as rabid	Immediate vaccination
Livestock, rodents, rabbits, squirrels, chipmunks, rats, mice, guinea pigs, hamsters, gerbels	N/A	Almost never require anti-rabies vaccine.

PML (Progressive Multifocal Leukoencephalopathy)

1. A slow virus (a papovavirus)
2. Seen in *AIDS, lymphoma, leukemia*
3. Affects the *CNS white matter* in an otherwise non-specific pattern
4. *Hemiparesis, visual field deficits, and cognitive impairment* are common presenting findings; aphasia, ataxia, and/or cranial nerve deficits can also develop.
5. Rapid clinical progression is common, and *death usually occurs within six months* of the diagnosis

MEASLES (Rubeola)

1. Prodromal URI symptoms common
2. Oral *Koplik's spots* are seen *before* the skin rash. Pathognomonic of measles, Koplik's spots are blue-gray lesions on a red base that appear on the buccal mucosa, usually adjacent to the second molars.
3. May cause encephalitis
4. *Staph aureus and H. Flu are the most common 2° bacterial infections*, and are, in fact, more common than 1° measles pneumonia.

RUBELLA

1. **Clinical**: fever, transient erythematous rash, posterior cervical LN, and arthralgia.
2. Pregnant women should not be given the vaccine since may cause congenital defects. Remember, it is a *live* vaccine (refer to section on vaccines later in this chapter)
3. For the same reason, women of child-bearing age should be warned not to become pregnant for 2-3 months following vaccination.

4. ✪ *Rubella titre and pregnancy…*

   a) If indicates immune→no treatment necessary
   b) If shows non-immune→follow patient for evidence of clinical rubella and recheck titre in 2-3 wk→if hasn't ↑d and no clinical signs→no treatment necessary.
   c) If, on the other hand, patient has seroconverted or she shows clinical signs of rubella→a *therapeutic abortion* should be considered

HEPATITIS B POST-EXPOSURE PROPHYLAXIS FOR ADULTS ✪ :

EXPOSED PERSON	EXPOSURE SOURCE		
	HBsAg +	**HBsAg -**	**STATUS UNKNOWN**
Unvaccinated	HBIG + Vaccine	Vaccine	Test source for HBsAg
Vaccinated	If exposed person has anti-HBs ≥10→No tx; If < 10→HBIG + 1 dose of vaccine.	No Tx	If exposed person has anti-HBs ≥10→No tx; If < 10→ 1 dose of vaccine.

DDX OF NIGHT SWEATS
1. Pulmonary TB
2. Lymphoma
3. Brucellosis; abscess; endocarditis
4. Alcoholic withdrawal
5. Nocturnal hypoglycemia
6. Nocturnal dyspnea
7. Nightmares

REMEMBER, AMONG THE MOST COMMON CAUSES OF FUO* ARE:
1. Malignancy
2. TB
3. Abscess

* *FUO is defined as temps > 38.3°C seen during a febrile illness that lasts > 3weeks and no specific diagnosis after 1 week of outpatient investigation or 3 days of inpatient investigation.*

DIRECT MICROSCOPY IN INFECTIOUS DISEASE
1. *Acid-fast* bacteria to Ziehl-Neelsen staining→mycobacteria species
2. *Weakly acid-fast* organisms
   a. Nocardia (aerobic)
   b. Actinomyces Israelii(anaerobic)
3. *Dark-field* examination→Treponema pallidum
4. *Silver Methenamine* stain→Pneumocystis carinii
5. *India ink* stain (CSF)→Cryptococcus neoformans
6. *Gram-negative diplococci within leukocytes* (endocervical/urethral swab)→N. gonorrhea
7. *Inclusion bodies within urethral epithelial cells*→Chlamydia trachomatis
8. Pyogenic meningitis in adults:

CSF gram stain	Presumptive diagnosis
Gram +	Strep pneumonia meningitis
Gram -	Meningococcal meningitis

THE BACTERIA

PSEUDOMONAS AERUGINOSA
1. Common organism leading to **infections complicating burns**
2. Cause of **malignant otitis externa in diabetics**. The term "malignant" is added when *P. aeruginosa* penetrates the epithelium overlying the floor of the external auditory canal at the junction between bone and cartilage and invades underlying soft tissue, cartilage, and cortical bone.
   - Pseudomonas aeruginosa and *Staph aureus* are the most common causes of otitis externa among patients in general
   - P. aeruginosa is also the cause of acute diffuse otitis externa (aka **swimmers ear**). {Remember, pseudomonas is a flagellated organism—you're not the only one who likes the water!}

3. May cause **ecthyma gangrenosum in neutropenic patients** with bacteremia

SALMONELLA TYPHI→TYPHOID FEVER
1. Fever
2. Relative bradycardia
3. Rose spots (50% of pts)

BORDETELLA PERTUSSIS

1. Responsible for whooping cough in children and cases of prolonged bronchitis in older children and adults
2. May cause ↑↑Lymphocytes
3. Treatment with Erythromycin

CHLAMYDIA PSITTACOSIS

1. Most patients with psittacosis have a history of contact with birds, e.g. poultry workers cleaning out bird cages, but as many as *3/4ths of patients are simply exposed to through their own pets.*
2. Chlamydia psittaci infection of humans most commonly presents as *fever of abrupt onset, severe headache, and dry cough* in a patient with a recent history of bird exposure; however, rigors, sweats, and myalgias are also seen in most patients.
3. Labs: The white cell count is usually normal, but the differential may show toxic granulation or a left shift; *AST ↑ in nearly half* of patients; *hyponatremia* common.
4. Serology via the complement fixation test is the test traditionally used to make the diagnosis. It is the most widely available but unfortunately cannot differentiate among the Chlamydial species. Paired acute and convalescent sera should be obtained at least two weeks apart, and a fourfold rise in antibody levels is significant.
5. *Doxycycline and TCN* are the drugs of choice.

LEGIONNAIRES' DISEASE

1. Clinical: → *"Lung Liver Lytes Loose BMs"*

    ➢ Lung → **bilateral patchy infiltrates; relatively nonproductive cough;** Patients with community-acquired Legionnaires' disease are much more likely than patients with pneumonia from other causes to be admitted to the ICU upon presentation.
    ➢ Liver → **HYPONATREMIA**, hypophosphatemia
    ➢ Lytes →**LFTs increase**
    ➢ Loose BMs → **diarrhea**

2. Weakness, malaise, **HIGH FEVER**, **cough**, and, relative bradycardia.
3. The most common risk factors for Legionnaires' disease are cigarette smoking, chronic lung disease, advanced age, and immunosuppression.
4. *Laboratory Diagnosis:*
    a. Gram stain of respiratory secretions commonly reveals numerous neutrophils but no organisms
    b. ✓ **URINE ANTIGEN-1** ; Antigen in urine is detectable 3 days after the onset of clinical disease, even if specific therapy has been started; furthermore, urinary antigen persists for several weeks after antibiotic therapy.
    c. ✓ Ab with IFA (Indirect fluorescent Ab) test; **≥ 1:256 or a 4-fold ↑ is pos.**
    d. Sensitivity and specificity: sputum cultures > urine antigen testing and DFA staining of the sputum > antibody titres
5. *Treatment*: Another clue to recognizing this disease is *failure to respond* to β-lactams (PCN or cephalosporins) or aminoglycosides. Treatment options include → *erythro ± rifampin; fluoroquinolone; or azithromax*

PASTEURELLA MULTOCIDA

1. *Cat* (>dog)modes is the #1 mode of transmission
2. Pen G best, but Amox or Augmentin fine

CAPNOCYTOPHAGIA (aka 'DF-2')

1. *Dog* (> > cat) bites
2. Give Augmentin or Clindamycin
3. May cause bacteremia in immunosuppressed patients, splenectomized patients, and alcoholics.

CAT SCRATCH DISEASE	vs.	BACILLARY ANGIOMATOSIS
Immunocompetent host		*Immunosuppressed* host(e.g. AIDS)
Bartonella henselae (and A. felis)		Bartonella henselae (and quintana)
Self-limited		*Progressive/recurrent*
(spontaneous resolution in 2-4mo)		*Erythro or Doxy ±prophylaxis*

CLOSTRIDIUM BOTULINUM ('BOTULISM')

☞ Neurotoxin interferes with presynaptic Ach release, causing the 6D's→Dilated fixed pupils; Diplopia; Dysarthria; Dysphagia; Dry tongue; Descending paralysis.

NEISSERIA GONORRHEA

1. Gram negative diplococci
2. Look out for the 20 y.o. man or woman with **fever + swollen knee**
3. >80% of women are asymptomatic; only 2% of men asymptomatic.
4. Disseminated gonorrhea most likely to occur in menstruating females; 2 phases…
   a) **Bacteremic phase**: tenosynovitis; skin lesions; joint cultures negative
   b) **Nonbacteremic phase**:monoarticular arthritis of knee/wrist/ankle; joint cx pos
5. Remember, if a patient has a history of **recurrent** Neisseria infections, s/he probably has a deficiency in late complement components (C5-8). This is **best screened for with CH50**
6. Patients with GC should also be empirically treated for Chlamydia because of the high risk of co-occurrence. This can be accomplished with any number of available regimens (see "Treatment of STDs" later in this chapter for details)

NEISSERIA MENINGITIS

1. Gram negative diplococci
2. Presentation: **fever, ↓BP, DIC, palpable purpura (purpura fulminans)**
3. Treatment→**PenG;** *Don't wait for cultures if you suspect!*
4. *Prophylaxis* for exposure (close contact): Options→
   a) **Cipro 500mg PO once**
   b) **Rifampin 600mg q12h x 4 doses**
   c) **Ceftriaxone 250mg IM x 1**

ASEPTIC MENINGITIS

1. Many causes, but *usually viral*

2. Usually *self-limited*

3. *CSF pleocytosis (↑monos)*, negative bacterial cultures

LISTERIA MONOCYTOGENES

1. Small, gram +, motile rod;

2. Causes aseptic meningitis/bacteremia in neonates, ***immunosuppressed (e.g. lymphoma) and pregnant women***;

3. Associated with consumption of contaminated milk, ice cream, undercooked hot dogs

4. Rx→Amp + Gent

BACTERIAL MENINGITIS → EMPIRIC TREATMENT (Based on initial gram stain)		
CSF GRAM STAIN	**MOST LIKELY ORGANISM**	**EMPIRIC TREATMENT**
Gram + cocci	Strep Pneumonia	Vanco + Ceftriaxone ± dexamethasone
Gram-neg cocci	N. Meningitidis	Pen G
Gram + bacilli	Listeria Monocytogenes	Amp + Gent
Gram - bacilli	H. flu, coliforms, Pseudomonas	Ceftazidime + Gent

RISK FACTORS FOR MENINGITIS	
Alcoholism	Strep; Klebsiella
Asplenia	Strep; H. flu; Neisseria meningitides
CSF rhinorrhea	Strep
HIV infection	Listeria; crypto; toxo; CMV
Immunosuppression (general)	Listeria; cryptococcus
Otitis/sinusitis/mastoiditis	Strep. (pneumoniae); H flu
Sickle cell anemia	Strep; Salmonella; H flu

GENERAL CSF PATTERNS AND THEIR DISEASE CORRELATES	
CSF	**USUAL SOURCE**
PMNs, low glucose	Bacterial meningitis
Lymphocytes, low glucose	Fungal or TB meningitis
Lymphocytes, normal glucose	Viral meningitis

IMPORTANT INDICATIONS FOR STEROIDS IN MENINGITIS

- ❖ To control the inflammation in adults with acute bacterial meningitis
- ❖ TB meningitis
- ❖ Altered mental status or other signs of elevated intracranial pressure

DDX OF FEVER + PURPURA
(**"MERSA"** might also help you recall endocarditis & sepsis; use ∀ as upside-down A)

- ➢ M eningococcemia
- ➢ E ndocarditis
- ➢ R MSF
- ➢ S epsis
- ➢ ∀asculitis

BRUCELLOSIS

- ➢ Brucellosis is a well-documented cause of _fever of unknown origin_ with varied and nonspecific symptoms.
- ➢ Patients tend to have a multitude of complaints, often without objective findings except fever. Physical findings, when present, are usually limited to minimal _lymphadenopathy and occasionally hepatosplenomegaly_.
- ➢ Virtually any organ system can be involved with brucellosis; most commonly however:
    - ▪ Osteoarticular, especially _sacroiliitis_ — 20 to 30 percent.
    - ▪ Genitourinary, especially _epididymoorchitis_ — 2 to 40 percent of males
- ➢ An important problem is that Brucella sp. tend to be _slow growing_ which can lead to erroneous results. Cultures generally become positive between 7 and 21 days but may take up to 35 days. So, if you suspect it, ask the lab to hang on to the cultures for a longer period.

- ➢ _Persons at risk_— _Acquired via contact with animal tissues or after ingestion of unpasteurized milk or cheese._
    1. Farmers; dairymen; livestock handlers; meat packers
    2. Veterinary surgeons
    3. Those who ingest unpasteurized dairy products, mostly, however, from sheep/goats in Italy/Greece/France/Mexico.

- ➢ _Presentation_—
    1. Fever, chills
    2. Headache
    3. Back pain
    4. Arthralgias
    5. Orchitis
    6. Cough
    7. Hepatomegaly/Splenomegaly
    8. Endocarditis

➤ *Diagnosis*
  1. <u>Cultures</u> of *blood* or other sites, especially *bone marrow or liver* biopsy specimens
  2. Serology

➤ *Treatment: 2 accepted regimens:*
  ✓ <u>Doxycycline</u> 100 mg PO twice daily for six weeks <u>plus streptomycin</u> 1 gram IM daily for the first 14 to 21 days.
  ✓ <u>Doxycycline</u> 100 mg PO twice daily <u>plus rifampin</u> 600 to 900 mg PO (15 mg/kg) once daily for six weeks.
  ✓ A brucella vaccine for human use is *not* currently available in the United States.

MYCOPLASMA PNEUMONIAE ('Walking Pneumonia')

1. Community-acquired pneumonia, esp in **young** patients
2. Cold agglutinin production ± **hemolytic anemia**
3. **Erythema multiforme**, **Stevens-Johnson** Syndrome
4. Non-specific musculoskeletal and/or GI upset
5. Neurological effects—**Guillain-Barre**, cranial nerve palsies, polio-like syndrome, **aseptic meningitis**.
6. **Mononeuritis multiplex**
7. **Erythromycin** is the drug of choice in the young patient with fever/dry cough/patchy bilateral **interstitial** infiltrates, and relatively benign exam. Don't give PCN.

DIPTHERIA

1. The term 'diphtheria' derives from the Greek word for *leather* which refers to the tough *pharyngeal pseudomembrane* that is the clinical hallmark of infection)
2. It is an acute, communicable disease caused by the Gram positive bacillus Corynebacterium diphtheriae.
3. The most important clinical form of infection involves the respiratory tract. Respiratory diphtheria can affect any part of the respiratory tree. Up to two-thirds of cases are *tonsillopharyngeal*. Patient's may also have cutaneous involvement.
4. *The more the pseudomembrane spreads from the tonsillopharyngeal area, the greater the systemic toxicity.*

5. **Toxin-mediated systemic complications**:

   a. *Myocarditis* → ST-T wave changes and 1st degree AV block; but also advanced heart blocks, arrhythmias, CHF, and circulatory collapse when more severe.
   b. <u>Polyneuritis</u> → Neurologic toxicity is unusual in mild disease but develops in up to three-fourths of patients with severe diphtheria.

      (1) *Local* neuropathies (paralysis of the soft palate and posterior pharyngeal wall) are followed by …
      (2) *Cranial* neuropathies (usually oculomotor and ciliary, followed by facial or laryngeal paralyses)

(3) *Peripheral* neuritis develops weeks to months later. This polyneuritis picture can span the clinical spectrum from mild weakness to *respiratory muscle paralysis to total paralysis.*

(4) the *severity of disease is directly related to the time* between the onset of symptoms and administration of antitoxin *and to the severity of pharyngeal membrane formation* and therefore toxin production.

6. Diagnosis is established by culture or fluorescent Ab staining of pharyngeal swab specimen.

7. *Isolate the patient and treat with antitoxin.* Patients with diphtheria need to be placed on respiratory droplet isolation for respiratory tract disease and contact isolation for cutaneous disease.

8. While *Erythromycin or PenG* do not alter the course of disease, they do *prevent transmission* to susceptible hosts. *Close contacts should be evaluated and treated with Abx if culture results are +, and Td toxoid should be given.*

ACTINOMYCES ISRAELII

1. Anaerobic, gram +, branching, filamentous
2. Sulfur granules, or clumps of filaments, seen on pathology
3. May present with
   a) Paramandibular infection with a *chronic draining sinus usually preceded by dental extraction*
   b) *Chest wound infection*
   c) *Pulmonary abscess*
   d) *Rib destruction*
4. Can cause brain abscess more rarely
5. Check anaerobic culture for diagnosis

NOCARDIA

1. Aerobic, gram +, branching, filamentous
2. An opportunistic infection (usually occurring in immunosuppressed)
3. Presents as chronic pneumonitis and lung abscess
4. In patients with chronic pneumonia who develop neurologic symptoms→r/o Nocardia brain abscess.

KEY TICK-BORNE DISEASES *("B aLERT" !)*

1. **Ba**besiosis (*below*)

2. **L**yme (see rheum chapter)

3. **E**rlichiosis (*below*)

4. **R**MSF (*below*)

5. **T**ularemia (*below*)

RICKETTSIAL INFECTIONS

1. All these infections have an **insect vector**, *except for* Q fever

2. They all yield a **rash**, *except for* Q fever and Erlichiosis (below).

3. **Rocky Mt. Spotted Fever (RMSF)**→Erythematous and hemorrhagic macules and papules **begin peripherally** (wrists/forearms, ankles) **and spread centripetally** (to arms, thighs, trunk, face). Fever, H/A, myalgia common symptoms. Rash usually begins on the 4th day of the fever. ↓Na+ is seen in half the cases. RMSF is **not seen in the Rocky Mt. States** (Go figure!), but is most common in the **mid-Atlantic states (i.e. MD, VA, NC, and Geogia)**; transmitted by the American **dog tick**, Dermacentor variabilis. History of tick bite given in >80% of cases. Doxycycline 100 IV or PO BID x 7days.

4. **Q fever** may develop hepatitis and pneumonitis and is seen in meat packers

5. **Erlichiosis**

    a) Spring and Summer, more common

    b) 'Spotless RMSF' (no rash), with fever, H/A, malaise, relative bradycardia

    c) ↓WBC, ↓platelets, ↑LFTs

    d) Self-limited, usually, yet treated with TCN since deaths have been reported

    e) Sometimes see morulae (Latin for "mulberry": the appearance of the cytoplasmic inclusion, a vacuolar cluster of Giemsa-stained ehrlichiae in phagocytes) are frequently seen in the *granulocytic* type (as opposed to monocytic type)

2 FORMS OF ERLICHIOSIS:			
Type of Erlichiosis	**Vector (colloquial)**	**Vector (formal)**	**Predominant Distribution**
HME (Human Monocytic Erlichiosis)	Star tick	Amblyomma Americanus	Southeast
HGE (Human Granulocytic Erlichiosis)	Long-Legged Black tick	Ixodes Scapularis (re may also carry Lyme and Babesiosis)	Northeast

> ***Pearl***: A recent rash, especially during warm weather, in a patient with severe H/A, stiff neck, and fever suggests Lyme disease, RMSF, or erlichiosis. Viral meningitis may also be considered in this setting.

TULAREMIA

- ✓ Tularemia is a zoonosis caused by a small, facultative gram-negative intracellular coccobacillus, Francisella tularensis.

- ✓ <u>Abrupt onset</u> of fever, chills, headache, and malaise, after an incubation period of 2 to 10 days.

- ✓ 60 to 80 percent of cases present with <u>ulceroglandular disease</u> with fever and a <u>single erythematous papuloulcerative lesion with a central eschar</u>. The skin lesion is accompanied by <u>tender regional lymphadenopathy</u>.

- ✓ Patients with ulceroglandular disease usually report recent handling of an animal (*suspect tularemia in cases with rabbits/<u>rabbit hunting</u>*), an animal bite (especially cat bites) , or have had exposure to potential vectors, particularly ticks. Affected patients typically present

- ✓ Normal to <u>slightly</u> ↑ WBC <u>(normal diff)</u> and ESR; serology can confirm at 2 weeks. The diagnosis of tularemia is usually confirmed serologically by tube agglutination or <u>ELISA</u>.

- ✓ <u>Streptomycin</u> is the drug of choice, achieving a 97 % cure rate with no relapses. <u>Streptomycin</u> is given at a dose 10 mg/kg IM every 12 hours for 7 to 10 days.

BABESIOSIS

- ➤ "Malaria-like" protozoa on thick and thin smears—Babesia; in RBC they are often located peripherally, thus commonly mistaken for P. falciparum, esp the ring forms of P. falciparum; *however*, the brown pigment deposits are seen in P. Falciparum only and Babesiosis may reveal characteristic "tetrads (the parent and "daughter" cells).

- ➤ Parasitizes erythrocytes of *rodents and cattle*→Ixodes Scapularis/I. Dammini ticks (which also transmit Lyme disease to humans from rodents) ingest Babesia while feeding and multiply within the tick's gut wall→tick bites human.

- ➤ Most cases occur in the *NE coastal areas*: Nantucket, Martha's Vineyard, Cape Cod, Rhode Island, Eastern Long Island, Shelter Island, Fire Island; and CT.

- ➤ **Clinically**, initial symptoms are non-specific and include constitutional symptoms + fever, rigors, H/A, abdom pain, dark urine, photophobia, conjunctival injection, sore throat, and cough.

- ➤ **Hematologically,** may see → Hemolytic anemia, ↓ haptoglobin, ↑ retic count, normal to ↑ WBC, ↓ platelets, + direct Coombs test, petechiae/ecchymoses, HSM; also may see ↑ BUN/Cr

- ➤ *In healthy individuals* → usually a *<u>mild illness</u>* and recover on their own

- ➤ *In asplenic or immunocompromised pts*→can see *<u>overwhelming infection</u>*

  - ☞ *<u>Clinda + quinine</u>; ± exchange transfusions* (see next)

☞ **Exchange transfusion** — Exchange transfusion is often used as adjunctive therapy in selected patients including those with:

- Immunodeficiency such as HIV
- Severe hemolysis
- B. divergens infection
- High-level parasitemia (>10 percent)

POST-SPLENECTOMY INFECTIONS
1. Strep Pneumoniae
2. H. Flu
3. Neisseria Meningitidis
4. Capnocytophaga (DF-2)
5. *Babesiosis*
6. *Malaria*

MALARIA
1. Transmitted by the bite of the Anopheles mosquito
2. Plasmodium is the parasite and has 4 species:
   a) P. *vivax*→Chloroquine + Primaquine
   b) P. *ovale*→Chloroquine + Primaquine
   c) P. *falciparum*→Chloroquine; if resistant to Chloroquine then→ PO Primaquine or Azithromax; if too ill for PO, then give IV Quinidine
   d) P. *malariae*→Chloroquine
3. **Presentation**
   a) High Fever→may see seizures
   b) Normochromic, normocytic anemia 2° to…
   c) Hemolysis→Hemoglobinuria→*blackish* urine
   d) Low BP/Shock/DIC
   e) Low glucose (poor prognosticator)
   f) Coma 2° to encephalopathy

4. Diagnosis made by examining *thick and thin smears*.

5. **Prophylaxis…**
   a) The CDC is now warning that *chloroquine is no longer an effective means of malaria prophylaxis in most areas*.
   b) CDC recommends mefloquine (Lariam®), doxycycline, or Malarone® (atovaquone + proguanil)
      1. **Mefloquine** should be started 1-2 wks prior to travel and be continued for 4 weeks following one's return.
      2. **Doxy** is as effective as mefloquine and can be used in areas with mefloquine resistance.
   c) Remember, **mefloquine** is *contraindicated* for patients on β-blockers
   d) Patient should be advised to take 3 tabs at once of pyrimethamine-sulfadoxine should fever develop in areas endemic for malaria.

OSTEOMYELITIS

1. Staph aureus is the #1 cause of acute hematogenous osteomyelitis and the #1 organism in chronic osteomyelitis; suspect salmonella of course in sickle cell disease.
2. Vertebral osteomyelitis
   a) Staph aureus and Gram neg bacilli
   b) MRI best imaging modality since may also show adjacent epidural abscess

SYPHILIS

SENSITIVITY OF VDRL IN 1°, 2°, LATENT, AND 3° SYPHILIS:

- 1° syphilis→ Positive in 80%; reliably negative within 2 years of successful treatment
- 2° syphilis→ Positive in 99%
- Latent syphilis→Positive in 70% (may remain + for long periods despite successful tx)
- Neurosyphilis→CSF positive in 50% (i.e. 50% false negative rate)

LATENT SYPHILIS

➢ Begins at **the end of the first untreated episode of secondary syphilis**
➢ divided into early and late latent substages.
  o **Early latent** syphilis is defined as the period **within the 1st year** after the onset of disease
  o **Late latent** syphilis is **after the first year** and is no longer infectious.

CHOOSING THE MOST APPROPRIATE TEST IN SUSPECTED SYPHILIS

- **PRIMARY (recent) exposure**
  o Darkfield exam of the 1° chancre
  o FTA-ABS is the first test to become positive

- **SECONDARY Syphilis**
  o Darkfield exam if skin/mucosal lesions present
  o VDRL

- **SCREENING** (pregnant women, prostitutes, contacts of cases)
  o VDRL
  o If positive→check FTA-ABS

- **FOLLOW-UP AFTER THERAPY**
  o VDRL at 3,6,12 months
  o If titre hasn't ↓d after 12 mo→retreat

- **EXCLUSION OF NEUROSYPHILIS**
  o CSF FTA-ABS (rules out if negative)

DIAGNOSTIC SIGNIFICANCE OF SYPHILIS SEROLOGY

	FTA-ABS +	FTA-ABS -
VDRL +	Syphilis	False Positives
VDRL -	Early, Latent, Late, or Treated Syphilis; False -	True Negatives

Early syphilis = (primary or secondary)
Late syphilis = tertiary

TREATMENT OF SYPHILIS DEPENDS ON THE STAGE AND IS SURPRISINGLY SIMPLE:

1° (painless chancre)→**Benzathine** PCN G 2.4 Million Units IM **x 1**

2° (maculopapular rash; condyloma lata; F/malaise/hepatitis/mucosal patches or erosions in mouth→ **Benzathine** PCN G 2.4 Million Units IM **x 1**

Latent (defined as positive serology but no clinical disease)

> **Early** (<1y)→ **Benzathine** PCN G 2.4 Million Units IM **x 1**
> ---
> **Late** (>1y or situation in which 1° infection was unrecognzied)→
> **Benzathine** PCN G 2.4 Million Units IM **weekly x 3**

3°/Neurosyphilis (may be either asymp plus a positive CSF VDRL **OR** symptomatic)→
PCN G 2-4M units **IV q4h x 10-14 days**→FOLLOWED BY…
Benzathine PCN G 2.4 Million Units IM **weekly x 3**

- *Follow sequential serum and CSF VDRL titres.*

THE JARISCH- HERXHEIMER REACTION

> Fever, chills, myalgias, headache, tachycardia, and sometimes hypotension, occurring 1-6 hours after initial therapy for syphilis.

> Seen in half of patients with primary syphilis, nearly all patients with secondary syphilis, and a quarter of those with early latent disease.

> Associated with a release of various cytokines into the plasma and rapid clearance of spirochetes from the blood, either during a *spontaneous crisis or in response to antibiotic treatment.*

> Positively correlated with the density of spirochetes in the blood at the time of treatment.

> The onset comes within 2 h of treatment, the temperature peaks at about 7 h, and defervescence takes place within 12 to 24 h.

> The reaction is self-limiting and usually easily treated with bedrest and antipyretics

IMPORTANT GRAM-STAINS:

1. **Gram + cocci**
   a. Staph
   b. Strep

2. **Gram - cocci (Neisseria species)**
   a. NM
   b. NG
   c. Moraxella Catarrhalis (aka Branhamella Catarralis)

3. **Gram + bacilli**
   a. Clostridium
   b. Bacillus species (e.g. B. cereus; B fragilis)
   c. Corynebacterium
   d. Actinomyces israeli
   e. Gardnerella vaginalis
   f. Listeria monocytogenes

4. **Gram - bacilli**
   a. Enterobacteriaceae (E. Coli, Proteus, Klebsiella, Salmonella, Shigella)
   b. Pseudomonas aeruginosa
   c. H. flu (actually a 'coccobacillus')
   d. Campylobacter jejuni
   e. Brucella

5. **Acid-fast bacilli (AFB)**
   a. Mycobacteria
   b. Nocardia asteroides (weakly acid-fast)

STREPTOCOCCAL INFECTIONS

3 MAIN CLINICAL GROUPS OF STREPTOCOCCI

☞ **STREP PYOGENES ("Beta-hemolytic" Strep)**

Acute invasive suppurative effects
- ✓ **Impetigo**
- ✓ **Cellulitis**
- ✓ **Pharyngitis**

Other acute sequelae
- ✓ **Scarlet fever**
- ✓ **Erysipelas**

Late non-suppurative sequelae
- ✓ **Rheumatic fever**
- ✓ **Poststreptococcal glomerulonephritis**

☞ **STREP PNEUMONIAE**
- ✓ Pneumonia (esp. community-acquired lobar)
- ✓ Otitis
- ✓ Meningitis

☞ **STREP VIRIDANS**—a broad term that includes (among others)

S. FAECALIS (enterococci)
- ✓ UTI
- ✓ Infective endocarditis (notoriously PCN-resistant)

S. BOVIS (enterococci)
- ✓ Infective endocarditis (exquisitely PCN-sensitive)
- ✓ Remember, if + BC in infective endocarditis→✓ colonoscopy for ca

CHARACTERIZATION OF STREPTOCOCCI

A. Classification by **LANCEFIELD ANTIGEN GROUPS:**

➢ **Group A Strep (Pyogenes)**
➢ **Group D Strep, e.g. Strep Bovis**→endocarditis→Treatment is PenG or Ceftriaxone, OR (if intermed sensitivity to PCN)→PenG + Gent
➢ **Enterococcus**--PCN is bacteriastatic, not bacteriacidal; resistant to all cephalosporins
  - ▪ E. faecalis→PCN G; add Gent for endocarditis or meningitis
  - ▪ E. faecium→No Abx regimen proven efficacious; multi-drug resistant (PCN, Aminoglycosides, and Vanco)

B. Classification by in vitro **HEMOLYSIS:**

➢ **α-hemolytic:**

  - ▪ Strep Viridans→#1 cause of non-IVDA native valve endocarditis (Staph aureus #1 if IVDA and usually affects the tricuspid valve)→Treatment same as for Strep Bovis
  - ▪ Pneumococci

➢ **β-hemolytic** = Strep Pyogenes

  - ▪ N.B. Strep Pyogenes and Pneumococcus rarely cause endocarditis

CLINICAL CORRELATIONS OF STREPTOCOCCAL INFECTIONS

1. Untreated Group A Strep *pharyngitis predisposes to development of rheumatic fever*
2. Remember, Strep A *throat **and skin** infections→post-strep glomerulonephritis*
3. *Prompt antibiotic therapy does not appear to prevent the development of post-strep glomerulonephritis, as compared to rheumatic fever following throat infection.*

RHEUMATIC FEVER

1. Acute Rheumatic Fever occurs only after **Group A Strep pharyngitis**, and never after Strep skin infections.

2. Preventable by antibiotic therapy (PCN best) **within 7 days of onset of strep throat**. Monthly IM PCN or daily PO PCN or Erythromycin are used.

3. Due to **cross-reactive anti-heart Abs stimulated by Group A strep**

4. Major and Minor Jones Criteria: **"S.A.F.E.R. C.A.S.E.S."** …
   (must have 2 major or 1major + 2 minor criteria to make the dx)

<u>Minor</u>	<u>Major</u>
Sore throat	Carditis
Arthralgias	ASO titre↑
Fever	Syndenham's chorea
EKG changes;↑ ESR	Erythema Marginatum
Rheumatic History	SQ nodules

5. **Rheumatic fever** is generally considered to be **an inflammatory disorder of connective tissue—an autoimmune response to untreated Group A β-Hemolytic Strep (GABHS) pharyngitis in a genetically predisposed host.**

6. *Clinical manifestations usually appear 1-3 weeks after the onset of pharyngitis.*

7. Although this self-limited, multisystem disease can affect heart, joints, brain, and cutaneous, and SQ tissues, **cardiac damage** *is the only potentially chronic debilitating effect. Carditis occurs in about 50%* of cases. Endocardial involvement with auscultatory evidence of MR or AI is required for diagnosis. Mild MR occurring as the sole cardiac manifestation during the acute attack will often disappear. AI occurring during the attack leads to permanent damage in 90% of patients.

8. *Migratory polyarthritis occurs in about 70%* of patients, characteristically shows rapid relief with ASA (usually within 48h) and *never* causes *permanent* joint damage.

9. **Treatment** is with an IM injection 1.2 M units benzathine Pen G.

10. ASA remains the anti-inflammatory of choice and should be started as soon as the diagnosis is suspected.

11. *Rheumatic fever* **may recur with subsequent GABHS infections**. Such recurrences can be prevented by appropriate **secondary prophylaxis** → PCN IM or PO (*or* Sulfadiazene or Eythromycin if pen-allergic). Generally speaking, continue prophylaxis for 5-10 years following the acute episode.

DURATION OF SECONDARY PROPHYLAXIS:	
Patient Type	**Duration**
Rheumatic fever with carditis and residual heart disease	≥10y since last episode or ≥ until age 40, whichever is longer
Rheumatic fever with carditis but no residual heart disease	10y or well into adulthood whichever is longer
Rheumatic fever without carditis	5y or until 21yo, whichever is longer

IMPORTANT INDICATIONS FOR VANCOMYCIN
1. Bacterial endocarditis—PCN allergy and prosthetic valve involvement
2. Enterococcus faecalis
3. MRSA
4. PCN-Resistant Strep Pneumoniae
5. Pseudomembranous colitis

IMPORTANT INDICATIONS FOR METRONIDAZOLE
1. Abscesses
2. Amebiasis
3. Anaerobic infections
4. Gardnerella vaginitis (Bacterial vaginosis)
5. Giardiasis
6. Trichomoniasis

CLASSIFICATION OF QUINOLONE ANTIBIOTICS:		
Classification	**Agent**	**Antimicrobial spectrum**
First generation	Nalidixic acid (NegGram®) Cinoxacin (Cinobac®)	Gram-negatives (but no Pseudomonas)
Second generation	Norfloxacin (Noroxin®) Lomefloxacin (Maxaquin®) Ofloxacin (Floxin®) Ciprofloxacin (Cipro®)	Gram-negatives (including Pseudomonas for Cipro), some gram + (Staph aureus but not Strep pneumoniae) and some atypicals
Third generation	Moxifloxacin (Avelox®) Sparfloxacin (Zagam®) Gatifloxacin (Tequin®) Levofloxacin (Levaquin®)	Same as for 2nd gen plus expanded gram + coverage (Pen-sensitive and Pen-resistant Strep pneumoniae) + expanded activity vs. atypicals
Fourth generation	Trovafloxacin (Trovan®)	3rd gen + broad anaerobic coverage

QUINOLONE INTERACTIONS:
May increase: 1) warfarin effects; 2) cyclosporine levels; 3) theophylline levels; 4) QTc if used concomitantly with class IA and III antiarrhythmics; 5) risk of CNS stimulation and convulsions when used with NSAIDs; and 6) serum digoxin levels (Tequin®).

TETANUS PROPHYLAXIS IN WOUND MANAGEMENT (32nd ed. Sanford Guide)

History of Tetanus Immunization	Dirty, Tetanus-prone Wound		Clean Minor Wounds	
	TD[1,2]	TIG	Td	TIG
Unknown or < 3doses*	Yes	Yes	Yes	No
≥3 doses**	No[3]	No	No[4]	No

* *"YES" to all except clean TIG !*
** *"NO" to all !*

1. Td=Tetanus & diptheria toxoids adsorbed (adults)
   TIG=Tetanus Immune Globulin
2. Yes if wound > 24 hours old
   For children < 7yo, DPT (DT if pertussis vaccine contraindicated)
   For persons ≥ 7 yo, Td preferred to tetanus toxoid alone
3. Yes if over 5 years since last booster
4. Yes if over 10 years since last booster

MECHANISMS OF VACCINE ACTION

1. **Toxoids:**
   a) Tetanus
   b) Diptheria
   c) Botulism

2. **Recombinant vaccines:**
   a) Hep B
   b) Cholera

3. **Pooled surface proteins:**
   a) Strep Pneumococcus
   b) H. Flu B (HiB)

4. **Attenuated (live) organisms**, **CONTRAINDICATED in PREGNANT OR IMMUNOCOMPROMISED pts!**
   a) Polio
   b) M, M, and R (all three)
   c) BCG
   d) Yellow fever
   e) Rabies
   f) VZV (Varicella-Zoster)

5. **Killed organisms:**
   a) Influenza B
   b) Hep A
   c) Typhoid
   d) Pertussis

ENDOCARDITIS ANTIBIOTIC PROPHYLAXIS In Patients With Underlying Heart Disease:

Prophylaxis Recommended	Prophylaxis *NOT* Recommended
Cardiac conditions	Negligible Risk
High risk	ASD (*secundum*;=right axis deviation)
Prosthetic valves	MVP without MR
Prev bacterial endocarditis	Physiologic/functional/
Cyanotic congenital heart disease	or innocent heart
Moderate risk	murmurs
IHSS	Pacemakers
MVP with regurgitation, or	IADs (implantable automatic
thickening of MV leaflets	defibrillators)
Dental	
Extractions	
Periodontal procedures	Routine cavity filling with local anesthesthetic
Respiratory	
Rigid Bronchoscopy	Flexible bronchoscopy
Tonsillectomy/Adenoidectomy	
GI	
Sclerotherapy of esoph varices	TEE
Dilatation of esoph stricture	EGD without biopsy
ERCP with biliary tract obstruction	
Biliary tract surgery	
GU	
Prostate surg; cystoscopy	Vag hysterectomy/delivery; C sx

✪ **IMPORTANT RULES OF THUMB:**
- Most congenital heart disease *(except → secundum ASD and primum ASD/VSD/PDA ≥6mo post-surgical repair)* requires antibiotic prophylaxis.
- **MVP with incompetence/murmur** needs antibiotic prophylaxis.

OCCURRENCE OF INFECTIVE ENDOCARDITIS (In ↓ing Order)

1. Primary (40%)→**Strep Viridans**

2. Previous Rheumatic Valve Damage (30%)→Strep Viridans

3. Congenital Heart disease (10%)

4. **Prosthetic valve (10%)→Staph Epidermidis**

5. IVDA (10%)→Staph Aureus; Tricuspid valve

6. **Colon Ca→Strep Bovis**

TREATMENT

1. **Native valve endocarditis**

    a) Strep Viridans→Pen G ± Gent

    b) Enterococci→Treatment depends on resistance to PCN/Aminoglycs/Vanco

    c) MSSA→Nafcillen (or oxacillen) + Gent

    d) MRSA→Vancomycin

    e) HACEK organisms (fastidious, slow-growing, Gram neg bacilli: **HACEK group organisms** = gram-negative organisms that tend to grow slowly over weeks. **H**emophilus, **A**ctinobacillus, **C**ardiobacterium, **E**ikenella, and **K**ingella) → Ceftriaxone

    f) Culture negative→Treatment depends on the specific causal organism (i.e. Q fever, bartonella, brucellosis, psittacosis, or fungi)

2. *Empiric* **therapy (culture pending) for NATIVE VALVE endocarditis**→ (PCN *or* Amp *or* Naf *or* Ox) + Gent; Vanco & Gent if Pen-allergic.

3. *Empiric* **therapy for PROSTHETIC VALVE** endocarditis→Vanco + Gent + Rifampin

4. **Culture positive prosthetic valve** infection→Surgical consult *PLUS*

    a) Staph epidermidis (usually a contaminant on BC) →Vanco + Gent + Rifampin

    b) MSSA→Nafcillen + Gent

    c) MRSA→ Vanco + Gent

    d) Strep Viridans→same as for native valve above

    e) Candida or Aspergillus→Ampho B ± Fluconazole

INDICATIONS FOR SURGERY IN INFECTIVE ENDOCARDITIS

1. Massive vegetations seen on echo

2. Persistent bacteremias/fevers despite optimal medical mgmt

3. Prosthetic valve involvement

4. Refractory CHF, esp with AI

5. Repeated septic emboli

6. Suspected extensive valve ring infection

7. Hemolysis

8. Conduction disturbances (associated with abscess)

TREATMENT OF STDs (PER SANFORD GUIDE AND CDC)

STD	TREATMENT GUIDELINES
Chancroid	Azithromycin single dose of 1g PO; or Ceftriaxone 250mg IM x1; or Erythro 500 qid x 1 week
Chlamydia trachomatis	Azithromycin single dose of 1g PO; or Doxy 100 BID x 1 week
GC, uncomplicated	Cipro 500 PO x1 or Ofloxacin 400 PO x1 or Ceftriaxone 125 IM x 1 or Cefixime 400 PO x 1
HSV, genital, primary	Acyclovir 400 TID x 10d; or Famvir 250 TID x 5-10d; or Valtrex 1000 BID x 10d
Lymphogranuloma Venereum (LGV)	Doxycycline 100 BID x 3 weeks
Syphilis	See section on Syphilis, since treatment depends on stage of disease.
Trichomonas vaginalis ('Trich')	Metronidazole 2g PO x 1; contraindicated in 1st trimester preg

VAGINITIS—3 MAIN TYPES:

VAGINITIS	CLINICAL FINDINGS	TREATMENT
Candida albicans	'Cottage cheese curds'; no odor; pruritic; common after Abx and in obese or diabetics.	Fluconazole 150 PO x1; or intravaginal azole
Trichomoniasis	Yellow, purulent discharge; 'Strawberry cervix' seen on culposcopy 2° petechia seen; Dx usu. by wet mount	Metronidazole 2g PO x 1; contraindicated in 1st trimester pregnancy; must also treat sexual partner
Gardnerella vaginalis ('Bacterial Vaginosis)	Malodorous "fishy" smell after adding KOH ('whiff test'); 'clue cells' on wet mount.	Metronidazole 2g PO x 1 less effective than PO or intravaginal dosing x 5-7 days

EPIDIDYMITIS: THE *RULE OF THUMB*:

$\Rightarrow$ Men <35=Chlamydia or GC$\rightarrow$ Treat as for **GC + Chlamydia** (see STD table above)

$\Rightarrow$ Men >35=**E. Coli** usually$\rightarrow$Treat with TMP-SMX or Ciprofloxacin.

DERMATOLOGIC INFECTIONS COMMON IN AIDS:

1. **Herpes Zoster** (shingles)→VZV
2. **Oral hairy leukoplakia** →EBV and usually seen in advanced AIDS. Treatment is acyclovir / antivirals (*Note*: this is **not the same as "oral leukoplakia"**, which is related to HPV, smoking, smokeless tobacco, alcohol, and syphilis. Candida can invade oral leukoplakia secondarily, and it is considered a premalignant lesion for squamous cell ca)
3. **Molluscum contagiosum**→Discrete, solid, skin-colored papules that are only 1-2 mm in diameter, have **central umbilication**
4. **Bacillary angiomatosis** (vascular papules or nodules caused by **Bartonella** (Rochalimaea) henselae and quintana and transmitted by cats or ticks)→Erythromycins or Doxycycline for treatment

LABORATORY CHARACTERIZATION OF GENITAL ULCERS

1. **Positive dark-field exam**→1° syphilis

2. *H. Ducreyi* on microscopy→**Chancroid**

3. **Donovan bodies** on microscopy→**Granuloma inguinale (Donovanosis); caused by *Calymmatobacterium granulomatis*** [1° Rx=Doxy or Bactrim x 3 weeks; alt Rx=Ery or Cipro also x 3 weeks]

4. *Chlamydia* on culture/serology→**LGV** (Lymphogranuloma venereum)

5. Herpes simplex on viral cultures

6. **Negative microbiology→consider Behcet's/Reiter's** syndrome

AMINOGLYCOSIDE TOXICITY

➢ The **nephrotoxicity is almost always reversible**; NSAIDs, Vanco, Ampho enhance
➢ The **ototoxicity** is almost always **IRreversible**; loop diuretics enhance
➢ Mg, K+, Ca : wasting

FUNGAL INFECTIONS

COCCIDIOIDES IMMITIS
1. **San Joaquin Valley, California**
2. **Central Arizona**
3. Dissemination most likely to occur in males, esp Filipino and blacks
4. Primary infection is pneumonitis; see dry cough, fever, and pleural effusion
5. E. Nodosum may be seen
6. Hilar adenopathy common
7. Diagnosis by complement fixation (titre ≥ 1:4)
8. PO Fluconazole (Diflucan®) is the treatment

HISTOPLASMOSIS

1. **Ohio and Mississippi River valleys**
2. Associated with cleaning chicken coops/bird nesting areas→exposure to **bird droppings**.
3. Patients are usually **immunocompetent**
4. Colonic involvement in AIDS
5. 2 forms:
   a) Primary (acute) form→resembles flu/URI
   b) Chronic cavity disease→Bilateral upper lung distribution, similar to TB
6. Itraconazole, Ampho B are the treatment options depending on severity/immune status.

BLASTOMYCOSIS

1. Affects lungs, skin, bone, and prostate/epididymis/testes
2. **Cutaneous** is most common clinical form
3. Itraconazole or Ampho B depending on severity

- **The major advantage of Itraconazole over Fluconazole is its greater activity against Aspergillus, Sporothrix, Histoplasmosis, and Blastomycosis.**

ASPERGILLOSIS THE FOUR PATTERNS OF PULMONARY INFECTION

1. Saprophytic infections (2° infection in necrotic tissue)

2. **Chronic Necrotizing Aspergillosis**→ especially in *preexisting pulmonary bullous disease*—e.g. TB or ankylosing spondylitis)→look for **ASPERGILLOMA** (fungal ball)
   a) Anti-fungal therapy not helpful
   b) Surgery for patients with hemoptysis

3. **ABPA** (Allergic Bronchopulmonary Aspergillosis)

   ➢ *ABPA is a syndrome of severe, refractory asthma in which hypersensitivity to aspergillus found in the lung.leads to severe, refractory asthma with central bronchiectasis and recurrent pulmonary infiltrates.*

   ➢ **Diagnosis:**
      i) *Clinical presentation*
         a) Presents as **asthma** with wheezing and brown mucus plugs
         b) Commonly seen in asthmatics who have been stable on chronic maintenance
         c) therapy and suddenly ***breaks through***.May cause sinus and pulmonary infection in neutropenic patients
         d) **Migratory pulmonary infiltrates**
         e) Presentation of chronic granulomatous disease in a young patient may be an Aspergillus infection.
      ii) Aspergillus precipitans in blood

iii) Wheal-and-flare (immediate Type 1) skin test reactivity
iv) ↑ Total IgG in blood
v) **↑ Total IgE ≥ 1000** and Aspergillus-specific Ab
vi) **Peripheral blood ↑eos ≥ 8 %**
vii) + Sputum culture for Aspergillus (beware, though, since it is a frequent colonizer)

✪ **TREATMENT IS STEROIDS.**
✪ **THERE IS NO ROLE FOR ANTIFUNGALTHERAPY IN ABPA.**

4. **Invasive Bronchopulmonary Disease**
   a) Prolonged neutropenia predisposes, especially in
      i) AML
      ii) CLL
      iii) Hodgkin's
   b) Ampho B or itraconazole

CRYPTOCOCCUS NEOFORMANS

1. Most infections occur in **immunosuppressed** patients (as opposed to Histo)

2. *Similar* to Histo, however, **pigeon droppings** may play a role

3. **Meningitis** is most common form of infection, and if C. Neoformans is isolated from anywhere→must ✓ the CSF

4. Treatment
   a) Non-meningeal, Non-AIDS→Ampho til response, then Fluconazole; or Fluconazole alone
   b) *Meningitis*, Non-AIDS→Ampho B + Flucytosine til afebrile & culture neg, →then PO Fluconazole; or Fluconazole alone
   c) HIV+/AIDS (usually *meningitis*)→Ampho B + Flucytosine→then PO Fluconazole indefinitely

CANDIDA

1. Immunosuppressed + infected intravenous catheters→Candidemia

2. IVDA→can see Candida albicans (and other Candida species) endocarditis

3. Hepatic candidiasis seen commonly in neutropenic patients following bone marrow transplant.

4. Causes oral & esophageal candidiasis in immunosuppressed

5. Ampho B / Fluconazole

SPOROTRICHOSIS

1. An ulceronodular dermatosis caused by Sporothrix schenckii, a fungus commonly found in *soil, and usually affecting gardeners*, farmers, florists, lawn workers. Chronic nodular lymphagitis and regional lymphadenitis are concomitant
2. Pulmonary infection may lead to empyema, chronic pneumonitis, cavities

MUCOR

1. Caused by Rhizopus, Zygomycetes
2. *DKA* or immunosuppressed + Mucormycosis→rhinocerebral infections
3. Diagnosis based on finding **black, necrotic lesions** around the eyes, nose, soft/hard palates;
4. Biopsy confirmatory.
5. *Ampho B + surgical debridement*

PARASITIC INFECTIONS

GIARDIA.

1. Recognize it as a potential pathogen in **white water rafting trips**; be able to recognize it's microscopic appearance.

2. Clinical: sudden onset of **watery diarrhea, bloating, flatulence**

3. The treatment is **metronidazole**.

AMEBIASIS

1. **AMEBIC LIVER ABSCESS**

   a) *Right* lobe effected in 90% of cases
   b) *Males* affected in 80% of cases
   c) *Single* abscess seen in 70% of cases; the fluid on aspiration has been said to resemble "chocolate syrup" or "anchovy paste".
   d) *Normal LFTs*, usually.

   • You can *remember these* by recalling, "**Ame** is looking for a **normal, single, male, Mr. Right**"!

   e) Stools may contain cysts and may be difficult to distinguish from leukocytes.
   f) Patients with hepatic abscess usually don't have the diarrhea

2. Bloody diarrhea when colonic involvement (discrete "flask-shaped" ulcers)

3. Serology, using complement fixation testing is positive in >90%

TOXOPLASMOSIS

1. Acquired from eating undercooked meat or exposure to <u>**cat**</u> feces

2. *Disorders in the normal host:*

   a) **Mono-like syndrome**

   b) **Ocular toxoplasmosis**

      i) Usually the result of congenital infections

      ii) Characteristic lesion is focal necrotizing retinitis tht initially appears in the fundus as yellowish-white, elevated, cotton patches with indistinct margins, usually on the posterior pole

      iii) Presents with blurred vision, scotoma, pain, photophobia

      iv) *Treatment: Pyrimethamine + Sulfadiazene + Leucovorin (folate); Steroids indicated if lesions involve the macula or optic nerve head*

   c) Congenital toxo (part of the TORCH syndrome)

3. *Disorders of the immunodeficient patient*

   a) Brain lesions (often difficult to ddx with CNS lymphoma, since both give ring-enhancing lesions)

   b) Myocarditis

   c) Pneumonia

HIV PRIMER

ANTIRETROVIRAL TREATMENT REGIMENS/COMBINATIONS:

Nucleoside Reverse-Transcriptase Inhibitors (NRTI), aka 'Nucleoside Analogues':

Group "**A**" drugs
1. Zidovudine (ZDV or AZT)—Retrovir®
2. Stavudine (d4T) —Zerit®

Group "**B**" drugs
1. Didanosine (ddI)   —Videx®
2. Zalcitabine (ddC) —HIVID®
3. Lamivudine (3TC)—Epivir®

Non- Nucleoside Reverse-Transcriptase Inhibitors (NNRTI):
('Non-Nucleoside Analogues')
1. Nevirapine (Viramune®)
2. Delavirdine (Rescriptor®)
3. Efavirenz (Sustiva®)

Protease Inhibitors (PI)
1. Saquinavir (Invirase®; Fortovase®)
2. Indinavir (Crixivan®)
3. Ritonavir (Norvir®; Kaletra)
4. Nelfinavir (Viracept®)
5. Amprenavir (Agenerase®)

☞ **Most experts recommend initiating triple combinations as follows→**
2 NRTI's ("A" + "B") *plus either* **a (NNRTI or PI).**
☞ **Triple therapy as such is _also_ recommended for 4 weeks following a**
needle stick injury from an individual known to be HIV+.

⇒ *Adding one "A" drug to one "B" drug prevents additive toxicities.*

HAART (Highly Active AntiRetroviral Therapy)
➢ Comprised of ≥ 3 antiretroviral meds used in combo
➢ Acceptable combinations suppress HIV virus to undetectable levels.
➢ All HAART regimens contain 2 NRTIs, along with an agent from a different class.
➢ *Recommended regimens include*:
  o 2 NRTIs + 1 PI
  o 2 NRTIs + 1 NNRTI
  o 2 NRTIs + Ritonavir + another PI (eg Saquinivir)

✓ The following *specific* combinations of HAART are currently considered *strongly recommended* initial regimens: (1 choice each from columns 1 and 2):

Column 1	Column 2
• Efavirenz	ddI + 3TC
• Indinavir	d4T + ddI
• Nelfinavir	d4T + 3TC
• Ritonavir + Indinavir	ZDV + ddI
• Ritonavir + Saquinavir	ZDV + 3TC

✓ The *following combinations should be avoided* (2° to overlapping toxicity or reduced efficacy):

- Stavudine (d4T) + **Z**DV → *Remember*: 4Z (4 z extra point!)
- dd**C** + dd**I** → *Remember*: CI (as in the commonly used abbreviation for **C**ontra**I**ndicated)
- **In**dinavir + **sa**quinavir → *Remember*: INSAne to use together
- **3**TC + d**4**T → *Remember*: 3,4

➢ **When to INITIATE HAART in ASYMPTOMATIC Individuals:**

CD4 COUNT (cells/mm^3)	VIRAL LOAD (copies/mL)		
	<5000	5000-30,000	>30,000
<200	+	+	+
200-350	+	+	+
>350	-	±	+

❖ In general, then, HAART should be offered to individuals with CD4 *≤ 350 or plasma HIV RNA levels > 30,000*.

❖ In general, *symptomatic* patients, *whatever* their CD4 count or viral load, *should receive* HAART.

SCHEDULED TREATMENT INTERRUPTIONS

➢ Viral suppression with ARTs removes the stimulus for ongoing endogenous immune suppression. The rationale of STI is that once the immune system has recovered to some degree, interrupting treatment allows ongoing HIV replication to stimulate the immune response to naturally suppress HIV replication.

IMPORTANT PRESCRIBING POINTS for Selected NRTIs, NNRTIs, and PIs:

NRTIs

➤ Abacavir (ABC)
  - *Febrile hypersensitivity*—resolves spont'ly within a few days of discontinuing. Attempting to rechallenge the patient with this same drug after resolution of this reaction is absolutely *contraindicated.*
  - *Hypertriglyceridemia*

➤ Didanosine(ddI)
  - *Pancreatitis; painful peripheral neuropathy*
  - Interacts with ketokonazole, calcium carbonate
  - Do not use with ddC 2° overlapping toxicity

➤ Lamivudine (3TC)
  - Best tolerated NRTI; synergistic with AZT →Combivir®; when add 3TC + AZT + abacavir (ABC)→ Trizivir®
  - Side effects uncommon

➤ Stavudine (d4T)
  - *Painful peripheral neuropathy = #1 side effect*
  - Do not use with AZT (↓ each other)

➤ Zidovudine (AZT) (ZDV)
  - *Bone marrow suppression, asthenia; headache* is the symptom patients complain about the most
  - The *myopathy* that is frequently seen with AZT isn't seen before 6 months of use.
  - Anemia in 30-40% of AIDS patients
  - Penetrates the CNS and may effective for HIV dementia and thrombocytopenia

NNRTIs

➤ Delavirdine
  - *Maculopapular rash*
  - Drug interactions: may ↑ sildenafil (Viagra®) levels; avoid concomitant use of simvastatin or lovastatin

➤ Efavirenz
  - Due to its ability to get into the CNS → *dizziness/drowsiness/trouble concentrating or sleeping/vivid dreams/etc. The drowsiness can manifest as a "hangover" the morning after the first dose.* This can be prevented by having the patient take it between 6-8pm, NOT at bedtime, so that the patient sleeps through the worst of it.
  - Drug interactions: can ↓ opiates/indivavir/rifabutin; can ↑ ritonavir; monitor anticonvulsants and warfarin carefully.

➤ Nevirapine
  - *Maculopapular rash (esp in women; most common in the 1st month of therapy), hepatotoxicity*

PROTEASE INHIBITORS

- ➢ Amprenavir

  - o A sulfonamide
  - o *Perioral paresthesias*
  - o High-fat meal can ↓ absorption

- ➢ Indinavir

  - o *Nephrolithiasis* (therefore encouraged to <u>*drink plenty of water*</u>), thromocytopenia, alopecia, hyperglycemia
  - o Food significantly decreases absorption

- ➢ Nelfinavir

  - o Most bothersome side effect, reported in 1/3 of patients is *diarrhea*; responds well to Imodium®.

- ➢ Ritonavir

  - o Most potent PI, yet the least well-tolerated
  - o *Circumoral/peripheral paresthesias, paraguesia*
    - ▪ Fewer side effects at low dose, so generally used in low-dose combination with other PIs.

  - o *Key drug interactions*:
    - ▪ ↓ theo levels; ↓ efficacy of oral contraceptives

    - ▪ Beware of serotonin syndrome in patients taking fluoxetine (Prozac, Serafem) with the ritonavir

    - ▪ Additional meds to avoid with many of the PIs: simvastatin, lovastatin, rifampin, clozapine, midazolam, triazolam, DHE and other ergot derivatives (add amiodarone and quinidine for ritonavir; and with ritonavir, rifampin is actually OK)

    - ▪ Cytochrome P450 enzyme inducers--such as phenobarb, carbamazepine, dexamethasone, phenytoin, and St. John's wart--↓ the efficacy of ritonavir.
      - • *Avoid use of St. John's wart with all PI and NNRTI.*

- ➢ Saquinavir

  - o Generally well-tolerated with the most common side effect being GI.
  - o The newer soft-gel form of saquinivir is more efficacious than the earlier hard–gel form (poor absorption), but has ↑ side effects that include:
    - ▪ ↑ glu, ↑ chol, ↑ TG
  - o Drug interactions: may ↑ rifampin/triazolam, midazolam, and ergots

INSTITUTING CHANGES IN HAART

> *Criteria for Treatment Failure*
> - o >400-500 viral copies/mL after 16-20 wks of treatment
> - o >40-50 viral copies/mL after 20-24 wks of treatment
> - o Repeated detection of virus after initial suppression to undetectable levels
> - o Persistently declining CD4+ cells on 2 occasions

> *How to Change* ✪
> - o Ideally, all agents should be changed in cases of treatment failure. However, *at least 2 of the 3 or 4 drug regimens should be changed to new drug classes*, one of which should be an NNRTI if not already part of the regimen being changed
> - o Consider resistance testing

> It is acceptable to change a single agent if patients are unable to tolerate a specific agent of course.

POST-EXPOSURE PROPHYLAXIS ✪

> Start within a few hours (not days!) of exposure

> **4 week regimen should include 2 NRTIs:** Use zidovidine + lamivudine (Combivir), lamivudine + stavudine, or stavudine + didanosine.

> > ✓ **If there is an ↑ risk for HIV transmission, a third drug (usu indinavir or nelfinavir) should be added**, eg in cases involving deep puncture wounds or large volumes of blood from symptomatic patients.

> > ✓ F/u in 2 weeks for toxicity eval/side effects
> > - o Half of healthcare workers report side effects, causing more than 1/3 of them to stop post-exposure prophylaxis.

> > ✓ Antibody testing should be done immediately post exposure to check baseline, and again at 6 wks, 12 weeks, and 6 months.

ZIDOVIDINE PERINATAL TRANSMISSION PROPHYLAXIS ✪ (AIDS Clinical Trial Group 076 study)

> ✓ *Reduces risk of HIV transmission to infant by 66%*

Antepartum	Starting as early as possible after <u>14 weeks</u> and continuing up to delivery, ZDV 200mg tid OR 300mg bid
Intrapartum	During labor, load ZDV 2mg/kg IV over 1h → then continuous infusion at 1mg/kg IV until delivery.
Postpartum	<u>Starting 8-12h after delivery</u>, oral administration of ZDV to the newborn as syrup at 2mg/kg q6h for 1st 6 wks of life

✪ MAY STOP PROPHYLACTIC OR MAINTENANCE THERAPY IN HIV WHEN...

     ✓ PCP   →   CD4> 200 x 3-6 months with viral load reduction over that period
     ✓ MAI   →   CD4>100 x 3-6 months with viral load suppressed at 3-6 months
     ✓ CMV   →   CD4>100 x 3-6 months

✪ GI DISEASE IN AIDS

1. HSV, CMV, and Candida esophagitis

2. **Histoplasma capsulatum**—colonic involvement; diagnosis by culture; treatment is ampho or itraconazole

3. **MAI** (mycobacterium avium intracellulare) can cause a voluminous diarrhea and is often associated with additional fever, abdominal pain, and weight loss.

4. **Cryptosporidium**—Voluminous, watery diarrhea. In immunocompromised hosts, especially those with AIDS, diarrhea can be chronic, persistent, and remarkably profuse, causing clinically significant fluid and electrolyte depletion. Stool volumes may range from 1 to 25 L/d.no therapy *proven* efficacious, although in AIDS patients may try treating with paromomycin.

5. **Microsporidia**— Affects the small intestine, causing diarrhea; albendazole is the primary treatment of choice.

6. **Isospora belli**- Diagnosis via oval oocysts in the stool seen with modified Kinyoun acid-fast stain. Primary treatment choice is TMP-SMX (160/800 mg qid for 10 days and then bid for 3 weeks) for treatment.

7. **Entameba histolytica**→Metronidazole; see amebiasis.

8. **Giardia lamblia**→Prominent early symptoms include diarrhea, abdominal pain, bloating, belching, flatus, nausea, and vomiting. Although diarrhea is common, upper intestinal manifestations such as nausea, vomiting, bloating, and abdominal pain may predominate. Associated with camping trips; "white-water rafting"; questions involving "Venezuela"(!); treatment is metronidazole

9. **Cyclospora**--Some patients may harbor the infection without symptoms, but many with cyclosporiasis have diarrhea, flulike symptoms, and flatulence and burping. The diagnosis can be made by detection of spherical 8- to 10-um oocysts in the stool. These refractile oocysts are variably acid-fast and are fluorescent when viewed with ultraviolet light microscopy.

10. **Blastocystis hominis**→ Role as a pathogen is controversial; no controlled rx trials

11. Remember also: When see **Hairy Leukoplakia**→must R/O HIV

12. In **CMV** infection, viremia does not necessarily correlate with organ involvment; therefore, cultures are often of no use in this setting.

IMPORTANT ADDITIONAL NOTES ON HIV

- ➤ Zidovidine should be included as part of an ART regimen for all HIV-positive pregnant women

- ➤ Remember CD4 counts <u>below 50/mm³</u> confer an ↑ risk for MAI and CMV.
  - o Suspect MAI with counts below 50, *fever, weight loss, abdominal pain, anemia,* and often voluminous diarrhea
  - o If you see *"floaters"* in a question → patient has CMV retinitis!

- ➤ The CDC now permits discontination of various prophylactic agents used in HIV opportunistic disease (eg PCP, MAI, CMV, toxo) when CD4 > 200 along with dramatic reductions in viral load.

- ➤ The average risk of seroconversion is 1/300 <u>(0.3%)</u> after a needlestick contaminated with HIV-infected blood, and 1/1111 <u>(0.09%)</u> after a mucous membrane exposure to HIV-infected blood.

- ➤ Remember, ***TMP-SMX also*** reduces the frequency of *toxoplasmosis*, and vice versa, so that patients who are being treated for Toxo with ***sulfadiazene-pyrimethamine*** are protected against PCP and do not need additional prophylaxis against PCP.

- ➤ Patients receiving **dapsone** should be ***tested for G6PD deficiency***.

- ➤ Diagnostic procedure of choice in <u>**PCP**</u> is sputum induction. Send for <u>**silver methenamine stain**</u>. If negative → bronchoscopy.

- ➤ **INDICATIONS FOR <u>STEROIDS</u> WHEN INITIATING TREATMENT FOR PCP:**
  - ✓ $PaO_2 < 70$
  - ✓ A-a gradient > 35

- ➤ For **PCP**, if the patient is **not acutely ill, is able to take PO meds, & PaO2 >70,** recommended treatment is:

  - ✓ Dapsone 100 qd + TMP (no SMX) @ 5mg/kd x 21d ; *OR:*
  - ✓ TMP-SMX-DS 2 tabs tid x 21d

- ➤ Remember, **AIDS Cholangiopathy** is essentially a sclerosing cholangitis that presents with RUQ pain and alk phos elevations out of proportion to the AST and ALT. Microsporidia, cryptosporidia CMV are chief culprits.

- ➤ ***<u>Rifampin should not be administered concurrently with protease inhibitors or nonnucleoside reverse transcriptase inhibitors</u>. Rifabutin is an alternative. <u>Even then</u>, rifabutin should not be given with saquinivir or delavirdine.***

APPENDIX

Table 1.   **PROPHYLAXIS VS. <u>FIRST EPISODE</u> OF OPPORTUNISTIC DISEASE IN HIV:**

<u>ORGANISM</u>	<u>INDICATION</u>	<u>DRUG OF CHOICE</u>	<u>ALTERNATIVES</u>
PCP	CD4 <200 or oropharyngeal candidiasis	Bactrim DS QD Bactrim SS QD	• Dapsone/Pyrimethamine/Leukovorin; • Pentamidine (aerosol); • Atovaquone;
MTB			
INH-Sensitive	• PPD ≥5mm; or • Prior +PPD without Rx; or • Contact with active TB case	INH + B6 Rifampin + Pyrazinamide (PZA)	Rifabutin +/- PZA
INH-Resistant	Same; and High prob of exposure to INH-Resistant TB	Rifampin + PZA	Rifabutin +/- PZA
MDR-TB (INH and Rifampin-Resistant)	Same; plus high prob. of exposure to MDR-TB	see section on MDR-TB	see section on MDR-TB
Toxoplasmosis gondii	IgG Ab to Toxoplasma and CD4<100	Bactrim DS	• Dapsone + Pyramethimine + Leucovorin • Atovaquone ± Pyramethamine + Leucovorin
MAI	CD4<50	Azithromycin; or Clarithromycin	Rifabutin ± Azithromycin
VZV	Significant exposure to chickenpox or shingles for patients who have no history of either condition or, if available, neg VZV Ab	Varicella zoster immune globulin (VZIG) as 5 vials IM given ≤ 96h post-exposure	None
Strep pneumoniae	All patients	Pneumovax	None
Hep A	All susceptible (anti-HAV-negative) patients with chronic Hep C	Hep A vaccine: 2 doses	None
Hep B	All susceptible (anti-HBc-negative) patients	Hep B vaccine: 3 doses	None
Influenza	All patients annually	Whole or split virus as IM	Rimantidine; or Amantadine

Table 2. PROPHYLAXIS TO PREVENT <u>RECURRENCES</u> OF OPPORTUNISTIC DZ IN HIV AFTER RX FOR ACUTE DZ.

<u>ORGANISM</u>	<u>DRUG OF CHOICE</u>	<u>ALTERNATIVES</u>
PCP	Bactrim SS or DS	• Dapsone; *or* • Dapsone + Pyimethamine + Leucovorin; *or* • Aerosolized Pentamidine; *or* • Atovaquone
Toxoplasmosis gondii	Sulfadiazine + Pyrimethamine + Leucovorin	• Clindamycin + Pyrimethamine + Leucovorin; *or* • Atovaquone + Pyrimethamine + Leucovorin
MAI	Clarithromycin + Ethambutol ± Rifabutin	Azithromycin + Ethambutol ± Rifabutin
CMV	Ganciclovir; Foscarnet	Cidofovir + Probenicid; *or* Fomivirsen
Cryptococcus Neoformans	Fluconazole	Ampho B; *or* Itraconazole
Histoplasma Capsulatum	Itraconazole	Ampho B
Coccidioides immitis	Fluconazole	Ampho B
Salmonella species (non-typhi)	Ciprofloxacin	(other active antibiotic ok)
RECOMMENDED ONLY FOR FREQUENT OR SEVERE SUBSEQUENT EPISODES:		
HSV	Acyclovir; or Famciclovir	Valacyclovir
Candida (oropharyngeal; esophageal; or vaginal)	Fluconazole	Itraconazole or ketoconazole

Table 3. **IMPORTANT DRUG-DRUG <u>INTERACTIONS</u> IN <u>PROPHYLAXIS</u> OF OPPORTUNISTIC DZ:**

<u>AFFECTED DRUG</u>	**<u>CULPRIT DRUG</u>**	**<u>EFFECT</u>**	**<u>RECOMMEDATION</u>**
Atovaquone	Rifampin	↓	Avoid this combo or ↑ atovaquone dose
Clarithromycin	Ritonavir	↑	No adjustment necessary if normal renal function; adjust if creat clearance <30
Clarithromycin	Nevirapine	↓	Effect of MAI prophylaxis may be ↓'d, so monitor closely
Ketoconazole	Antacids, didanosine (ddI), H2-receptor antagonists, proton-pump inhibitors	↓ absorption	Avoid using ketoconazole with pH-raising agents or use another antifungal
Quinolone antibiotics	Didanosine, antacids, iron products, calcium products, sucralfate	↓	Give quinolone ≥2h prior
Rifabutin	Fluconazole	↑	Monitor rifabutin toxicity such as uveitis, nausea, & neutropenia
Rifabutin	Efavirenz	↓	↑ Rifabutin dose to 450 mg QD
Rifabutin	Ritonavir, saquinavir, indinavir, nelfinavir, amprenavir, delavirdine	↑	Contraindicated with hard-gel saquinivir and delavirdine; Use ½ dose with indinavir, nelfinavir, amprenavir; Use ¼ dose w/ ritonavir

INFECTIOUS DISEASE & HIV

Table 4.

HIV-RELATED DRUGS WITH OVERLAPPING TOXICITIES

(Table 19 of "The Living Document", Aug 13, 2001, abbrev, CDC/MMWR; www.hivatis.org)

BONE MARROW SUPPRESSION	PERIPHERAL NEUROPATHY	PANCREATITIS	NEPHROTOXICITY	HEPATOTOXICTY	RASH	DIARRHEA
Cidofovir	Didanosine	TMP-SMX	Adefovir	Delavirdine	Abacavir	Didanosine
TMP-SMX	Isoniazid	Didanosine	Aminoglycosides	Efavirenz	Amprenavir	Clinda
Dapsone	Stavudine	Lamivudine	Ampho B	Fluconazole	TMP-SMX	Nelfinavir
Flucytosine	Zalcitabine	Pentamidine	Cidofovir	INH	Dapsone	Ritonavir
Gancyclovir		Ritonavir	Foscarnet	Itra/ketoconazole	NNRTIs	Lopinavir
Hydroxyurea		Stavudine	Indinavir	Nevirapine	Sulfadiazene	Ritonavir
α interferon		Zalcitabine	Pentamidine	NRTIs		Atovaquone
Primaquine				PIs		
Pyimethamine				Rifabutin/rifampin		
Ribavirin						
Rifabutin						
Sulfadiazene						
Zidovudine						

Table 5. **IMPORTANT <u>ADVERSE</u> EFFECTS OF <u>ANTIRETROVIRALS</u>:**

DRUG	COMMON ADVERSE EFFECTS
NUCLEOSIDE REVERSE TRANSCRIPTASE INHIBTORS (NRTI)	
Zidovidine (**AZT**) (Retrovir®)	Anemia
Didanosine (**ddI**) (Videx®)	*Pancreatitis; peripheral neuropathy*
Zalcitabine (**ddC**) (Hivid®)	Neuropathy
Stavudine (**d4T**) (Zerit®)	Painful peripheral neuropathy
Lamivudine (**3TC**) (Epivir®)	Rare
Abacavir (**ABC**) (Ziagen®)	*Hypertriglyceridemia*; rash, fever
Non-Nucleoside Reverse Transcriptase Inhibtors (NNRTI)	
Nevirapine (Viramune®)	Rash
Delavirdine (Rescriptor®)	Rash
Efavirenz (Sustiva®)	*Altered mental status*
PROTEASE INHIBITORS	
Ritonavir (Norvir®)	GI upset, paresthesias
Indinavir (Crixivan®)	*Nephrolithiasis*
Saquinavir (Fortovase®)	Nausea
Nelfinavir (Viracept®)	Diarrhea
Amprenavir (Agenerase®)	Nausea

6. DERMATOLOGY

✪ SKIN DISEASE AS A MANIFESTATION OF MALIGNANCY...

1. **Acanthosis nigricans** (not just DM and obesity!)→ GI malignancy, esp gastric, ovarian.

2. **Actinic keratosis**→Squamous cell carcinoma

3. **Café au lait spots**→ Von Recklinghausen's disease

4. **Dysplastic nevus**→Malignant melanoma

5. **Epidermal cysts, fibromas, lipomas**→Gardner's syndrome

6. **Flushing, telangiectasias**→Carcinoid tumors

7. **Mucosal hyperpigmentation** (esp. lips)→ Peutz-Jeghers syndrome

8. **Necrolytic erythematous rash**→Glucagonoma

9. **Erythroderma**→ Sezary syndrome (rare variant of cutaneous T-cell lymphoma, aka mycosis fungoides), mycosis fungoides

10. **Dermatomyositis** (esp. steroid-resistant form in adults)→Many types of cancers, esp ovarian/gastric/lung ca.; look for heliotrope rash/Gottron's papules/violaceous erythematous rash

11. **Post-proctoscopic periorbital 'pinch' purpura**→Myeloma with 2° amyloidosis

12. **Acquired ichthyosis**→Hodgkin's Disease

13. **Hirsutism**→PCO (Polycystic Ovary Syndrome); adrenal or ovarian tumors (2° to androgen excess)

14. **Erythema gyratum repens**→Classically associated with breast ca

15. **Sweet's syndrome** (acute febrile neutrophilic dermatosis)→AML; Sweet's syndrome is characterized by painful plaque-forming inflammatory papules and associated with Fever, arthralgias, and peripheral ↑WBC. Note, the fever/arthralgias/splenomegaly/ ↑WBC is similar to Still's Disease

16. **Generalized pruritis**→May be indicative of lymphoma

17. **Tylosis (palmar/plantar keratoderma)**→Esophageal carcinoma;

18. **Pemphigus**→Thymoma ± myasthenia gravis

19. **Bullous pemphigoid**→Has not been associated with any underlying malignancy

20. **Ashleef spots**→Tuberous sclerosis (also associated with mental retardation, seizures, and renal angiomyolipomas)

DERMATOLOGY & SKIN_{NY} NOTES

✪ **CUTANEOUS SIGNS OF SYSTEMIC DISEASE...**

1. **Pyoderma Gangrenosum**→*IBD* (UC> Crohn's); *Rheumatoid Arthritis*

2. **Heliotrope rash** (periorbital discoloration)→*Dermatomyositis*

3. **Lupus Pernio** (erythematous swelling of the nose) and Erythema Nodosum→*sarcoidosis*

4. E. Nodosum + Fever + arthralgias + bilateral hilar LN→=**Lofgren's Syndrome**, with which acute *sarcoidosis* may present; usually a self-limited process of less than 6 month's duration

5. **Pseudoxanthoma elasticum** (yellow xanthomatous papules seen on the abdomen/groin/ neck/axilla→ ↑ risk of CVA, MI, PVD, MVP, angioid streaks in the retina

6. **Ehlers-Danlos syndrome** (skin hyperextensibility + joint hypermobility) →↑ risk of angina, PVD, MVP, GI bleed

7. Hereditary hemorrhagic telangiectasia **(Osler-Weber-Rendu)**=cutaneous and mucosal telangiectasias → associated with nosebleeds, GI bleeds, pulmonary AVMs, and CNS angiomas

8. **Acrodermatitis enteropathics** →*Zinc deficiency* ± alopecia, diarrhea

9. **Dermatitis herpetiformis** (immune-mediated bullous disease)→*Celiac disease*

10. **Apthous ulcers**→*Celiac disease; Crohn's disease; Behcet's disease; Reiter's Syndrome; HIV*

11. **Mucosal/Labial hyperpigmentation**→*Peutz-Jeghers syndrome* (no ↑ risk of developing ca)

12. **Erythema Chronicum Migrans**→*Lyme Disease*

13. **C.R.E.S.T. (variant of scleroderma)**=Calcinosis cutis; Raynaud's phenomenon; Esophageal dysmotility; Sclerodactyly; and Telangiectasias

14. **Livido Reticularis**; this is a mottled bluish (livid) discoloration of the skin that looks like a net. It is not a diagnosis per se, but more a reaction pattern to vasculitis syndromes, drugs, atheroemboli. Causes include *SLE, polyarteritis nodosa, and cholesterol embolization.* Treatment options include: alpha blockers, calcium channel blockers, and ACE inhibitors

15. **Morphea** (discrete sclerotic plaques with white shiny center)→*Scleroderma*

16. **Eosinophilic Fasciitis** (tightly bound thickening of skin and underlying tissues)→*Scleroderma*

17. Erythematous macular-papular eruption of trunk/palms/soles after BMT→**GVHD**

18. **Necrobiosis lipoidica diabeticorum** (yellow-brown atrophic telangiectatic plaques on the shins)→*Diabetes Mellitus*

19. **Pretibial Myxedema** (pink- and skin-colored papules, plaques, and nodules, usually occurring on the shins)→Graves' disease. Do not confuse this dermatologic myxedema with the myxedema associated with Hypothyroidism ("Myxedema coma")

20. **Toxic Epidermal Necrolysis and Stevens-Johnson Syndrome**→mucocutaneous usually *drug-induced* skin tenderness and erythema, followed by extensive exfoliation

21. **Janeway lesions**→ Infective endocarditis. *Nontender*, hemorrhagic, infarcted macules and papules on the fingers, palms, soles; they represent septic emboli. While **Osler's nodes** are also seen in infective endocarditis and have a similar distribution, they are, by contrast, *tender* and represent arteriolar intimal proliferation with extension into the capillaries.

22. **SSSS (Staphylococcal Scalded-Skin Syndrome)**-A Staph aureus *toxin-mediated* painful, tender, diffuse erythema that is followed by desquamation and occurring mainly in newborns and infants under 2 yo

23. **Toxic Shock Syndrome**—Similar to SSSS, it is a Staph aureus *toxin-mediated* illness that causes Fever, Hypotension, generalized skin and mucosal erythema, and multisystem failure occurring in menstrual and nonmenstrual patterns

24. **"Salmon-colored"** rash + arthralgias + ↑ WBC + Fever + Splenomegaly→*Still's Disease* → think *RASH*: **R**ash, **A**rthralgias, **S**plenomegaly, **H**igh white count and temp.

25. **Cushing's Syndrome**→ "buffalo hump" (fat pad), purple striae (usu. on the abdomen), hirsutism, steroid acne

✪ CUTANEOUS MANIFESTATIONS IN INFECTIOUS DISEASE

1. **Keratoderma Blenorrhagicum** (vesicular rash on the palms/soles that crusts)→*Reiter's Syndrome* (other signs include conjunctivitis, uveitis, urethritis, and arthritis); rash known differently as **Circinate Ballinitis** if affects the glans penis.

2. **Ampicillen (or Amoxicillin) + Infectious Mono (EBV or CMV)**→ Almost all patients develop a Morbilliform rash, defined as an exanthematous (viral-like) drug eruption, often mimicking rash of measles.

3. **Measles**→A maculopapular rash that *spreads from the head down and resolves in the same order* after approximately 3 days.

4. **Rocky Mt. Spotted Fever (RMSF)**→Erythematous and hemorrhagic macules and papules *begin peripherally* (wrists/forearms, ankles) *and spread centripetally* to arms, thighs, trunk, face. Fever, H/A, myalgia typically accompany.

5. **Ecthyma Gangrenosum**→ A cellulitis with necrosis related to septic vasculitis. It begins with cutaneous infarction and progresses to large, ulcerated gangrenous lesions. The causative organism is *Pseudomonas Aeruginosa*; the patient is usually immunocompromised/neutropenic and bacteremia is common.

6. **Impetigo**→*crusted golden-yellow erosions* which become confluent on the nose, cheeks, chin, and lips 2° to Staph Aureus and Group A Strep (Pyogenes).

7. **Erysipelas**→ Red, painful cellulitis 2° to Staph aureus, but more commonly group A Strep. The margins of the cellulitis are raised, and the borders are sharply demarcated.

8. **Erysipeloid**→A violaceous erythematous cellulitis to the hand 2° to Erysipelothrix rhusiopathiae after handling saltwater fish, shellfish, meat, hides, poultry. (DDx is V. Vulnificus)

9. **Desquamation + Strawberry tongue**→*Scarlet fever* 2° to Group A Strep; Kawasaki disease may also give a Strawberry tongue + a Desquamating rash.

10. **Purpura Fulminans**→The cutaneous manifestation of DIC or *acute meningococcemia*; the less fulminant cases of meningococcemia may manifest as a more discrete petechial rash.

11. **Cat Scratch Disease**→caused by *Bartonella henselae* (formerly Rochalimaea henselae) and is a *benign, self-limiting* infection characterized by a primary skin or conjunctival lesion, following cat scratches or contact with a cat, and subsequent tender regional lymphadenopathy. Unlike Bacillary angiomatosis, also caused by Bartonella, antibiotics have not proved effective in treatment.

12. **Rosacea**—A chronic acneform disorder of the facial pilosebaceous units. ↑ capillary sensitivity to heat results in flushing and ultimately telangiectasia. Long-standing disease with edema and hyperplasia of the skin overlying the nose, cheeks, and forehead leads to *Rhinophyma.*

13. **Pityriasis Versicolor**→A chronic, asymptomatic scaling rash caused by the *hyphal* form of Pityrosporum ovale, characterized by well-demarcated scaling patches with variable hyperpigmentation, usually occurring on the trunk. Diagnosis confirmed by a + KOH prep. *It's other name is Tinea Versicolor.* Treatment is antifungals, like ketoconazole or itraconazole or topical azole creams, selenium sulfide, or propylene glycol.

14. **Pityriasis Rosea**—Distinctive rash that *begins as a "herald patch", usually on the trunk,* followed 1-2 weeks later with a generalized exanthematous eruption that resolves spontaneously after 6 weeks without therapy. More common in the *spring and fall.* May be 2° to picornavirus.

15. **Sporotrichosis**—An ulceronodular dermatosis caused by Sporothrix schenckii, a fungus commonly found in *soil, and usually affecting gardeners,* farmers, florists, lawn workers. Chronic nodular lymphagitis and regional lymphadenitis are concomitant.

16. STD's (chancroid, chancre, etc)→see ID lecture. However, should remember that *among the genital ulcers,* Chancroid, HSV, and Behc et's→ *are PAINFUL;* Syphilis (Syphi<u>LESS</u>), LGV, and Granuloma Inguinale→ *are painLESS*

DERMATOLOGY AND AIDS

1. **Kaposi's sarcoma**—oval papules or purplish plaques on the trunk, extremities, face, mucosa;

2. **Herpes Zoster** (shingles)→VZV

3. **Oral hairy leukoplakia** ✪ →EBV and usually seen in advanced AIDS. (This is ***not*** the same as "oral leukoplakia", which is related to HPV, smoking, smokeless tobacco, alcohol, and syphilis. Candida can invade oral leukoplakia secondarily, and it is considered a premalignant lesion for squamous cell ca)

4. **Molluscum contagiosum** ✪→Discrete, solid, skin-colored papules that are only 1-2 mm in diameter, have central umbilication

5. **Bacillary angiomatosis** ✪ (vascular papules or nodules caused by Bartonella (Rochalimaea) henselae and quintana and transmitted by cats or ticks)→Erythromycins or Doxycycline for rx.

2 TONGUE DISORDERS THAT LOOK HIGHLY ABNORMAL, BUT REQUIRE SIMPLE REASSURANCE...

1. **FISSURED** tongue (aka scrotal tongue)
2. **GEOGRAPHIC** tongue (migratory glossitis)

SQUAMOUS CELL CA

1. **RISK FACTORS** ✪ include:
   a) Solar/*Actinic keratosis*
   b) Ionizing radiation-induced keratosis
   c) Arsenical keratosis
   d) *Bowen's disease* (a solitary lesion as a slowly enlarging erythematous plaque with a sharp border, slight scaling, and some crusting); related to exposure to solar irradiation or topical arsenic.
   e) *HPV* (subtypes 5, 8, 48—see chart below)

2. *Hyperkeratosis* is an important feature of SCC; may see ulceration with a necrotic base.

3. Any persistent nodule, plaque, or ulcer, *especially if to* sun-exposed areas or to the lips/at areas of radiodermatitis/in old burn scars/to the genitalia should be examined for SCC.

4. Carries a *much greater risk of metastasizing* than does basal cell ca

A SUMMARY OF COMMON HPV TYPES AND CLINICAL FINDINGS			
Mucosal		**Cutaneous**	
6,11	Genital warts	1	Plantar warts
34,40,42	Anogenital warts; Intraepithelial neoplasia	2	Common warts
72,73	Oral papillomas in immunosuppressed pts	3	Flat warts
16,18,31,33	Anogenital malignancies	5,8	Benign warts; *Squamous cell carcinoma*
		36	Actinic keratoses
		48	*Squamous cell ca*
		49	Warts, actinic keratoses

BASAL CELL CA ✪

1. The *most common* type of skin ca
2. Nodular or ulcerative types with *"pearly white", "rolled-up" borders*
   - Nodular type may ulcerate and bleed
   - Superficial type has erythematous, scaling plaques that slowly enlarge
3. Malignant in its locally aggressive growth properties, but with *limited capacity to metastasize*.
4. *Sun exposure* is important in the development of this ca; arsenic exposure may also predispose.

IMMUNOLOGIC MECHANISMS OF DRUG-INDUCED SKIN REACTIONS

1. **Type I** reaction (immediate hypersensitivity): **Urticaria** commonly caused by…
   a) PCN; Sulfonamides
   b) ASA
   c) Contrast media

2. **Type II** reaction (cytotoxic): e.g. **Thrombocytopenic purpura (ITP)**—commonly caused by:
   a) Methyldopa
   b) Gold

3. **Type III** reaction (vaculitis): e.g. **Drug-induced lupus**—commonly caused by…
   a) Hydralazine, procainamide
   b) Sulphonamides
   c) PCN

4. **Type IV** reaction (delayed, cell-mediated hypersensitivity): **CONTACT DERMATITIS**
   ☞ Test with *patch testing (not to be confused with Prick testing, which is used to investigate respiratory allery to pollens and molds)*;

☞ ## IMPORTANT COMMON CAUSES TO KNOW:

a) The most common sensitizer in North America is the plant **oleoresin** found in poison ivy, poison oak, and poison sumac; other important common causes to know:

b) **Nickle**→*jewelry (eg earrings)*

c) **Nail polish** (*a common cause of* <u>*contact blepharitis*</u>)

d) **Paraphenylenediamine**→hair dyes/*cosmetics*

e) **PABA**→*sunscreens* (immunologically related to (b) above)

f) **Potassium Dichromate**→*cement, leathers, certain paints*

g) **Formaldehyde**→*cosmetics*/shampoos

h) **Parabens**→*cosmetics*

i) **Neomycin,** bacitracin

j) **Thiuram**→wearing *shoes containing rubber*

✓ Allergic contact dermatitis is common in patients with <u>*chronic venous insufficiency*</u>, and difficult to diagnose without a high index of suspicion since it often *mimics* stasis dermatitis or cellulitis. *More than 30 percent* (!) of patients with chronic venous insufficiency develop contact dermatitis to neomycin and 13 percent to bacitracin

CONDITIONS PREDISPOSING TO AMPICILLIN RASH:

1. EBV
2. CMV
3. CLL
4. Concurrent allopurinol treatment

✪ ## HEREDITARY ANGIONEUROTIC EDEMA (HANE)

☞ 2° to **C1 INH DEFICIENCY** <u>(deficiency of the C1 inhibitor; therefore C1 is</u> <u>*disinhibited*, and thus the symptoms)</u>

☞ Recurrent episodes of *nonpainful, nonpruritic*, and nonerythematous angioedema

☞ **NO URTICARIA** in angioedema due to C1 INH deficiency (remember, angioedema is generally considered a subset of urticaria)

☞ A *family history* and a marked increase in attacks at adolescence is highly suggestive of the inherited form. It is important to realize, however, that <u>*20 to 40 percent* of</u> kindreds represent *new, i.e. sporadic, mutations* in the gene and therefore lack a family history should not surprise you.

☞ *Symptoms*:
   o Affects *mucocutaneous junctions: lips/eyes/penis*
   o *Glottal edema* may complicate, esp if angioedema occurs in the context of *anaphylaxis*
   o Facial, truncal, and extremity edema is primarily a cosmetic problem.

- o Swelling of the bowel wall can result in severe abdominal pain, nausea, and vomiting. Such symptoms can mimic acute abdominal syndromes but are not associated with fever, peritoneal signs, or an elevated white blood cell count and resolves spontaneously in 48 to 72 hours.
- o Precipitating factors are not well understood although *mild trauma is associated with a flare in about 50 percent* of patients.
- o The attacks usually *begin in adolescence* and continue throughout life.

☞ *Treatment* → For the patient with known or suspected angioedema secondary to an *inherited or acquired* deficiency of C1-INH, the **attenuated androgens**, stanozolol (2 to 4 mg/day) or danazol (200 to 400 mg/day) may be useful as both *acute and prophylactic therapy by increasing the plasma concentrations of C1-INH* (via enhanced hepatic synthesis) *and C4*

✪ ACQUIRED C1-INH DEFICIENCY

☞ Acquired C1-INH deficiency is caused either by *excessive utilization*, usually in the setting of *malignancy*, or by an *autoantibody* to C1-INH. Among 22 patients in one series, 14 had *low-grade lymphoproliferative disorders*.

☞ The symptoms and signs of an attack are indistinguishable from those arising in inherited forms of the disorder. However, the lack of a family history and late age of onset suggest acquired C1-INH deficiency.

CHECK TOO FOR THESE MEDS WHEN YOU SEE ANGIOEDEMA

- ✓ *ACE inhibitors*; angiotensin II receptor antagonists
- ✓ NSAIDs
- ✓ Opiates

MELANOMA

➢ Most important prognosticator is **TUMOR THICKNESS! (BRESLOW LEVEL)**

➢ **5 SIGNS OF MALIGNANT MELANOMA...**

Asymmetry

Border is irregular—edges irregularly scalloped

Color—mottled (haphazard display of colors); may include shades of brown, black grey, red, and white

Diameter—greater than 6.0mm (roughly the size of a pencil eraser)

Enlargement—the patient's history of an ↑ in the size of the lesion

---

✪ The following **MARGINS** are recommended for **PRIMARY MELANOMA** :

IN SITU: → 0.5 cm
INVASIVE UP TO 1 mm thick→1.0 cm
1-4 mm thick→2.0 cm
>4 mm thick→ ≥ 2 cm.

> ## RISK FACTORS

Greatly ↑ risk…
1. Changing "mole" (from patient's history)
2. Presence of one or more atypical nevi or "dysplastic nevi" along with a family history of melanoma (mutations in p16 have been identified in up to half of such patients)

Moderatly ↑ risk…
1. One family member with melanoma (parent, sibling, child)
2. Sporadic dysplastic nevi
3. Congenital melanocytic nevi (risk directly proportional to size)

Slightly ↑d risk…
1. White skin, but especially poorly tanning skin
2. Red hair
3. Freckling
4. History of severe sunburn(s) as child

> ## STAGES of Malignant Melanoma

Stage I → Cutaneous lesion; no lymph nodes yet
Stage II → Lymph nodes now involved
Stage III → Distant mets

> Tumor thickness ✪ , defined by the **BRESLOW LEVEL**, measured in millimeters, <u>is the single most powerful prognostic factor for survival in patients with primary melanoma</u> (stage I and II). Tumor thickness is a continuous variable; no natural breakpoints can be identified above or below which survival changes dramatically. The **CLARK LEVEL,** which characterizes the tumor based on the depth of the tumor in relation to the skin layer, measures the histologic level of invasion and also correlates with survival, though not as well.

> Re: ***Moh's surgery*** is both diagnostic and therapeutic and involves essentially shaving off the lesion tier by tier until the margins are clear per the pathologist. Melanoma is not the only indication for Moh's surgery, which can be used in tumors involving cosmetically or aesthetically sensitive zones.

> Remember ***sentinel lymph node mapping*** is used for melanoma and is increasingly being used for breast ca (to spare the patient unnecessarily extensive lymph node dissections).

✪ AUTOIMMUNE BULLOUS DISEASES

BULLOUS PEMPHIGOID	vs.	**PEMPHIGUS VULGARUS**
Relatively benign		Can be life-threatening
IgG at *basement membrane*		IgG at *intercellular substance*
Titre of circulating IgG *does not* correlate with dz activity		Titre of IgG correlates to disease activity
Tense bullae		*Flaccid* bullae
Subepidermal		Intraepidermal
Tx: *less* immunosuppressive than PV		Tx: *more* immunosuppressive than BP

> ✪ **DERMATITIS HERPETIFORMIS**—Another autoimmune bullous disease; it is associated with **CELIAC DISEASE** (aka gluten-sensitive enteropathy). While the *diagnostic significance of a gluten-free diet (in celiac disease)* is critical, remember ✓ **ANTI-ENDOMYSIAL, ANTI-RETICULIN, AND ANTI-GLIADIN antibodies** to confirm the diagnosis. Immunofluorescent staining is less important in this bullous disease.

DIFFERENTIAL DIAGNOSIS OF PALPABLE PURPURA
1. *Vasculitis…*
   a) Hypersensitivity Vasculitis (Henoch-Schonlein Purpura, or HSP, is a type of HV associated with Ig A)
   b) Septic Vasculitis (ricketssial spotted fevers)
   c) Cryoglobulinemia
   d) Wegener's, PAN, Kawasaki disease
2. *TTP*
3. *Acute Meningococcemia* (DIC with Purpura Fulminans)
4. *Disseminated gonococcemia*

DDX OF DISCRETE HYPOPIGMENTED AREAS:
1. *Vitiligo; causes…*
   a) Hypo and hyperthyroidism
   b) Addison's or Cushing's
   c) SLE
   d) Alopecia Areata
2. *Tinea Versicolor* (Pityriasis Versicolor)
3. Tuberculoid Leprosy
4. *"Ash-leaf " spots* of tuberous sclerosis
5. *Morphea* (localized patches of scleroderma)

✪ DIAGNOSTIC SIGNIFICANCE OF FINGERNAIL EXAMINATION :

1. **Clubbing** →TB; bronchiectasis; lung ca; COPD

2. **Pitting**→**P**soriasis; alopecia areata

3. **Subungal splinter hemorrhages**→Infective endocarditis

4. **Telangiectasia, nailfold infarts**→ Collagen-vascular diseases

5. **"Half-and-half" (Terry's) nails**→ CHF; ↓*Albumin associated with cirrhosis*

6. **Koilonychia (spoon nails)**→Chronic Fe deficiency

7. **Onycholysis** (separation of the nail plate from the bed)→Thyrotoxicosis (esp when it affects only the ring finger); otherwise it can be seen in onychomycosis, trauma, and psoriasis

AND (as they say on Broadway) →*"DON'T FORGET YOUR <u>LINES</u>! "*...

8. <u>**Muehrcke's LINES**</u>→*Hypoalbuminemia associated with nephrotic syndrome.*

9. <u>**Mee's LINES (white bands)**</u>→Arsenic poisoning

10. <u>**Beau's LINES**</u> (Transverse furrows or ridges of the nail plate that develop after dz or chemo and caused by temporary arrest of nail plate function

✪ <u>**HERE'S THE ERYTHEMAS**</u> **AND THEIR CLINICAL SIGNIFICANCE** ...

1. E. **Nodosum**→see associated conditions below

2. E. **Chronicum Migrans (ECM)**→<u>Lyme Disease</u>

3. E. **Marginatum**→transient truncal rash in <u>Rheumatic Fever</u>

4. E. **Multiforme**-<u>Stephen Johnson Syndrome</u> (e.g.Dilantin, Sulfa, PCN, HSV, Mycoplasma)

5. E. **Gyratum Repens** (looks like the grain pattern of wood)→<u>Internal malignancy (e.g. breast ca)</u>;

6. **Necrolytic Migratory Erythema (NME)**→<u>Glucagonoma</u>

✪ <u>**ERYTHEMA NODOSUM**</u> **---ASSOC'D CONDITIONS → "L.U.M.P.S." (or "<u>B</u>LUMP<u>Y</u>S")**

L ofgren's syndrome; **L**ymphoma

U lcerative Colitis (& Crohn's)

M TB; mycoses

P arasites, **P**regnancy, **P**ills (OCPs)

S ulphonamides, **S**trep pharyngitis, **S**arcoidosis

+ <u>**Behcet's**</u> (defined as recurrent painful oral ulcers plus any 2 of the following: Ocular lesions; Skin lesions; Genital ulcers; and Pathergy test); + <u>**Y**</u>**ersinia** enterocolytica.

✪ <u>SKIN_{NY} NOTES</u>

Acanthosis Nigricans
- A diffuse, velvety thickening and hyperpigmentation of the flexural skin, chiefly in axillae and other body folds.
- 5 types:
  - Hereditary benign AN: no associated endocrine disorder
  - Benign AN: may be assoc'd with insulin-resistant states (DM, acromegaly, Cushing's, Addison's and hypothyroidism)
  - Pseudo-AN: Cx of obesity (which is also assoc'd with insulin resistance)
  - Drug-induced AN: OCPs, nicotinic acid (high dose)
  - Malignant AN: adenoca (2/3 gastric)

Erythema Nodosum
- Large, painful, erythematous SQ nodules
- Vast DDx including these impt ones:
  - Sarcoidosis
  - TB
  - Strep infection
  - Crohn's; UC
  - Yersinia enterocolitis
  - Coccidiomycosis/Blasto/Histo
  - Drugs (e.g. sulfonamides, gold, indomethacin, tegretol)
  - Hodgkin's Disease
  - Behcet's syndrome
  - Idiopathic (25%)

Sarcoidosis
- **Lupus Pernio**: extensive infiltration of the nose and cheeks by granulomatous inflammation.
- A chronic granulomatous inflammation affecting diverse organs, but presenting primarily as skin lesions, eye lesions, bilateral hilar LN, and pulmonary infiltrates.
- All races, but much more frequent in blacks
- Re: can cause E. nodosum
- Presentation: Fever, fatigue, weight loss, arrhythmia, dyspnea, neuropathy, renal stones, uveitis, arthralgia
- When seen with E. nodosum and arthritis, is referred to as *Lofgren's* syndrome
- The *Heerfordt* syndrome represents patients with fever, parotid enlargement, uveitis, and facial nerve palsy.

Squamous Cell Carcinoma
- Usually develops from a precancerous lesion or a carcinoma in situ, often on the lips and other sun-exposed areas
- Commonly hyperkeratotic with elevated, rolled-up margin
- Leukoplakia, arsenic, Bowen's disease (trunk or face-->SCC); radiation-induced keratoses; old burn scars
- Capacity to metastasize (3-4% rate) w/ lesions arising in solar keratoses having lowest potential for mets.
- A slowly enlarging, hyperkeratotic papulonodule originating from the vermillion border of the lower lip is characteristic. Remember, SCC of the lip has a higher incidence of metastasis than with other cutaneous sites of involvement. Wedge resection is the treatment of choice.

Dysplastic Melanocytic Nevi

- Acquired, circumscribed, pigmented lesions representing disordered proliferations of atypical melanocytes
- They may arise de novo or as part of a compound melanocytic nevus
- Autosomal dominant
- Considered *potential precursors or superficial spreading melanoma and markers for persons at risk for developing primary malignant melanoma* of the skin.
- Primarily in lighter skin races
- Unlike common aquired nevi, new lesions continue to develop over many years and after middle age.

Cutaneous T-Cell Lymphoma (**Mycosis Fungoides**)

- Lymph nodes and internal organs can become involved
- This is a malignancy of helper T cells (CD4+)
- Male: Female 27:1
- Can mimic psoriasis in its scaly plaque appearance and in its *dis*appearance with sunlight exposure
- Thin (1-micron sections) and cytophotometry (for aneu/polyploidy) often helpful.
- Check CXR for hilar LN; CT for retroperitoneal LN in more advanced dz.
- Px: median=5y from time of histological diagnosis

Sezary Syndrome

- A special variant of CTCL characterized by generalized *erythroderma*, *generalized LN*, and cellular infiltrates of *atypical lymphocytes* (Sezary cells) in the skin and the blood.
- Generalized erythema, scaling and thickening of the skin (erythroderma)
- Buffy coat classically contains 15-30% atypical lymphocytes, but may be normal.
- Palms and soles: diffuse hyperkeratosis
- Alopecia

Hypersensitivity Vasculitis--Palpable Purpura

- Manifests as "palpable purpura" on the skin
- AKA "allergic cutaneous vasculitis", "necrotizing vasculitis"
- May also be systemic involving kidneys/muscles/joints/GI tract/and peripheral nerves
- Idiopathic in 50%
- Noteworthy DDx
  - HSP (HV associated with IgA)
  - Serum sickness
  - Drug-induced reactions (e.g PCN, sulfa)
  - HepBand C; group A Strep; Staph Aureus
  - Neoplasms
  - SLE, RA, Sjogren's syndrome, cryoglobulinemia

Cryoglobulinemia

> Remember, *cryoglobulins are antigen-antibody complexes that precipitate when cooled.*

A. **Type I** (MONOCLONAL); non-inflammatory

- Associated with a single, *monoclonal* antibody
- Symptoms, if any, are usually related to **hyperviscosity**
    - H/As
    - Epistaxis
    - Raynaud's phenomenon
    - Ischemic ulcers; skin necrosis
    - Visual complaints

B. **Types II & III** (mixed types); inflammatory

- POLYCLONAL or "mixed" cryoglobulinemias (usually IgG and anti-IgG)
- Commonly associated with **autoimmune disorders and chronic infections (must know Hepatitis C)**
- The typical presentation for essential mixed dz is glomerulonephritis, arthralgias, hepatosplenomegaly, and lymphadenopathy in addition to skin involvement (*palpable purpura*; **cold-induced urticaria**; **skin ulcers**)
- *Associated with leukocytoclastic vasculitis on histology and are inflammatory--these therefore give "palpable purpura"*
- Over the long run, nephritis/**progressive renal disease** is a common complication
- Labs for essential mixed cryoglobulinemia include: hypocomplementemia, ↑ LFTs, and cryoglobulin titer
- Plasmapheresis temporarily lowers the level of globulins, removes the immune complexes, and improves symptoms. However, long-term management should include, if possible, control of the underlying disease that produces the abnormal globulins or immune complexes.
- Associated Raynaud's phenomenon and arterial occlusion have resulted in extensive necroses, hemorrhage, and ulcerations.

> Dx: clinical suspicion confirmed with detection of cryoglobulins
> Tx: NSAIDs, cytotoxic agents, plasmapheresis

von Recklinghausen's Disease (Neurofibromatosis):Café au lait spots

- Autosomal dominant disease of the skin,bone, nervous and endocrine systems
- 2 major forms:
    - NF1 (classic type): more common; *Lisch nodules* (95% cases over 6yo): pigmented hamartomas of the iris; dx via slit-lamp exam; chromosome 17; rare *unilateral* acoustic neuromas.
    - NF2: "central" or "acoustic" type; chromosome 22; *bilateral* acoustic neuromas are only NF2!
  - ◆ *Both types have café-au-lait spots and neurofibromas.*

Peutz-Jeghers Disease:

- Autosomal dominant
- GI polyps, esp. jejunal
- Polyps are usually hamartomas (juvenile polyps) having a low potential for malignant degeneration.
- Mucocutaneous pigmentation
- Blue/black macules mouth, lips & buccal mucosa & hands
- Bleeding, obstruction, diarrhea, intussusception
- Anemia
- Malignant potential

Hereditary Hemorrhagic Telangiectasia

- AKA Osler-Weber-Rendu sydrome
- HHT is an autosomal dominant dz affecting blood vessels, esp in the mucous membranes of the mouth and GI tract.
- Recurrent epistaxis common
- Hemoptyisis from pulm AVMs
- GI bleeds secondary to AVMs
- Tx: destruction of telangiectatic vessels using electrosurgery or laser surgery with pulse dye laser

Dermatomyositis

- DM is a systemic disease characterized by violaceous (heliotrope) inflammatory changes of the eyelids and periorbital area; erythema of the face, neck, and upper trunk; and flat-topped violaceous papules over the knuckles (Gottron's papules)
- Progressive proximal muscle weakness (e.g. difficulty rising from a chair without use of the arms)
- Photosensitivity
- Elevated CK or aldolase during acute phase
- It bears an association with polymyositis, interstitial pneumonitis, myocardial involvement and vasculitis
- Associated malignancies include: Breast, ovary, uterus, lung, colon, stomach
- Tx: steroids +/- azathioprine
- In adults, the risk of ca is 5-7x increased.
- In addition to the heliotrope rash and Gottron's papules and the photosensitivity, can also see:
    - ◆ Poikiloderma
    - ◆ Cuticular hypertrophy with punctate infarcts
    - ◆ Periungal telangiectasias
    - ◆ Calcinosis

Primary Systemic Amyloidosis

- So-called "pinch purpura" of the upper eyelid can appear as hemorrhagic papules after pinching or rubbing the eyelid.
- Equally uncanny, can also see post-proctoscopic periorbital purpura
- Waxy papuless, usually eyelids or perialar area
- Macroglossia
- Sclerodermalike
- Patchy alopecia
- Bullous eruptions
- Biopsy of normal skin, rectum, gingiva, SQ abdominal fat pad
- Other commonly clinical presentations: cardiac, renal, hepatic, GI, carpal tunnel
- Re: Type AL is primary; AA is secondary. Usually no derm findings in secondary type. Multiple myeloma increased with AL type.

Ichthyosis Vulgaris

- In adults, rhomboidal scales due to a generalized hyperkeratosis with xerosis, most pronounced on the lower extremities
- **Clinical Associations**:
  - *Hodgkin's* Disease; NHL
  - Atopy
    - Atopic dermatitis
    - Allergic rhinitis
    - Intrinsic asthma
  - Myeloma, Kaposi's sarcoma, lung/breast/cervical carcinomas
  - Sarcoid, hypothyroid, leprosy
  - Nicotinic acid
  - Essential fatty acid deficiency
  - AIDS

Sweet's Syndrome

- Aka "Acute febrile neutrophilic dermatosis"
- *Tender*, red plaques to face, upper trunk, extremities
- Association with AML and febrile URIs
- Fever
- Neutrophilia
- Dense dermal infiltrate of neutrophils
- Arthralgia
- Prompt response to steroids

Pemphigus Vulgaris

- Superficial blisters on non-inflamed skin
- Rupture leads to large erosions
- Age 50-70; increased in Jewish descent
- 60% initially present with oral lesions
- Oral lesions in 80-90% of all patients
- 6 mo interval b/w onset of oral lesions and dissemination to skin
- Pain, weakness, weight loss, dysphagia
- Nikolsky Sign: application of pressure to blister causes extension of bullae
- Associated with myasthenia, thymoma
- Penicillamine can induce it 6wks to 6 mo after d/c the drug
- Increased incidence of lymphoreticular malignancy.
- Autoantibodies to intercellular substance
- Intraepidermal blister
- Tx: steroids

Bullous Pemphigoid

- In contrast to the bullae of PV, which arise within the epidermis, and are fragile and flaccid, the bullae of BP are tense and intact
- Also in contrast to PV, this disorder is chronic only; PV can be acute or chronic.
- Also PV is usu 40-60yo; BP is 60-80
- Intertriginous areas common
- Arise from erythematous macules, urticaria
- Oral lesions in 1/3
- Circulating anti-basement membrane IgG antibodies detected in 70% of pts
- Titres do not correlate with disease activity.
- Peripheral eosinophilia may be seen
- No relationship to malignancy

Dermatitis Herpetiformis

- Chronic, recurrent, **intensely pruritic** vesicles, papules, or urticarial wheals
- Symmetric **extensor surfaces**, elbows, knees, scapula, buttocks
- Nearly always associated with *celiac sprue (gluten enteropathy); rare:* iodide ingestion; 30% have thyroid dz as well.
- Most common age 20-30
- *Circulating autoantibodies*-gotta know!
  - ◆ Anti-gliadin Ab
  - ◆ Anti-reticulin Ab
  - ◆ Anti-endomysial Ab
- Subepidermal *bullae*
- *Granular IgA* immunofluorescence pattern of infiltration in the skin
- *Increased incidence of lymphoma*, esp of the GI tract.
- Tx: Dapsone, sulfapyridine, or gluten-free diet

Pseudoxanthoma Elasticum

- Multiple, confluent, chamois-colored or yellow papules (pseudoxanthomas) creating a large, circumferential, pebbled plaque on the neck. Changes in the connective tissue lead to excessive folds on the lateral neck.
- Flexural areas, "plucked-chicken" skin
- Connective tissue disorder tha involves the elastic tissue in the skin, blood vessels (GI hemorrhage, HTN, claudication), and eyes (angioid streaks and blindness)
- Stomach and proximal small intestine
- Vascular calcification upper and lower extremities
- *Angioid streaks* in retina
- Ischemic cardiac and PVD
- MVP
- Angioid streaks, which are wider than blood vessels and extend across the fundus, represent rupture of Bruch's membrane secondary to elastic fiber defect

Ehlers-Danlos Syndrome

- Due to deficient synthesis of type III collagen
- Hyperextensible and fragile skin and hypermobility of the joints frequently to the point of dislocation
- MVP
- Eyes: myopia, presbyopia, blue sclera
- Severe bruising
- Thin skin
- Rupture of bowel, rupture of large arteries
- Gyn: miscarriage; PROM

Zinc Deficiency

- AE (Acrodermatitis Enteropathica) is a genetic disorder of Zn absorption
- Triad of acral dermatitis (face, hands, feet, anogenital area), alopecia, and diarrhea
- Nearly identical clinically with acquired Zn deficiency due either to dietary def. or other absorptive disorder
- Can present with psoriasiform dermatitis, anemia, and poor wound healing, and diffuse alopecia

Apthous Ulcers

- AKA "Apthous stomatitis" or "canker sores"
- "Apthous" from the Greek "ulcer"
- Most common in oropharynx (buccal and labial mucosa) and less common in esophagus, UGI and LGI tracts, and anogenital mucosa
- Multiple associated disorders, including
  - Behcet's disease
  - Cyclic neutropenia
  - HIV

Erythema Chronicum Migrans

- Primary Lyme disease
- Transmitted via bite of deer tick that is   infected with the spirochete borrelia burgdorferi
- Rapidly expanding ring
- Average duration 3 weeks
- Initial macule or papule enlarges within days of the bite to form an expanding annular lesion with a distinct red border and partially clearing middle. At times concentric rings form and a "Bull's eye" pattern is seen.
- Only 14% of pts report a hx of bite
- Removal of the tick within 18h may preclude infection.
- Prodrome: malaise, fatigue, lethargy, H/A, stiff neck, arthralgia, myalgia, anorexia,

Scleroderma

- Telangiectasias in a patient with **CREST** syndrome (**C**alcinosis cutis; **R**aynaud's phenomenon; **E**sophageal dysmotility; **S**clerosis; **T**elangiectasias)
- Aka Progressive Systemic Sclerosis or Systemic Sclerosis
- Limited or Diffuse

- *Limited* (60%):
  - Usually female
  - Long h/o Raynaud's phenomenon usually
  - Acrosclerosis
  - CREST syndrome and morphea fall here
  - systemic involvement may not appear for years
  - high incidence of anticentromere Ab

- *Diffuse*:
  - Relatively rapid onset; indeed diffuse
  - Anticentromere Ab uncommon, but Scl-70 in 30%
  - Internal organ involvement may be seen (heart, lungs, GI tract)

Livedo Reticularis

- A mottled bluish (livid) discoloration of the skin in a netlike (reticularis) pattern
- Appears/worsens with cold exposure
- It is not a dx per se, but a sign of other disease, including causes of:
  - Intravascular obstruction
    - *Atheroemboli*
    - *Cryoglobulinemia*
  - Vessel wall disease
    - Vasculitides (PAN, RA, SLE, ACLS, DM, DM,etc)
  - Drugs
- Sneddon's Syndrome: Extensive LR + HTN + CVAs or TIAs

Graft Versus Host Disease (GVHD)

- GVHD is an immune disorder caused by immunocompetent donor cells reacting vs. the tissues of an immunocompetent host
- Primarily in Allogeneic BMT (seen in 60-80% of successful engraftments)
- *Acute*:   Usually seen b/w 14-21 days post BMT
- *Chronic*:   >100 days post transplant; may arise from acute or *de novo*
- *Acute* manifestations: fever, jaundice, serositis, pulmonary insufficiency, TEN, diarrhea, liver dysfunction
- *Chronic*: May see: lichenoid eruptions and sclerodermatous changes; wasting; chronic liver disease; skin/joint contractures; permanent hair loss; xerostomia, xeropthalmia-->corneal ulcers-->blindness; malabsorption.
- Tx: steroids; cyclosporine; PUVA

Necrobiosis Lipoidica, Diabeticorum

- The lesion is a large plaque with an active yellow-orange to tan-pink, well-demarcated, raised, firm border. The central part of the lesion has resolved with atrophic changes of epidermal thinning and telangiectasias against yellow backrouind.
- 1/3 of NL patients have DM; 1/3 have abnormal glucose tolerance only; 1/3 have normal glucose tolerance
- A history of preceding trauma to the site can be a factor in the initial development; for this reason, NL is often present on the shins (>80%) and over the bony areas of the feet.
- The majority of individual have long-standing Type I DM
- The lesions are so distinctive that confirmation with biopsy is rarely necessary.
- Topical or intralesional steroids; if ulcerative, local wound care/excision as per usual.

Myxedema

- Myxedema results from insufficient production of thyroid hormones and can be caused by multiple disturbances, characterized by accumulation of water binding mucopolysaccharides in the dermis, resulting in thickening of facial features, doughy induration, and pale, waxy skin.
- This is not the same as the pretibial myxedema of thyrotoxicosis.
- Clinical findings confirmed by TSH levels (elevated)
- Untreated, long-standing hypothyroidism can progress to a hypothermic, stuporous state, ie myxedema coma, which may be fatal.
- Boggy, non-pitting edema
- Patchy alopecia; dry, coarse, brittle hair; loss of outer 1/3 eyebrows.

Infective Endocarditis:

Janeway Lesions
- *Nontender*, infarcted, erythematous or hemorrhagic papules of the palms or soles
- More common in ABE but occur in SBE

Osler's Nodes
- Violaceous, *tender* nodules on the volar fingers associated with minute infective emboli (ABE) or immune complex deposition (SBE)

Toxic Shock Syndrome: Desquamation

- An acute toxin-mediated illness caused by toxin-producing Staph aureus, characterized by rapid onset of *fever*, *hypotension*, generalized skin and mucosal *erythema then desquamation (1-2 weeks later; primarily palms, soles, fingers, toes)*, mental status changes, and *multisystem failure*, occurring in menstrual (re: tampons) and non-menstrual forms
- Characteristically, degree of mental status changes is out of proportion to the degree of hypotension.
- Implicated toxins: TSST-1 (most common), enterotoxin B
- In the U.S., almost all of the cases are among whites
- Affects mostly the young since 90% of individuals have antibodies to toxins in adulthood
- Common settings for TSS: menstruation, use of barrier contraceptives, puerpurium, septic abortion, nonOB/Gyn surg, thermal burns, insect bites, varicella lesions, surgical wounds
- Besides aggressive fluid resuscitation, pressors, etc…
- Antibiotics…
  - ✓ For Staph aureus → IV Nafcillin or oxacillin
  - ✓ For Streptococcus → Pen G IV + Clinda IV
- Pts in septic shock, ventilated with an undrainable focus of infection should be treated with IV IgG which contains high levels of antibody o TSS toxins

Stevens-Johnson Syndrome

- SJS and TEN are mucocutaneous drug-induced or idiopathic reaction patterns characterized by skin tenderness and erythema of skin and mucosa, followed by extensive cutaneous and mucosal exfoliation, and are potentially life-threatening due to multisystem involvement.
- SJS is considered a maximal variant of erythema multiforme; TEN is considered a maximal variant of SJS
- TEN: 80% have strong assn w/ drugs
- SJS: 50% are drug-associated; etiology often not clear-cut
- Most *frequent drug culprits*: sulfa, allopurinol, carbamazepine, aminoPCNs, phenylbutazone, piroxicam
- SJS: <10% epidermal detachment
- TEN: >30% epidermal detachment
- ***90% of patients have mucosal lesions***
- 85% have conjunctival lesions
- Both have fever & severe pain
- Mortality: 30% in TEN; 5% in SJS
- Tx as for pt with 3rd degree burns

Cushing's Syndrome

- 'Moon face', plethora
- Steroid acne (monomorphous with few or no comedones)
- 'Buffalo hump'; truncal obesity
- Striae, bruises
- Acanthosis nigricans
- Increased incidence of tinea versicolor
- HTN
- Carbohydrate intolerance
- Amenorrhea and hirsutism
- Steroid-related psychiatric d/o's
- Remember, Cushing's "disease" refers to a pituitary ACTH-producing adenoma
- Re: may be associated with oat cell from paraneoplastic ACTH.

Necrotizing Fasciitis

- Fulminant necrotic infection of the superficial and deep fascia
- The infection causes thrombosis of subcutaneous blood vessels and ultimately gangrene of underlying tissues
- Surgical dibridement and antibiotics are appropriate management

Measles

- Aka *Rubeola*
- Highly contagious usually childhood viral infection characterized by fever, malaise, coryza, photophobia, cough, conjunctivitis, pathognomonic *Koplik's spots* (cluster of tiny bluish-white papules appearing on or after 2nd day of febrile illness on buccal mucosa opposite premolar teeth)
- *Face, neck-->trunk, extrems in 2-3 days*; Rubella: face-->trunk in 1day
- Following immunization in 1963, incidence has decreased by 98%
- Spread by respiratory droplet aerosols (sneezing, coughing)
- Contagious from several days pre-rash to up to 5d post-rash
- *Hacking, barklike cough*

Rocky Mountain Spotted Fever

- Rash on 4th day of fever (range 2-6 days); sudden onset F/C, severe H/A
- Wrists, ankles, arms--> trunk ("centripetally", unlike measles), palms, soles
- Mac/pap to petechiae to purpura
- Tick bite, mid-to-late summer
- R. Rickettsii
- Rare in Rocky Mountain states!
- Most common in S. Atlantic states
- **W**ood tick=Dermacentor andersoni in the **W**estern US
- Dog tick--D. variabilis in East
- Only 60% give a h/o a tick bite
- Diffuse vasculitis, hyponatremia, thrombocytopenia
- Extensive cutaneous necrosis due to DIC occurs in 4%; these may become gangrenous
- Dx: Comp. fix. titre; Weil-Felix DFA of skin bx (false + in 30%) thus dx must be made clinically and confirmed later
- Tx: Doxy/TCN; chloramphenicol
- Only 3% of cases with RMSF present with the triad of rash, fever, and a h/o a tick bite
- On the 1st day of illness, only 14% of patients have the rash; during 1st 3d only 49% have the rash; 20% take 6 or more days to see the rash; 13% have no rash (true "spotless RMSF")

Exanthematous Drug Eruption: Ampicillen Rash

- Aka *morbilliform* drug reaction or maculopapular drug eruption
- Almost always on trunk, extremities
- May progress to exfoliative dermatitis , esp if drug is not discontinued
- Most common cultprits: PCNs, carbamazepine, allopurinol, sulfonamids, NSAIDs, INH, Erythromycin
- Nearly all patients with EBV or CMV *mono*, given Ampicillen or Amox, will develop this rash
- Over half of HIV-infected pts who receive sulfa drugs (e.g. Bactrim) develop eruption

Ecthyma Gangrenosum

- Pseudomonas aeruginosa
- Cutaneous infection → infarction → bulla → large ulcerated gangrenous lesion
- Considered a necrotizing cellulitis
- Usually solitary; may be multiple
- Therefore not surprising that it's often followed by P. aeruginosa bacteremia
- Most commonly seen in the setting of profoud prolonged neutropenia

Impetigo

- Staph aureus and Strep pyogenes (Group A Strep)
- These infections cause impetigo when epidermis is involved; ecthyma when extends into dermis
- Characterized by crusted erosions or ulcers
- Bullous subtype (bullous impetigo) is caused (80%) by phage 2 staph, which produce exotoxins, as discussed in SSSS
- Dx: Gram stain; culture; anti-DNAase serology detects prior group A strep
- Between 20-40% of normal adults are persistent carriers of Staph aureus
- Group A step usually colonizes the skin first and subsequently the nasopharynx.

Erysipelas

- Usually caused by group A strep
- Most common cause of virulent soft tissue infx in a healthy host, often w/o any obvious portal of entry
- A superficial type of cellulitis involving lymphatics
- Margin or lesion is raised, *sharply demarcated* from adjacent normal tissue; often painful
- Sites of predilection: face; lower legs; areas of preexisting lymphedema

Erysipeloid

- An acute but slowly evolving cellulitis occurring at sites of inoculation, most commonly the hands, and is often occupational, associated with handling fish, shellfish, meat, poultry, hides, and bones (essentially those who handle dead animal matter in their work).
- Aka 'Crab' dermatitis
- Erysipelothrix rhusiopathiae, a gram-positive rod is the cause
- Non-contagious
- "Erysipeloid" or "erysipelas-like" due to the painful, swollen lesion with sharply defined irregular raised border
- Enlarges peripherally with central fading
- Tx: PCN or Erythromcyin

Sporotrichosis

- A mycosis, sporothrix schenckii
- Characterized by ulceronodular formation at the inoculation site, chronic nodular lymphangitis (usually manifested as a streak up the arm), and regional lymphadenitis.
- Occupational exposure important: gardeners, farmers, florists, lawn laborers, agricultural workers, forestry workers, lab workers
- SQ inoculation by a contaminated thorn, barb, splinter, or other sharp object (lab)
- Disseminated infection can occur in an immunocompromised host.
- Tx: systemic antifungal therapy

Scarlet Fever

- **Pastia's lines:** Erythema may be accentuated in skin folds such as neck, axillae, groin, antecubital and popliteal fossae
- Group A strep infection to the tonsils, skin, or other sites
- Household members may be a streptococcal carrier
- Strawberry tongue; beefy red pharynx
- Rash appears within 1-3 days of infection
- Erythema first noted on trunk. Spreads to extremities. Palms, soles usually spared.
- Exanthem fades within 4-5 days and is followed by brawny desquamation on the body and extemities and by sheetlike exfoliation on the palms and soles
- Dx: Serologic tests detect immune responses to extracellular products (streptolysin O, hyaluronidase, DNaseB, NADase, and streptokinase) and cellular components (M protein, group A antigen)

Cat Scratch Disease

- A benign, self-limiting zoonotic infection that follows cat scratches or contact with a cat, and subsequent acute to subacute tender regional LN
- Bartonella henselae (formerly Rochmalimaea henselae)
- HIV-infected patients may develop bacillary angiomatosis.
- Nodes are usually solitary, moderately tender, and freely mobile. They are suppurative.
- WBC usually normal; ESR usually elevated.
- Dx: Warthin-Starry-stained sections of skin lesion , conjunctiva, or LN shows small, pleomorphic bacilli; Antibodies to B. henselae usually pos (>= 1:64); PCR 96% sensitive from aspirations of infected LNs.
- Self-limiting, so Abx usually unnecessary
- Occasionally, surgical drainage for LNs.

Rosacea

- A chronic acneiform disorder of the *facial* pilosebaceous units coupled with an *increased reactivity of capillaries to heat, leading to flushing and ultimately to telangiectasias*.
- Previously called acne rosacea but is unrelated to acne (though frequently coexists)
- Unlike acne vulgaris, *no comedones*!
- Peak incidence between 40-50 yo
- F>M (except for rhinophyma)
- Celtic peoples and southern Italians
  - **Stage I**: Papules, telangiectasias
  - **Stage II**: Pustules present
  - **Stage III**: Nodules present
- Tx: topical metronidazole or topical Abx; if these fail or for more severe dz, PO TCN or minocycline; if still those fail, then PO isotretinoin is an option

Rhynophyma

- Long-standing disease with edema and marked sebaceous hyperplasia of the tissues of the nose
- Successfully treated with surgery or laser surgery.

Pityriasis Versicolor (Tinea Versicolor)

- A chronic, asymptomatic scaling dermatosis associated with the overgrowth of the hyphal form of Pityrosporum ovale, characterized by well-demarcated scaling macules with variable pigmentation, occurring most commonly on the trunk.
- Gently abrasion of the surface accentuates the scaling; check KOH
- Classically, young adults;usu asymp
- High levels of cortisol increase susceptibility (e.g. Cushing's or exogenous steroids)
- Humidity predisposes (increased incidence in summer time)
- Tx: antifungals e.g. selenium sulfide or topical/systemic azoles (keto/itra)

Pityriasis Rosea

- A single "herald" patch first appears (80% of patients), typically on the trunk, followed 1-2 weeks later by a generalized secondary eruption most often to the trunk and proximal extremities
- The herald patch is typically an oval, slighlty raised plaque 2-5 cm, bright red, with a fine scale at the periphery; may be multiple.
- Ages 10-35 yo most common; etiology unclear
- More common in spring and fall in temperate climates
- Spontaneously remitting usually by 6 weeks
- Herald patch commonly misdiagnosed as ringworm

Oral Leukoplakia

- A sharply defined, white, macular or slightly raised area in the mouth that *cannot be rubbed off and persists* after the irritation (e.g. smoking) has been stopped for several weeks.
- Candida may secondarily invade.
- A *premalignant* lesion since is caused by exposure to the same agents that cause squamous cell ca: smoking, alcohol, chronic irritation/inlfammation, HPV-11 and HPV-16.
- About 10% of lesions can progress to malignancy. Leukoplakia on the *floor* of the mouth is serious , with over 60% showing either carcinoma in situ or invasive SCC *whereas buccal* involvement is almost always benign.
- Careful f/u is important with biopsies to r/o dyplasia or frank carcinoma.

Behcet's Syndrome

- Most recent diagnostic criteria include one basic major feature--*recurrent oral apthous ulcers--and 2 of the following features:* recurrent genital apthous ulcers; eye lesions (posterior uveitis); skin lesions (E. nodosum-like lesions, or cutaneous pustular vasculitis)
- Can see colorectal ulcerations
- Spontaneous thrombophlebitis
- *Positive pathergy test*: physician-placed oblique insertion of a 20-gauge needle under sterile conditions produces an inflammatory pustule at 24-48 h).
- HLA B5; otherwise etiology unknown
- Seronegative arthritis
- Erythema nodosum-like lesions (painful erythematous nodules on the arms and legs in 40%)
- Tx: *Apthous ulcers*: potent topical or intralesional steroids; thalidomide; colchicine; dapsone
    Systemic cx's: Prednisone with or without other immunosupps.

Kaposi's Sarcoma

- A multisystem vascular neoplasia characterized by mucocutaneous violaceous lesions and edema as well as involvement of nearly any organ.
- AIDS and immunosuppressed; also classic KS: elderly males of eastern European heritage (Mediterranean and Ashkenazi Jewish)--secondary malignancies occur in >35% of these; also African-Endemic KS that is not HIV-associated
- All types, M>>F
- Linked to HHV-8 or human herpesvirus type 8
- Types: macules; papules; plaques; nodules
- Almost all KS lesions are palpable, even macules.
- CDC case definition is that in a patient <60 yo, KS is an AIDS-defining condition if the patient has no other cause of immunodeficiency and is without knowledge of HIV Ab status.
- At autopsy of HIV-infected individuals with mucocutaneous KS, 75% have visceral involvement (bowel, liver, spleen, lungs)
- In HIV-associated KS, see LN involvement in half the cases
- GI involvement in KS rarely causes symptoms
- At time of dx, 40% of KS cases have GI involvement; 80% at autopsy.
- Pulmonary KS can cause bronchospasm, intractable cough, progressive respiratory failure, SOB.
- Pulmonary KS has a high mortality (median survival < 6 months) KS of the bowel/lungs is the cause of death in 10%-20% of AIDS patients
- The goal of treatment of KS is to control symptoms of the disease, not cure.
- Classic type usually responds well to radiotherapy.
- Immunosupressive drug-associated KS improves when drug dosages are reduced or d/c'd.
- HIV-associated KS usually responds to a variety of local therapies (radiotherapy; cryo; laser surgery; electrosurgery; excisional surgery); however, chemotherapy (intralesional; single agent; and combination) is indicated for extensive mucocutaneous involvement or visceral involvement.

Bacillary Angiomatosis

- A systemic infection caused by Bartonella species, occurring almost exclusively in HIV, characterized by cutaneous vascular tumors resembling Kaposi's sarcoma and symptomatic multisystemic infection, usually involving the liver (peliosis hepatis) and/or spleen (parenchymal bacillary peliosis)
- B. henselae and B. quintana.
- In immunocompetent individuals, B. henselae is also the agent of cat-scratch disease.
- Contact (bites, scratches) with cats bearing usually B. henselae
- Cutaneous lesions may be painful (as opposed to Kaposi's sarcoma, a dx for which it is frequently mistaken)
- Also in contrast to KS, the clinical picture can progress rapidly, e.g. in peliosis hepatis (where you can see N/V, F/C, and often marked elevations in LFTs) or Bartonella Bacteremic Syndrome with bacteremia, malaise, anorexia, weight loss, and progressively higher fevers.
- Dx options: culture of skin biopsy or blood; tissue silver stain; tissue PCR; increased GGTP seen in peliosis hepatis; anti-Bartonella Abs via IFA or ELISA
- HIV pts should avoid cats (esp kittens) to minimize risk of BA or toxoplasmosis
- Tx: 8-12 weeks of Abx: Ery, Azithromycin,Doxy, Cipro; often requires lifelong secondary prophylaxis in HIV due to relapses.

Molluscum Contagiosum

- Discrete, solid, skin-colored papules with central **umbilication**
- A pox virus
- Occur in children and sexually-active adults; **HIV**
- **Self-limited, HIV being the notable exception.**
- Mostly on face and upper body in children and HIV. Seen on the genitals in sexually active adults.
- R/O cryptococcus and histoplasmosis
- Transmission via skin-to-skin contact; spread by shaving in HIV
- Tx: curettage; cryosurgery; electrodessication.

Lichen Planus

- An inflammatory dermatosis involving skin and/or mucus membranes, characterized by flat-topped (Latin: planus, "flat"), violaceous, shiny, pruritic papules on the skin and milky-white papules in the mouth.
- Etiology is unknown
- Onset may be acute of insidious over weeks
- Distribution: wrists (flexor), lumbar region, eyelids, shins, (thicker, hyperkeratotic), scalp, glans penis
- 40-60% of patients have oropharyngeal involvement
- Types include: reticular; plaque; atrophic; erosive or ulcerative; bullous.
- Tx: *Local*: steroids (topical and intralesional); *Systemic*: steroids; systemic retinoids; cyclosporine; PUVA

Urticaria

- Urticaria and angioedema are composed of transient wheals (edematous papules and plaques, usually pruritic) and larger edematous areas that involve the dermis and SQ tissue (angioedema).
- Urticaria and angioedema can be classified as IgE-mediated, complement-mediated, related to physical stimuli (cold, sunlight, pressure→eg dermatographism) or idiopathic.
- HANE: hereditary angioneurotic edema *remember*: 1) no urticaria; 2) pillow-fights; 3) C1 inhibitor deficiency (85%) or dysfunction (15%) and low C4 despite nl C1,C3; 4) angioedema to face, extremities, larynx, bowel wall (painful)

Urticarial Vasculitis

- A multisystem disease with cutaneous lesions resembling urticaria, except that they **persist > 24 h, generally up to 3-4 days.**
- Leukocytoclastic vasculitis with fever, arthralgias, increased ESR
- May be seen in serum sickness; collagen vascular diseases; HepB; idiopathic
- Lesions may be associated with itching, burning; stinging sensation; pain; tenderness
- Other systems which may see involvement (in decreasing order: joints; GI; CNS; ocular; renal; LN
- Hypocomplementemia in 70%
- Dx: clinical suspicion confirmed by biopsy
- Etiology is thought to be immune complex disease, similar to cutaneous vasculitis
- Course: Chronic but benign

Paget's Disease of the Nipple

- A malignant neoplasm tha unilaterally involves the nipple or areola and simulates a chronic eczematous dermatitis (usually bilateral when involves nipples)
- It is associated with underlying intraductal ca of the breast
- 1-4% of all breast ca
- Sx: may be none; pruritis, pain, burning, discharge,bleeding, ulceration, invagination
- Typically a sharply demarcated, scaling plaque, and slightly indurated (eczema is not indurated)
- Mgmt: as per breast carcinoma

Tuberous Sclerosis

- Autosomal dominant disease resulting in hyperplasia of ectodermal and mesodermal cells and a disturbance in embryonic cellular differentiation.
- The principal early signs are the triad of seizures, mental retardation, and congenital hypopigmented macules of many sizes and shapes, one of which is the ash-leaf, usually 3-4cm
- Facial angiofibromata are pathognomonic but do not appear until year 3 or 4.
- Px: In severe cases, 30% die before age 5, and 50-70% by adult age
- Malignant gliomas are not uncommon.
- Other systems commonly involved: CNS, eye, heart, kidney.

Fissured Tongue

- Common, benign, asymptomatic
- Deep, corrugated-appearing, linear fissures or "valleys"
- Aka scrotal tongue
- Estimated to be 5% of the general pop
- The linear valleys do not involve the mucosal epithelium and are therefore not painful
- Persists and becomes more exaggerated through life
- Appropriate management is simple reassurance

Geographic Tongue

- As with fissured tongue, this morphology is benign and "management" is simple reassurance.
- Aka migratory glossitis; etiology is unknown
- Often mistaken for candidiasis.
- Areas of hyperkeratosis alternate with areas of normal pink epithelium, greating a geographic pattern.
- It is the most common of the psoriasiform lesions; seen in 2% of the general population.
- About 40% of these patients also have a fissured tongue

Nailfold Telangiectasias (nailfold infarcts)

- Capillary loops of the proximal nail fold become tortuous and dilated, presumably as a result of injury from repeated bouts of microangiitis and immune-complex deposition. Nail fold telangiectasias occur with varying degrees of severity. It is a characteristic feature of dermatomyositis but is also seen in SLE and occasionally in progressive systemic sclerosis.
- Some believe that a dx of connective tissue disease can be made by this finding alone.

Clubbing

- Clubbed fingers are the result of hyperplasia of the fibrovascular tissue between the nail matrix and the bony phalanx.
- The pathogenesis is unknown, but thought to be related to increased blood flow to these tissues.
- *Associated conditions include*:
  - Cardiac disease
    - Cyanotic heart disease
    - Endocarditis
  - Pulmonary disease
    - *Bronchiectasis*
    - *Tuberculosis*
    - Primary and metastatic *carcinoma;* mesothelioma
    - *Lung Abscess*
  - GI disease
    - IBD
    - Hepatic cirrhosis

Subungal Splinter Hemorrhages

- These brown or red streaks that represent splinter hemorrhages most often result from **trauma** to the nail and arise distally in the nail bed. Thye may, however, be a sign of **endocarditis** and arise in the midportion of the nail bed.

Terry's Nails ('Half & Half' Nails)

- The proximal 2/3rds of the nail plate is white, whereas the distal 1/3 shows the red color of the nail bed.
- May be a manifestation of CHF or hypoalbuminemia associated with hepatic cirrhosis.
- Found in 10% of patients with uremia of CRF. The color change does not correlate with the severity of the renal disease.

Koilonychia

- AKA "spoon nails"
- Caused by softening and thinning of the nail plate that results in concave or spoon-shaped nails.
- Seen in patients with long-standing iron-deficiency anemia or Plummer-Vinson syndrome (a combination of koilonychia, dysphagia from esophageal web, and glossitis affecting primarily middle-aged women).
- Other causes include Raynaud's syndrome, hemochromatosis, and physical or chemical trauma
- Also may be inherited as an autosomal dominant disorder

Onycholysis

- A separation of the nail plate from the nail bed. The separated portion is white and opaque, in contrast to the pink translucence of the attached portion.
- May be a sign of hyperthyroidism (Plummer's nails), especially when it affects only the ring finger.
- Also a very common nail condition that accompanies:
  - Onychomycosis
  - Trauma
  - Chemical exposure
  - Psoriasis

Beau's Lines

- The horizontal depressions across the nail plate are caused by a transient arrest in nail growth.
- A temporary growth arrest can occur during acute stress (e.g. high fever, shock, MI, PE) and will manifest as Beau's lines as the nail grows out. It is, therefore, possible to estimate the date of illness by the distance of the furrow from the proximal nail fold. As a rule of thumb, in an average patient, the nail plate takes 3-4 months to grow from its base to the distal edge.

Glucagonoma Syndrome: NME

- Characterized by superficial Necrolytic Migratory Erythema with erosions that crust and heal with hyperpigmentation, a beefy-red tongue, and angular cheilitis.
- Alpha cell tumor of the pancreas
- Flexural and frictional areas with blistering, hyperpigmentation
- Superficial skin necrosis, erosions/ crusts
- Central 1/3 face, groin, perineum & lower abdomen
- Hepatic mets have occurred in 75% of patients at the time of diagnosis.
- Course and prognosis depends on the aggressiveness of the particular glucagonoma.
- Surgical excision of glucagonoma is curative only 30% of the time because of persistent metastases (usually liver)
- The NME rash resolves or improves after tumor excision and is poorly responsive to medical treatment.
- Clinical: sore red tongue, angular cheilitis, weight ↓, anemia, glucose intolerance, neuropsych changes.
- R/O acrodermatitis enteropathica, Zn deficiency, essential fatty acid deficiencies, kwashiorkor, candidiasis, seborrheic dermatitis, atypical psoriasis
- Fasting plasma glucagon >1000 (normal 50-250 ng/L)
- CT/angiography: locates pancreatic tumor

Porphyria Cutaneous Tarda

- As the name implies, occurs mostly in adults
- Patients do not present with photosensitivity, but with complaints of "fragile skin", vesicles, and bullae, particularly on the dorsum of the hands, esp after minor trauma
- Dx confirmed by the presence of an orange-red fluorescence of the urine under Wood's lamp
- Unlike variegate and intermittent acute porphyrias, PCT lack acute, life-threatening attacks (abdominal pain, peripheral autonomic neuropathy, and respiratory failure)
- Periorbital and malar violaceous coloration, hyperpigmentation, and hypertrichosis on the face; bullae, crust, and scars on the dorsa of the hands
- *Primary causes* of PCT include: ***Ethanol & Estrogens***
- Most PCT patients are induced by drugs and are not hereditary
- DM, HepC, & AIDS can predispose
- Skin changes are of gradual onset
- Increased plasma iron (33-50%): there is increased hepatic iron in Kupffer cells and hepatocytes)
- Important in differentiating variegate porphyria (besides the lack of acute symptoms) is to check the stool for protoporphyrins (neg in PCT, + in VP)
- Tx: D/C offending agents; phlebotomy (qw or qow to Hbg<10) + low-dose chloroquine

Erythema Multiforme

- A reaction pattern of blood vessels in the dermis with secondary epidermal changes
- Erythematous *iris-shaped/target-shaped lesions* typically involving the extremities (esp *palms and soles) and the mucous membranes.*
- Mouth lesions are painful, tender
- *Drugs*: sulfonamides; phenytoin; barbiturates; PCN; allopurinol
- Following *HSV, Mycoplasma*
- Most severe manifestation is Stevens-Johnson Syndrome, which may be life-threatening and is usually drug-induced.

7. OPTHALMOLOGY, NEUROLOGY AND GERIATRICS

OPTHALMOLOGY

✪ **CHARACTERISTICS OF HYPERTENSIVE & DIABETIC RETINOPATHY**

__HTN__	__DM__
AV nicking	*Neovascularization (new vessel formation)*
Papilledema	*Microaneuysms*
Flame hemorrhages	*Dot and blot hemorrhages*
Silver/copper wiring	*Hard exudates (lipid deposits)*
	Soft exudates (cotton wool spots)

DIABETIC EYE DISEASE

✪ A. ___BACKROUND RETINOPATHY___

    1. "Dot and blot" intraretinal **hemorrhages**

    2. **Exudates** are either…

        (a) "Cotton wool" spots (microinfarcts of superficial retina); or

        (b) "Hard" exudates, from protein/lipids leaking from capillaries of deep retinal layers

    3. **Microaneurysms**

✪ B. ___PROLIFERATIVE RETINOPATHY___

- In 10-15%, **proliferative** retinopathy develops 2° to underlying retinal ischemia that leads to new vessel formation.

- *Complications of proliferative retinopathy to remember include:*

    (a) ___Vitreous hemorrhages___
    (b) ___Retinal detachment___
    (c) ___Neovascularization___

- Proliferative retinopathy may therefore present as *sudden monocular visual loss*

- Proliferative retinopathy is the chief cause of blindness ages 20-64

C. ___MACULOPATHY___ (chief cause of blindness in DM): edema/exudates/ischemia

D. And remember, there's an ↑frequency of cataracts and glaucoma in diabetics

✪ OVERVIEW OF KEY TERMS USED IN DIABETIC RETINOPATHY	
BACKROUND Retinopathy	**PROLIFERATIVE Retinopathy** *(mnemonic: "Nerves")*
Microaneurysms Dot and blot hemorrhages Cotton-wool exudates Hard exudates	**N**eovascularization **R**etinal detachment **V**itreous hemorrhage **S**car tissue (retinitis proliferans)

✪ ACUTE ANGLE CLOSURE GLAUCOMA vs. UVEITIS	
ACUTE ANGLE GLAUCOMA	**UVEITIS**
Painful eye with hazy vision and halos around lights Red (around the limbus) Pupil **dilated** Obv **increase** in intraocular pressure	Photophobia; ↓ vision; (posterior uveitis is more likely to be painless) Also red (around the limbus); esp in anterior uveitis **Constricted** pupil **Normal** intraocular pressure

B/L INO (Bilateral Internuclear Opthalmoplegia)

> Most commonly seen in MS

> ↓ ability for either eye to look medially (*when asked to look to the left or to the right*)

> However, because this is a problem originating in the MLF (medial longitudinal fasiculus) and not the pathway governing convergence, convergence remains intact *when patient is instructed to converge*.

MULTIPLE SCLEROSIS

> INO (*Intranuclear Opthalmoplegia*), ✪ esp. B/L {2° to involvement of the MLF which coordinates adduction of one eye & abduction of the contralateral eye by connecting contralateral third and sixth cranial nerve nuclei}. Convergence is preserved, which distinguishes INO from medial rectus palsy.

> *Optic Neuritis*
>   o Variable visual field loss
>   o Painful; pain worsens with eye movement
>   o 40% will ultimately develop it
>   o Usually unilateral, but may be B/L

> Blurry vision may be secondary to
>   o Diplopia (2° to INO)
>   o Optic neuritis

> Nystagmus

NYSTAGMUS

> While it is normal to have some degree of horizontal nystagmus on extreme lateral gaze, marked degrees of **horizontal** nystagmus are abnormal and are caused by conditions affecting the *vestibular apparatus or brain stem*.
> **Vertical** nystagmus is always abnormal and indicates problems at the *brain stem*.

SLIT LAMP

> Helps to visualize the layers of the cornea and the lens
> Often useful in identifying **Kaiser-Fleischer rings in Wilson's disease**.
> KF rings are the golden-brown copper deposits in Descemet's membrane in the periphery of the iris. These rings can usually be seen with the naked eye, but occasionally, remember, slit-lamp fundoscopy is needed.

MANAGEMENT OF CORNEAL ABRASION →After visualizing with focalized fluorescein uptake, treat with topical antibiotics and patch the eye until healed in a day or two.

SCHIRMER'S TEST ✪

> Important in diagnosing keratoconjunctivitis sicca syndrome
> Diagnostic evaluation of sicca syndrome includes measurement of tear flow by Schirmer's I test (less than 5mm in 5 min is considered positive). Other important ocular symptoms in Sjogren's include: dry eyes for more than 3 months, recurrent sensation of sand or gravel in the eyes, or use of tear substitutes more than 3 times per day.

HERPES ZOSTER OPTHALMICUS ✪

> The vesicular skin eruptions are in the distribution of the opthalmic division of the CN 5.
> Serious opthalmic complications are a real threat, especially when the *tip of the nose* is affected (which indicates involvement of the *nasociliary nerve* that also supplies the cornea). This is the so-called *Hutchinson's sign*.

SIGNIFICANCE OF THE CAVERNOUS SINUS—

> Receives the venous outflow from the orbit
> Carotid artery runs through it
> All the CNs entering the eye run thru or adjacent to it, ie CNs 2-6.
> The proximity of many of these CNs relative to the pituitary is significant in cases of hyperpituitarism and pituitary tumors and surgeries.
> Invasion of the cavernous sinus by a pituitary tumor usually affects the 6th nerve first, because it is more medial than the 3rd and 4th CNs. 6th nerve palso manifests with lack of abduction of the affected eye.
> Remember, $(LR_6SO_4)_3$ to remind you that CN6 innervates the Lateral Rectus; CN4 the Superior Oblique; and all the rest are innervated by CN3, including the all-imporant medial rectus.

RHEUMATOID EPISCLERITIS ✪

> *Inflammation of the episclera, the tissue which lies between the conjunctiva and sclera*
> *Episcleritis is the most common ocular complication of RA & indicates a poor prognosis.*
> *The **difference** between episcleritis and scleritis is that scleritis is deeper, more painful, and can result in vision loss. Both can be seen in collagen vascular dz's.*
> *May **also** be a feature of infections and granulomatous disorders*

ENDOCARDITIS:

1. Roth spots
2. Scleral & conjunctival hemorrhages

GRAVES' DISEASE ✪

2 types of ocular findings:

a) **Infiltrative findings** (*only Graves'*):
   (1) Proptosis
   (2) Optic neuritis
   (3) Opthalmoplegia (extraocular muscle dysfunction)

b) **Noninfiltrative Findings** (any thyrotoxicosis)
   (1) Lid lag
   (2) Lid retraction (exposure of the sclera above the iris is an early sign)

ARGYLL-ROBERTSON PUPILS ✪

> A feature of tertiary syphilis, but may also be seen in diabetes.
> Usually bilateral
> Argyll Robertson pupils are small, irregular and unresponsive to light, but they show an intact near response if the patient's visual acuity is intact.
> Also known as the "prostitute's pupil" because it "accommodates but does not react."

HORNER'S SYNDROME

> The triad of 1) ptosis; 2) miosis; and 3) anhydrosis
> Results from tumor infiltration of the inferior cervical sympathetic ganglion, most commonly from Pancoast tumor

PTOSIS CAUSED BY 3RD NERVE PALSY

> ✓ *Sparing of the pupil distinguishes diabetic 3rd nerve palsy from that caused by mechanical factors such as aneurysm or neoplasm*

PROGRESSIVE SUPRANUCLEAR PALSY ✪

> An early and diagnostic feature of PSP is difficulty in making "downgaze", ie trouble looking down! These patients commonly present with frequent falls despite adequate visual acuity. A second reason these patients suffer frequent falls is the loss of postural reflexes, esp. early in the course of the disorder.

> Mean age at onset is about 65 years

> Causes bradykinesia and rigidity

> Conspicuous abnormalities of voluntary eye movements (especially vertical gaze), dementia, pseudobulbar palsy (=exaggerated jaw jerk and gag reflexes), and axial dystonia distinguish it from Parkinson's disease.

> There is little or no response to antiparkinsonian drugs.

> The importance of the diagnosis lies in the poor prognosis: patients die in a relatively short time from progressive neurologic disease, whereas Parkinsonian patients will survive for many years with only moderate disability and intact mental function.

PAPILLEDEMA

> Seen in cases of ↑d intracranial pressure whether from …
> - Malignant HTN
> - Intracranial mass or
> - Pseudotumor cerebri.

> Remember, LP is contraindicated with intracranial mass-associated papilledema as opposed to pseudotumor cerebri.

BENIGN INTRACRANIAL HTN (aka Pseudotumor Cerebri) ✪

> An unexplained disorder occurring mainly in pregnant, obese, young and middle-aged women producing headache and papilledema

> Increased intracranial pressure on LP yet no local structural cause.

> Long-term consequences include blindness from optic nerve atrophy

> Dx is made on LP and the CT is used to exclude other pathology.

> Treatment included weight reduction, diuretics, occasionally a shunt, and optic nerve decompression

A/V CROSSING AND A/V NICKING

> Normally, remember, the veins are darker and wider than the accompanying arterioles, having a ratio of 3:2 in diameter. At times the vein will appear to be deflected away by the crossing artery; this is not abnormal, but when the veins narrow and appear darker on either or both sides of the AV crossing, this signifies a HTN/atherosclerotic state of the retinal vasculature.

CMV RETINITIS ✪

➢ The most common serious ocular complication of AIDS.

➢ Prior to the availability of highly active antiretroviral therapy (HAART), CMV retinitis occurred in 21 to 44 percent of patients with AIDS. However, the incidence of CMV retinitis has decreased by more than 50 percent since HAART became available.

➢ "Ketchup and cheese" is most often the term used to describe the appearance, referring to hemorrhagic and necrotic retinopathy, respectively, of CMV infection common in AIDS

➢ Also referred to as a "pizza pie" appearance

➢ Remember, CMV is typical at CD4 counts $< 50/mm^3$

➢ Clinical: blurring or loss of central vision; scotomata ("blind spots"); photopsia ("flashing lights"); also look for "floaters" in the question; retinal detachment can result in acute visual loss.

➢ Retinal detachment, which occurs in approximately one-quarter of patients treated with antiviral therapy, is one of the major causes of vision loss in patients with CMV retinitis.

➢ Treatment options: gancyclovir, foscarnet, and cidofovir

CHLOROQUINE RETINOPATHY

➢ Typical "bull's-eye macula" because of damage to the retinal pigment epithelium; central vision is severely affected.

CENTRAL RETINAL ARTERY OCCLUSION

➢ Result from emboli to the central retinal artery

➢ A cherry-red fovea may be seen

➢ Emboli are composed of either cholesterol (Hollenhorst plaque), calcium, or platelet-fibrin debris

➢ While there are a variety of sources for these emboli, look especially at the ipsilateral carotid as well as the heart, esp if there is Afib, h/o MI, or wall motion abnormalities (dys/hypo/akinesia)

KEY CAUSES OF A SUDDEN LOSS OF VISION

PAINLESS

1. Central retinal artery occlusion (cherry red fovea)
2. Retinal artery embolism (amaurosis fugax → *patients may describe progressive visual loss, "like a shade" coming down*)
3. Retinal detachment
4. Vitreous hemorrhage (eg in proliferative diabetic retinopathy)
5. Giant cell arteritis (temporal arteritis)

PAINFUL

1. Optic neuritis
2. Acute (closed angle) glaucoma (blurred vision; red eye; dilated, non-reactive pupil)
3. Trauma

WARNING <u>SIGNS</u> AND SYMPTOMS FOR URGENT OPTHALMOLOGIC REFERRAL:

Ocular Finding:	Associated Conditions:
Severe Eye Pain	Uveitis, scleritis, angle-closure glaucoma (ACG) microbial keratitis, iridocyclitis
Photophobia	Iridocyclitis, keratitis, ACG
Impaired vision/loss of vision	Uveitis, scleritis, ACG, microbial keratitis, iridocyclitis
Corneal abnormalities	Corneal laceration, ACG, microbial keratitis
Pupillary abnormalities	Uveitis, ACG
Anterior chamber abnormality	Intraocular foreign body, hyphema, hypopyon, corneal perforation, ACG

OTHER <u>CONDITIONS</u> THAT WARRANT OPTHALMOLOGIC REFERRAL:

1. Acute or chronic motility disorder
2. Central retinal artery or vein occlusion
3. Chemical or alkali burn
4. Corneal ulceration or abrasion that does not heal within 48 h
5. Diabetic retinopathy
6. Endopthalmitis
7. Herpetic corneal lesions
8. Hyphema (blood in anterior chamber)
9. Macular degeneration
10. Orbital cellulitis
11. Penetrating trauma
12. Retinal detachment

NEUROLOGY

Commonly Asked Material:

1. Recognize the clinical presentation of **acoustic neuroma** (schwannomas involving the 8th cranial nerve which grow slowly and produce hearing loss and tinnitus as most common symptoms).

2. Know the triad of **Meniere's Disease** is vertigo, tinnitus, and hearing loss that is progressive and sensorineural. 30% are bilateral. You need not have all three to make the diagnosis, but the vertigo *must* be present.

3. In patients with **recurrent unilateral hemiparesis as TIA/CVA**, remember especially to study the contralateral carotid artery.

4. Remember, **warfarin** is more effective than ASA for preventing stroke in patients with A Fib, but is not better than **ASA** for preventing stroke in patients without A Fib, so choose aspirin first for the prevention of recurrent noncardioembolic strokes.

5. Recognize a case of **isolated peroneal neuropathy** (foot drop, etc)

6. Recognize a case of **3rd nerve palsy**. Remember: $(LR_6SO_4)_3$; 3rd nerve is to the medial rectus.

7. **Multiple Sclerosis**, remember, is secondary to inflammatory demyelination (which later scars to form a plaque) in the white matter of the brain (most frequently periventricular), brain stem, or spinal cord. This can lead to an otherwise healthy person presenting with exacerbations and remissions of any combination of the following symptoms: opthalmoplegia/unilateral loss of vision/diplopia/vertigo/ataxia/dysathria/paresthesias/paralysis/emotional lability.

8. Remember (B→O→M):   **B**otulin→presynaptic
                                  Organophosphate poisoning→synaptic
                                  Myasthenia Gravis→postsynaptic.

9. Botulism: **Remember the <u>6 D's</u> →**

           Eyes →   D ilated, fixed pupil
                       D iplopia

           Tongue → D ysarthria
                       D ysphagia
                       D ry tongue

           And…   D escending paralysis

10. Recognize **MYASTHENIA GRAVIS** (often heralded by such *cranial nerve findings as diplopia; dysarthria; dysphagia; dyspnea; and fatiguability*) and be able to differentiate it from **Eaton Lambert Syndrome** {discussed later; ELS often *associated with small cell lung* ca; proximal muscle weakness}; also know that ***thymoma→10% develop Myasthenia Gravis. Tensilon test for dx. Physostigmine or pyridostigmine for treatment***.

11. **GUILLAIN-BARRE SYNDROME**:
    ➢ Half the patients have *mild respiratory or GI infection 1-3 weeks prior*
    ➢ Severe rapidly progressive, symmetrical polyneuropathy with pronounced proximal muscle weakness; resp weakness critical (don't forget to *check Negative Inspiratory Pressures and Vital Capacities* frequently)

12. Know these important **INDICATIONS FOR MRI** for the boards:

    ➢ *Cancer patient with back pain* ± neuro symptoms

    ➢ Suspected *neural claudication* (i.e. spinal stenosis; back pain worse with walking, etc)

    ➢ Percussion tenderness over spine in a *suspected septic discitis* as well as *paraspinal abscess*.

    ➢ Know that pain is the most common initial presenting symptom in cancer patients with *imminent cord compression*.

    ➢ *Suspected avascular necrosis, e.g. of the femoral head in patients on chronic steroids, sickle cell patients*, etc.

13. Classic case of **Normal Pressure Hydrocephalus**(triad of **A**taxia, **I**ncontinence, **D**ementia)

14. Recognize a case of **MERALGIA PARESTHETICA**. This is *the most common pure sensory mononeuropathy*, resulting from *compression of the lateral cutaneous nerve* of the thigh as it passes through the inguinal ligament. It presents with *numbness or burning sensation over the lateral thigh; sometimes, prolonged standing or walking can provoke the symptoms. Weight loss can help, but in many cases, its spontaneously subsides.*

15. Recognize a case of **DIABETIC AMYOTROPHY** → *weakness, atrophy, and pain affecting the pelvic girdle and thigh muscles* [it's all in the name: "a…trophy" of the "myo"(muscles)]

16. **Seizures**. Know that seizure disorder is a clinical not an EEG diagnosis and that a normal EEG does not R/O seizure disorder. EEG is simply an adjuvant tool in the diagnosis. Know also that head trauma is chief cause of focal sz in young adults, as opposed to brain tumor/vascular dz in older patients. Know that Valproic Acid may cause neural tube defects and that Tegretol/Dilantin/Phenobarb can all make OCPs less effective.

17. Similarly, in **anticonvulsant blood levels**, remember:
    ➢ Therapeutic levels represent only average bell-shaped curves.
    ➢ Anticonvulsant dose should never be changed based on blood levels alone.
    ➢ Toxicity is a clinical, not a laboratory, phenomenon.

18. **POLYMYALGIA RHEUMATICA**: elderly patient with aching/pain and stiffness of neck/upper back/shoulders/upper arms/hip girdle; can see fever; anorexia; weight loss; Remember: no muscle weakness (that's myositis!)

19. Recognize a classic case of **Pseudotumor Cerebri**: high opening pressure on LP; MS changes; fundoscopic changes; etc.
    ➤ Lumbar puncture is dangerous and contraindicated when papilledema is due to *intracranial mass*, but is safe in pseudotumor cerebri.

20. Recognize a case of **Classic Migraine** and **Migraine Equivalent**.

    ➤ *Classic Migraine*: N/V; photophobia; visual (scintillations, scotomas) and paresthetic (manual, perioral) neurologic symptoms prior to H/A.
    ➤ *Migraine Equivalent*: recurrent attacks of neurologic dysfunction that mimic the migraine alone, but do not culminate in headache.
    ➤ Remember, migraines (and cluster H/As) are typically unilateral, as opposed to tension H/As, which can be either unilateral or bilateral
    ➤ *Cluster headaches*: severe; unilateral; often at the same time each day assoc'd with at least one of the following: conjunctival injection; lacrimation; nasal congestion; rhinorrhea; forehead/facial swelling; miosis; ptosis; eyelid edema. They occur qod to 8x/d over a 3-6 week period (and therefore the name).

21. **ESSENTIAL TREMOR**: be able to DDx it from Parkinson's tremor:
    ➤ Essential Tremor: hands/head/voice tremor→*can treat with propranolol or even a bit of ETOH*.
    ➤ Parkinson's Tremor: there's no head involvement.

22. Know that **SUBARACHNOID HEMORRHAGE** can present with *meningismus and and incomplete 3rd nerve palsy* (secondary to aneurysmal expansion); in up to 50% of cases, alert patients with aneurysm may have a small sentinel bleed with warning headache.

23. Recognize a case of **ALS (AMYOTROPHIC LATERAL SCLEROSIS)**: *tongue fasciculations*; weakness; atrophy; progressive limb weakness affecting *distal more than proximal* areas and esp. affecting the *small muscles of the hand*; *upper and lower motor neuronal involvement*. Characteristically, *bowel and bladder functions remain unaffected*.

NEUROLOGY NOTES

✪ THE DISTRIBUTION OF SELECTIVE CVAs & THEIR SIGNS	
DISTRIBUTION	**SIGNS**
Anterior Cerebral Artery	Contralateral face & extremities (for boths sensory & motor deficits)
Lacunar	Internal capsule → pure <u>motor</u> hemiparesis Thalamus → pure <u>sensory</u> Posterior internal capsule + thalamus →sensorimotor Pons → dysarthria, clumsy hand
Middle Cerebral Artery	Aphasia; contralateral hemiparesis
Vertebral/basilar arteries	**A**mnesia, **a**taxia, **d**iplopia, **d**ysphagia, **d**ysarthria, **v**ertigo, **v**isual field defects (*think*: "**ADV**anced" diagnosis); Ipsilateral face & contralateral extremities for both sensory & motor deficits, if any

CARDIOEMBOLIC SOURCES OF ISCHEMIC CVA	
Major Risk Factors	**Minor Risk Factors**
A Fib	MVP
Mitral Stenosis	Severe mitral annular calcification
Prosthetic valve	Patent foramen ovale
Recent MI	Atrial septal aneurysm
LV thrombus	Calcific AS
Atrial myxoma	LV regional wall abnormalities
Infectious endocarditis	
Nonischemic dilated cardiomyopathy	
Nonbacterial thrombotic endocarditis	
Sick sinus syndrome	

CONTRAINDICATIONS TO tPA FOR ACUTE ISCHEMIC STROKE ✪

1. *≥ 3 hours from stroke onset*
2. Seizure at stroke onset
3. Uncontrolled HTN at time of treatment
4. Recent (within 3 months) previous CVA, serious head trauma, or intracranial/intraspinal surgery
5. Evidence of intracranial hemorrhage; suspicion of SAH (subarachnoid hemorrhage); h/o intracranial hemorrhage; active internal bleeding;
6. Intracranial neoplasm, AVM, or aneurysm
7. *Current use of anticoagulants, an INR > 1.7*, or PT > 15 seconds
8. *Platelet count < 100,000*

Causes of Continued Clinical Deterioriation Following an Apparently Completed CVA
1. Continued Emboli
2. Extension of infarct
3. Hemorrhage into infarct
4. Worsening cerebral vasospasm/edema
5. Improper diagnosis (e.g. vasculitis or tumor)

DIFFERENTIAL DX OF HORNER'S SYNDROME
1. Lateral medullary syndrome
2. Pancoast tumor
3. Shy-Drager syndrome
4. Sympathectomy
5. Syringomyelia

PTOSIS
1. Complete unilateral→3rd nerve palsy
2. Partial unilateral
    a) Horner's syndrome (ptosis, meiosis, anhydrosis)
    b) Congenital (#1 cause in the healthy adult)
    c) Partial 3rd nerve palsy

3. Bilateral→muscle disease
    a) Myotonic Dystrophy
    b) Myasthenia Gravis

RAMSAY-HUNT SYNDROME ✪
1. Varicella-zoster of the geniculate ganglion of CN 7
2. **May see** *herpetic vesicles in the external ear* **canal (classic), + TM involvement/vertigo/nystagmus/deafness/facial paralysis**

LATERALIZATION IN NYSTAGMUS AND CONJUGATE DEVIATION

1. *Nystagmus*

    - **Vestibular lesion**→nystagmus is greatest on looking *away from* the lesion
    - **Cerebellar lesion**→nystagmus is greatest on looking *towards* the lesion.

2. *Conjugate Deviation*

    - **Hemispheric stroke**→eyes deviate *towards* the side of the lesion (and away from the hemiplegic extremity/ies)
    - **Epileptogenic focus during seizure**→eyes deviate *away from* the side of the nidus.
    - **Brainstem disease**→eyes deviate *away from* side of lateral pontine lesion (and toward the hemiplegic extremity/ies)
    - **Caloric testing** in patients with intact brainstem/labyrinth→Eyes deviate *towards* the ear that is irrigated with the cold water.

Remember, **nystagmus** from <u>central</u> causes is *vertical*. *Peripheral* etiologies lead to *horizontal or rotational* nystagmus.

PHYSICAL EXAM IN HEARING LOSS

1. Weber's Test→Tests using lateralization
2. Rinne's Test →Tests using conduction differences

INTERPRETING WEBER'S TEST

1. Lateralizes to deaf side in *conduction deafness* (e.g. otosclerosis)
2. Lateralizes to normal side in *nerve deafness* (e.g. acoustic neuroma)

INTERPRETING RINNE'S TEST

1. Bone conduction > Air conduction on the affected side in *conduction deafness*
2. Air conduction > Bone conduction on both sides in *nerve deafness*

   or, (if you really like misery)…

Rinne Test
- Holding the tuning fork against the mastoid process, the patient indicates when s/he can no longer hear the sound. At that point the tuning fork is changed to just outside the auditory meatus to see if the sound can be heard again. *Normal hearing patients and patients with sensorineural hearing loss* hear the sound longer through air than through bone, noted as "AC>BC" (air conduction > bone conduction). In a *conductive hearing loss*, bone conduction becomes ≥ air conduction, **paradoxically**. This results is reported as an "abnormal Rinne" or "reversed Rinne".

Weber Test
- Holding the tuning fork on the middle of the patient's forehead, the patient is asked, "Where do you hear this the loudest?" The sound **localizes** *toward the side with conducting loss (toward the worse-hearing ear) or away from the side with a sensorineural loss (toward the better hearing ear)*. The Weber test is only useful if there is an asymmetric hearing loss. If hearing is symmetric, the patient perceives the sound in the middle of the forehead.

<u>UPPER MOTOR NEURON Lesions</u> vs.	<u>LOWER MOTOR NEURON Lesions</u>
↑ Tone ± clonus	↓ Tone
↑ DTRs	↓ DTRs
Babinski (extensor plantar response)	No Babinski
Absent abdomenal reflexes	
	Fasciculations
	Atrophy

__REFLEX (DTR)__	→	__NERVE ROOT__
Biceps (supinator jerk present)		C6
Triceps reflex		C8
Abdominal reflex		T7-12
Cremasteric reflex		L1/2
Patellar reflex		L3/4
Achilles reflex		S1
Anal reflex		S3/4

> ➢ If you see **unilateral wasting of the small hand muscles**, think of either an *ulnar nerve* lesion or a *T1 nerve root* lesion, such as might be caused by a bronchogenic carcinoma.

✪ __Peripheral Neuropathy__   →   __CN involvement__

Diabetes	CN 3,4,6
Guillain-Barre	CN 6,7
Sarcoidosis	CN 7
Diptheria	CN 9

✪ __Aneurysm__   →   __CN involvement__

ICA at the cavernous sinus	CN 3-6
Opthalmic artery	CN 2
PCA (post communicating)	CN 6

DIAGNOSTIC LIMITATIONS OF THE EEG

1. Cannot exclude epilepsy
2. Cannot exclude focal pathology
3. Cannot suggest structural nature of focal pathology
4. Cannot be used to assess the adequacy of antiseizure medication
5. In determining brain death, if brain stem reflexes are present OR if they are persistently absent, there is no need to order an EEG.

DETERMINATION OF BRAIN DEATH

1. Sufficient cause—must exclude hypothermia and sedative overdose

2. Absent gag/corneal/cough reflexes

3. Fixed pupils

4. Loss of oculovestibular and oculocephalic reflexes

5. No response to painful stimuli, except for spinal reflexes

6. No spontaneous respiratory movements after ventilator disconnected and patient observed for 5 minutes with oxygen supplied via tracheal catheter.

✪ INTERPRETIVE PATTERNS IN EMG (ELECTROMYOGRAPHY)

1. Myasthenia Gravis→ *decremental response* to repetitive ('tetanic') stimulation

2. Myasthenic syndrome (Eaton-Lambert Syndrome)→ *incremental response* to such stimulation.

3. Myotonia→'**Dive-bomber**' EMG (*high frequency* action potential discharges)

4. Polymyositis→**Fibrillation** (brief *low-amplitude* action potentials due to 'denervation hypersensitivity' at the motor end plate)

> ✪ On exam, **ELS can be differentiated from Myasthenia Gravis** since ELS patients derive ↑ strength from repeated activity, while Myasthenic patients get weaker.

WHEN IS IT APPROPRIATE TO MONITOR ANTICONVULSANT LEVELS?

1. Suspect non-compliance
2. Renal or hepatic disease
3. Poor seizure control
4. Suspected toxicity
   a) **Phenytoin**
      (1) Gingival hyperplasia
      (2) Hirsutism
      (3) Nystagmus →ataxia→drowsiness
      (4) Osteomalacia
      (5) Arrthmias/Hypotension in IV use
   b) **Carbamazepine**
      (1) Drowsiness (esp if used with phenytoin)
      (2) Leukopenia
      (3) SIADH
      (4) Anticholinergic effects (structurally similar to tricyclics)
   c) **Valproic Acid**
      (1) Tremor
      (2) Hair Thinning
      (3) ↑appetite/weight gain; ankle edema

   - *Note all 3 of the above may cause drowsiness and ataxia*

5. 2nd drug added which could potentiate or diminish its activity.

CONDITIONS PREDISPOSING TO CEREBRAL ANEURYSMS

1. Polycystic Kidney Disease
2. Essential HTN
3. Aortic Coarctation
4. Ehlers-Danlos Syndrome
5. Renal Artery Stenosis due to FMD (fibromuscular dysplasia)
6. Wegener's/PAN/SBE

PREDOMINANT VERTEBRAL LEVELS IN SPECIFIC DISORDERS

Cervical Cord
- Syringomyelia
- Siphylitic myelitis

Thoracic Cord
- Anterior spinal artery thrombosis
- Pott's disease (TB)
- Subacute Combined Degeneration (B12 deficiency)

Thoracolumbar
- Transverse Myelitis
- Metastases

Lumbosacral
- Tabes Dorsalis

MYASTHENIA GRAVIS ✪

➤ MG is an acquired weakness of the skeletal muscle that is due to autoimmune _acetylcholine receptor antibodies_ interfering with normal acetylcholine stimulation at the postsynaptic membrane at the neuromuscular junction.

- Characteristically, the _weakness increases during repeated use_ (as opposed to Eaton-Lambert Syndrome, where it improves), and the patient typically complains of _weakness that increases as the day progresses._

- _Anterior mediastinal mass_ (when thymoma associated)

    - In the absence of a tumor, the available evidence suggests that up to 85 percent of patients experience _improvement after thymectomy_, and, of these, about 35 percent achieve drug-free remission. However, the improvement is typically delayed for months to years.

    - It is the _consensus_ that thymectomy should be carried out in all patients with generalized MG between the ages of puberty and at least 55 years.

- _Diplopia and ptosis_ are common initial complaints

- _Weakness in chewing is most noticeable after prolonged effort, as in chewing meat;_ facial muscle weakness

- Easy fatiguability
- Recurrent aspiration pneumonias (2° to difficulty in swallowing)
- If weakness of respiration becomes so severe as to require respiratory assistance, the patient is said to be in _myasthenic crisis_.

➤ Diagnostics ✪

- _Acetylcholine receptor antibodies_ have a 90% sensitivity (70% in ocular myasthenia)

- _Tensilon test_ (short-acting acetylcholinesterase inhibitor edrophonium)→ in MG, usually see improvement of symptoms at the bedside in a minute or so.

- EMG→should see a _decremental response to repetitive stimulation ('post-tetanic inhibition')_

➤ Treatment
  o PO <u>acetylcholinesterase inhibitors</u>, like neostigmine (Prostigmin®) or pyridostigmine (Mestinon®)
  o High-dose <u>steroids</u> for severe attacks
  o <u>Plasmapheresis</u> for severe, life-threatening cases.

Parkinson's Disease (SMART)...
S huffling gait
M asked facies
A kinesia
R igidity (cogwheel)
T remor

POINTS TO REMEMBER WITH PARKINSON'S DISEASE ✪

- PD is a *clinical* diagnosis
- Drug therapy should be initiated only when symptoms have a negative impact on the patient's ability to function.
- **NEW GUIDELINES** (*Neurology (2001; 56 suppl 5)*)
  ➤ Start with levodopa-sparing **dopamine agonists** to reduce the likelihood of dyskinesias New guidelines emphasize *dopamine agonists as INITIAL therapy* in most symptomatic patients. Dopamine agonists are *less likely to cause the motor problems seen with levodopa and may even have neuroprotective benefit*
  ➤ They *can delay the need for levodopa* for many years
  ➤ Mirapex® (preamixpexole) and Requip® (ropinirole) are *more selective dopamine agonists than bromocryptine or pergolide*
    ▪ Remember, the major hypothalamic <u>inhibitory factor for prolactin is dopamine</u>, which is of course, used in the treatment of prolactinomas to decrease the PRL level. Prolactin excess is often associated with galactorrhea (and/or hypogonadism). Therefore, if a patient develops galactorrhea after coming off of bromocryptine or other dopamine agonist, check for prolactinoma that may have developed during treatment and may have been masked.
  ➤ **Levodopa**, while the most effective treatment, can wear off over the long term and even cause dyskinesias. It is *best as initial treatment in patients over 70 and those with dementia or significant cognitive impairment*. For younger patients it can be added after dopamine agonists no longer provide symptomatic relief.
    ➤ A patient's failure to respond to one dopamine antagonist does not mean that s/he will not benefit from another.
    ➤ Remember, Levodopa (L-Dopa) is the most effective drug for PD; it is generally used in combination with carbidopa (Sinemet CR®)
  ➤ *Tolcapone*, one of the newer agents, inhibits dopa metabolism in plasma and allows higher amounts of L-Dopa to cross the blood-brain barrier without increasing the L-Dopa dose.
  ➤ *Anticholinergics* are the oldest group of PD medications and most effective in persons with tremor-predominant disease.

> ➤ Consider *surgery* for the patient only after medical therapies fail to confer benefit. Palliative surgeries, such as pallidotomy and thalamic Deep Brain Stimulation (electrode implant excellent for severe tremors) as well as so-called "restorative" surgeries, such as fetal mesencephalic cell transplantation are a few of the surgical options available to such individuals.

ACUTE NEUROLOGICAL SIDE EFFECTS OF TYPICAL ANTIPSYCHOTIC MEDICATIONS		
REACTION	**CLINICAL FEATURES**	**MANAGEMENT**
Acute dystonia	Spasm of tongue, throat, face, jaw, eyes, or back muscles	Injectable benztropine or Benadryl®, followed by PO anticholinergics or benzodiazepines
Akathisia	Motor restlessness, inability to stay still	If possible, ↓ the dose of the antipsychotic; add β-blockers, benzos, or anticholinergics
Pseudoparkinsonism	Bradykinesia, rigidity, resting tremor, flat affect, etc.	Add anticholinergics or amantadine; diphenhydramine and lorazepam may also be effective

VERTIGO

- **_Vestibular neuronitis_** is felt to be 2° to viral infection to the vestibular nerve/ vestibular apparatus and usually lasts a few weeks

- ✪ **_BPV_** (Benign Positional Vertigo) is a vertigo brought about by specific head positions and the most common presenting complaint is vertigo on *rolling over in bed*, e.g. in getting out of bed in the morning, and *turning the head*, e.g. while changing lanes. Remember that Nylen-Bárány maneuver is often checked to confirm. When vertigo is reproduced, the test is positive.

- **_Labyrinthitis_** may be the result of bacterial or viral infection.

- **_Vestibular ototoxicity_** *(2° drugs)* is usually a more chronic condition, accompanied by disequilibrium and hearing loss.

DDX OF VERTIGO

CENTRAL
1. Basilar Migraine
2. Cerebellopontine angle neoplasm
3. Multiple Sclerosis
4. Posterior fossa tumor
5. Vertebrobasilar ischemia

PERIPHERAL
1. Medications
2. Motion sickness
3. Benign Positional Vertigo (BPV)
4. Vestibular Neuronitis
5. Labyrinthitis
6. Meniere's Disease
7. Trauma

UNDERSTANDING TERMS IN ABNORMAL MOTOR KINETICS:

MOVEMENT	TONE	RATE	DESCRIPTION	MISCELLANEOUS
Ballism	0	Rapid	Abrupt, irregular, large amplitude	Proximal muscle
Chorea	1+	Rapid	Jerky, irregular, no rhythm	Distal muscle; semi-purposeful; seen in Huntington's and Wilson's diseases.
Athetosis	3+	Slow	Snake-like/writhing	Digits/hands/tongue; purposeless
Cogwheel rigidity	5+	N/A	Intermittent, unintentional resistance to passive motion	Commonly seen in Parkinson's Disease

PROGRESSIVE SUPRANUCLEAR PALSY ✪
1. A key differential in Parkinson's Disease
2. It resemble Parkinson's in most ways, except :
    a) There is usually no resting tremor in SNP
    b) Patients with SNP can have a vertical gaze palsy, particularly on downward gaze, so often present with frequent falls.

CLINICAL FEATURES OF COMMON TREMORS			
Feature	**ESSENTIAL**	**PARKINSONIAN**	**CEREBELLAR**
Best seen	With certain postures	At rest	With action
Frequency (cycles/s)	4-12	4-6	3-5
Aggravated by	Stress, anxiety	Stress, walking	Action
Relieved by	Alcohol	Action	Rest
Associated features	Voice, head, chin tremors	Rigidity, bradykinesia, gait	Dysarthria, ataxia, nystagmus
Disabling	Can be	Unusual	Yes
Common Cause	Familial	Idiopathic	Various

MULTIPLE SCLEROSIS
1. Consider MS when patient presents with periodic alterations in vision (e.g. central vision blurring), as well as sensory-motor skills.
2. Common optic findings include
    a) Diplopia (usually 2° to INO, or internuclear opthalmoplegia)
    b) Optic neuritis (pain on ocular movement)
    c) Nystagmus

3. Patients frequently note ↑ exacerbations in hot weather
4. Diagnosis is usually made when clinical suspicion leads to an MRI, which <u>shows</u> <u>plaques in the white matter</u>, esp the *periventricular white matter*; corpus callosum is a frequent site of involvement.
5. ✓ the CSF for *oligoclonal bands*: > 2 is abnormal.
   ✓ the CSF for *myelin basic protein*: ≥ 70% in acute cases.

KEY SYMPTOMS

- ➢ Bowel/bladder/sexual dysfunction
- ➢ Cognitive Deficits
- ➢ Depression; mood lability
- ➢ Fatigue; weakness
- ➢ Impaired mobility
- ➢ Pain; sensory changes
- ➢ Lhermitte's sign → sense of electric shock-like sensations when flexing the neck
- ➢ Spinocerebellar tract involvement
  - ▪ Intention tremor
  - ▪ Ataxic gait
  - ▪ Scanning speech
- ➢ Spasticity
- ➢ Visual Changes

CLAUDICATION-2 TYPES ✪

CLAUDICATION VERSUS PSEUDOCLAUDICATION		
Feature	**CLAUDICATION** *(vascular)*	**PSEUDOCLAUDICATION** *(neurogenic →spinal stenosis)*
Bilateral	Occasionally	Usually
Etiology	Vascular	Spinal
Onset	On exertion	Standing, walking
Quality	Crampy, achy	Sharp paresthesias
Relieved by	Standing still	Sitting down, leaning forward
Walking distance	Constant	Variable

SIGNS AND SYMPTOMS OF INCREASED INTRACRANIAL PRESSURE

1. Throbbing intermittent pain
2. Nausea and vomiting
3. Visual impairment
4. Papilledema
5. Decreased level of consciousness
6. Abnormal gait
7. Lateral rectus paresis

Further Evaluation (LP/CT/MRI) should be considered when any of the following are present:

1. Immunosuppressed patients
2. Most intense/painful H/A the patient has ever experienced
3. Any subacute H/A occurring with changing pattern of intensity
4. Any H/A associated with neurological deficits
5. Headaches appearing for the first time after age 50
6. Associated fever or stiff neck
7. Associated papilledema or cognitive deficit
8. H/o recent head trauma, change in mental status, focal neurologic deficit, progressive global symptoms, or high risk of bleeding

DIAGNOSTIC FEATURES OF HEADACHES

Migraine *without* Aura (aka <u>*Common*</u> Migraine)

- Pain distribution predominantly on one side of the head
- Pulsating and throbbing quality to the pain
- Moderate to severe intensity
- Sensitivity to light and sound
- Durations typically 4-72h if untreated
- Similar headaches in the past

Migraine *with* Aura (aka <u>*Classic*</u> Migraine)

- As above, plus an aura (visual warning of scintillating scotomata or fortification spectra)
- Aura duration typically < 60 min
- Aura onset typically 1-2 h before the H/A
- Alternatively, aura alone without subsequent H/A development (acephalgic migraine or migraine equivalent)

PRODROMAL SYMPTOMS OF MIGRAINE WITH AURA	
Clinical descriptor	**Meaning**
"Alice in Wonderland" syndrome	Visual and auditory hallucinations
Fortification spectra	Zigzag pattern resembling the facade of a fort
Hemianopia	Partial visual field loss
Paresthesias	Burning, prickling, tingling, or tickling sensations
Photopsia	Flashing lights
Scotomata	Blind spots
Teichopsia	Bright shimmering or wavy lines

EPISODIC TENSION H/A

- Distribution generally B/L
- Pressing, squeezing, or band-like (throbbing during physical exertion)
- Mild to moderate in intensity
- Sensitivity to light or sound
- No nausea
- Duration from 30min-7days
- <15 headache days/month

CHRONIC TENSION H/A

- As above, but ≥15 headache days/month
- Nausea may be present during intense or prolonged H/A

EPISODIC CLUSTER H/A

- Severe unilateral orbital, supraorbital, or temporal pain
- Duration 15-180 min (if untreated)
- Associated with at least one ipsilateral autonomic sign: (e.g. conjunctival injection, lacrimation, nasal congestion, rhinorrhea, sweating, miosis, ptosis, or eye edema)
- Frequency of attacks from 1 QOD - 8 QD
- Cycles last from 7days to 1 year and are separated by pain-free periods lasting ≥14days

CHRONIC CLUSTER H/A

- As above, except that cycles last >1year or are separated by remissions lasting < 14 days

GERIATRICS

URINARY INCONTINENCE ✪			
TYPE	**PRESENTATION**	**ASSOCIATED FINDINGS**	**PATHOPHYSIOLOGY**
STRESS	Small amounts of leaking with stress (*coughing, sneezing, laughing, or physical activity* such as bending)	Multiparity; Estrogen deficiency Prior urethral procedure or radiation	*Urethral* hypermobility; *internal sphincter deficiency*
URGE	*Sudden*, uncontrollable need to void resulting in loss of large amount of urine; *nocturia* and frequency also common	*Motor urgency:* CNS-related (CVA, Alzheimer's Dz, Parkinson's Dz, MS); spinal cord pathology; *Sensory urgency:* local bladder pathology or sudden ↑ in bladder volume (diuretic or glycosuria)	*Abnormal bladder contractions*; due to *detrusor instability* in a large % of these patients.
OVERFLOW	Poor stream, straining, dribbling, although may present similar to urge or stress incontinence	*Obstruction* (BPH, fecal impaction, tumor); *Chronic bladder overdistension* (such as from DM or detrusor areflexia)	**Bladder** *overdistension*

MEDS ASSOCIATED WITH URINARY INCONTINENCE:		
CLASS	**MECHANISM OF ACTION**	**TYPE OF INCONTINENCE**
α **agonists;** β **blockers**	$\uparrow$ tone of internal sphincter leading to *obstruction*	Overflow
α **blockers**	$\downarrow$ tone of internal sphincter leading to *leakage*	Stress
Anticholinergics; and Calcium channel blockers	$\downarrow$ bladder *contractions*	Overflow
Diuretics	Brisk filling of the bladder	Urge
Sedatives/hynotics/opiates/alcohol	Produce confusion; $\downarrow$ bladder contractions Depress central inhibition of micturition	Functional overflow

Agents that $\downarrow$ Bladder Contractility and Are Therefore Useful in URGE Incontinence	
AGENT	**ACTION**
ANTICHOLINERGICS (use limited by $\uparrow$side effects) ▪ Atropine ▪ L-Hyoscyamine ▪ Propantheline	Antagonize muscarinic receptors of the bladder, causing relaxation
ANTICHOLINERGIC + ANTISPASMODICS ▪ Oxybutinin (**Ditropan®, Ditropan XL®**) ▪ Dicyclomine (Bentyl®, etc.) ▪ Flavoxate (**Urispas®**) ▪ Tolterodine (**Detrol®**)	Additional smooth muscle relaxing properties
TCAs (drugs of choice for *mixed incontinence*) ▪ Amitriptylline (Elavil®) ▪ Doxepin (Sinequan®) ▪ Imipramine (Tofranil®)	Both anticholinergic and α-agonist effects
CCBs ▪ Nifedipine	Relax muscles through calcium influx blockage into cells; also probably anticholinergic effect

Agents that ↑ Urethral Resistance and are Therefore Useful in <u>STRESS</u> Incontinence:	
AGENT	**ACTION**
α-agonists • Ephedrine • Phenylpropanolamine	Affect symp innervation to the proximal urethra, causing ↑ pressure
TCAs	Both anticholinergic and α-agonist effects
Estrogen (hormone replacement therapy)	Thought to improve vaginal and urethral vascularity and tone

THE EFFECT OF AGE ON VARIOUS LABS ✪		
↑ WITH AGE	**↓ WITH AGE**	**NO EFFECT WITH AGE**
Alk phos	Serum albumin	Bilirubin
Uric acid	Serum Mg	AST, ALT, GGTP
Total cholesterol	PaO2	pH, PaCO2
HDL	Creat clearance	Serum creatinine
Triglycerides	T3, TSH	T4
Fasting blood glucose; 1h postprandial glucose; 2h postprandial glucose	WBC	Hgb, Hct, platelets, RBC indices
ESR	Vit B12	
	CPK	

✪ SLEEP PATTERNS ASSOCIATED WITH NORMAL AGING

- ☞ No change in sleep requirements
- ☞ ↑ Nocturnal awakenings
- ☞ ↑ Sleep latency
- ☞ ↓ Deep sleep
- ☞ ↓ REM sleep
- ☞ ↓ Sleep efficiency
- ☞ Advanced sleep-wake cycle (earlier bedtime and arising time)

NARCOLEPSY
- ➢ Abnormal REM sleep regulation leads to...
  - o *Excessive daytime sleepiness with involuntary daytime sleep episodes*, disturbed nocturnal sleep, and *cataplexy* (sudden weakness or loss of muscle tone without loss of consciousness that is elicited by emotion) are the most common symptoms of narcolepsy.
  - o *Hypnagogic hallucinations* occur upon falling asleep
  - o *Hypnopompic hallucinations* and *sleep paralysis* occur upon awakening

MIXED URGE/STRESS INCONTINENCE
✓ 1/3 of incontinent older women have *mixed urge/stress incontinence*. The most appropriate initial management is behavioral therapy with pelvic muscle exercises and bladder training.

CATARACTS
✓ Know that older pts with cataracts can have normal visual acuity and yet have various types of functional visual impairment, such as *nighttime glare and disorders of depth and contrast perception often associated with falls even in the face of normal visual acuity*, which is therefore inadequate to assess the total impact of a cataract on vision.

ANEMIA
✓ Know that the presence of mild anemia associated with low serum Fe and TIBC strongly suggests *Anemia of Chronic Disease*.

SUBCORTICAL DEMENTIAS
✓ e.g. Parkinson's Dz; low-pressure hydrocephalus; M.I.D (multi-infarct dementia)
✓ Characterized by *prominent motor* abnormalities and *by changes in mood, personality, impulse control, and difficulty with planning.*

CORTICAL DEMENTIA
✓ e.g. Alzheimer's Dz
✓ characterized by disturbances in higher cortical functions that include language, calculation, visuospatial skills, and praxis (ability to follow commands)

CAPACITY
✓ Recognize that patients with dementia can still make some of their own decisions, even if e.g., they may be legally incompetent to manage their own financial affairs. Patients with dementia are frequently found by physicians, nurses , and social workers to be **capable of making their own decisions**. So, for example, if you had such a patient with Advance Directives, these directives do not go into effect until he or she is no longer able to make her own decisions, so her current, expressed wishes should be adhered to, even if there is disagreement among family members.
✓ Remember, a person's current wishes (if pt has capacity) preempt his or her **Advance Directives**, which in turn preempt (if there is no capacity) the wishes of a previously designated **Health Care Proxy**. When all else fails and we have none of the aforementioned, the physician can exert **Substituted Judgment**.
✓ "Consult the hospital ethics committee" is usually not the answer. They want *you* to know these basic principles.

MULTI-DISCIPLINARY APPROACH
✓ On the exam it is important to recognize this in developing a care plan early in the hospital course for a frail older person who is functionally impaired.

DELIRIUM

- Be able to recognize that the sudden change in behavior of a patient with dementia and multiple medical problems may be the onset of delirium, which requires a thorough medical evaluation.
- Remember this Mnemonic for the causes of "*DELIRIUM*": **D**rugs—**E**lectrolyte imbalance—**L**ow pCO_2—**I**nfection—**R**elapsing fever—**I**njury to brain—**U**remia—**M**etabolic (liver damage)
- Keep in mind the key differences between Cortical Dementia and Delirium:

FEATURE	DEMENTIA	DELIRIUM
Onset	Insidious	Sudden
Duration	Chronic	Acute
Speech	OK	Slurred
Attention	OK	Impaired
Perception	OK	Hallucinations common
Mood/affect	Apathetic/loss of impulse control	Fear/suspiciousness often present

HALLUCINATIONS

- ✓ Visual—often organic in origin; e.g. delirium
- ✓ Auditory—usually inorganic in origin; think of schizophrenia

MAJOR DEPRESSION—DIAGNOSTIC CRITERIA:

- ✓ At least 5 of the following occurring each day during a 2 wk period, representing a change from previous function: (#1 or #2 is a required criterion) and not due to medication or other condition:
    1. Depressed mood most of the day
    2. Anhedonia
    3. Unintended change in weight or appetite
    4. Insomnia/Hypersomnia
    5. Psychomotor agitation/retardation
    6. Fatigue or loss of energy
    7. Feelings of worthlessness or inappropriate guilt
    8. Diminished ability to think/concentrate/make decisions
    9. Recurrent thoughts of death or suicide

REHABILITATION

- Be able to recognize the most appropriate management of hospital discharge of a severely functionally impaired older patient who need rehab to recover functional ability.
- e.g. to an extended care facility, such as a nursing home with an on-site facility or a hospital based transitional care or rehabilitation unit.
- Often the hospital's emphasis is on an expedient discharge to the first nursing home with an available bed when the patient has rehabilitation potential.

8. ALLERGY & IMMUNOLOGY

SYMPTOMS AND SIGNS OF ANAPHYLAXIS
1. Bronchospasm; laryngeal edema
2. Diffuse erythema
3. Hypotension
4. Nausea & Vomiting
5. Sense of warmth
6. Urticaria/Angioedema

TREATMENT OF ANAPHYLAXIS
1. Epinephrine .3ml of 1:1000 s.c.
2. Antihistamines to block the effects of further histamine release, control hypotension & reduce swelling.
3. Diphenhydramine (Benadryl®) IM/IV & continue PO x 48h q6h to prevent recurrence.
4. IV fluids, especially NS or plasma expanders for signs hypotension.
5. Corticosteroids-- while no help for acute attack, they diminish subsequent reactions.
6. Tracheostomy, O2, Aminophylline as needed

MAIN CAUSES OF ANAPHYLACTIC REACTIONS
1. 75% due to PCN
2. 15% due to *Hymenoptera* stings (bees, yellow jackets, hornets, wasps)
3. Reactions to latex and foods account for much of the rest

- Remember, when a patient is allergic to PCN, s/he is usually allergic to the beta-lactam ring. *Other beta-lactam antibiotics* include cephalosporins, monobactams, and carbapenams.
- In patients who are allergic to PCN, approximately 5% will develop an allergic reaction if challenged with a cephalosporin.

- ✪ Main cause of *__Anaphylactoid__* reactions is *__Radiocontrast Media__* (75% of cases)
- ✪ Remember, anaphylactoid reactions resemble anaphylaxis reactions in most ways, except they *are not mediated by specific Ab (e.g. Ig E)*
- ✪ Because they are not mediated by IgE, skin tests are useless

---

RADIOCONTRAST MEDIA REACTIONS ✪
1. Anaphylactoid reaction 2° to high osmolality of contrast media
2. No Ig E involved
3. No association with shellfish allergy or iodine
4. If patient had a bad reaction in the past, s/he has a 20-35% risk of a similar reaction on reexposure to these media.
5. A combination of Prednisone/Diphenhydramine/Ephedrine can prevent ~90% of these reactions. Lower osmolar media are also better received.

CAUSES OF ANAPHYLACTOID REACTIONS ✪

1. Radiocontrast media
2. Medications (ASA or NSAIDs; narcotics; protamine vancomycin)
3. Dialysis
4. Physical stimuli (cold, exercise)
5. Plasma expanders
6. Transfusion reactions

✪ IMMUNE REACTIONS—Types I, II, III, and IV		
TYPE	**MEDIATORS**	**EXAMPLES**
I **Immediate hypersensitivity** (*wheal-and-flare*)	Specific IgE antibody	*Allergic rhinitis Anaphylaxis; asthma urticaria*
II **Cytotoxic**	Cytotoxic cells or specific Ab plus complement	*Goodpasture's Graves' disease Myasthenia Gravis Immune hemolytic anemia and thrombocytopenia*
III **Immune complex** (*Arthrus rxn*)	Specific IgG/M which complexes with circulating Ag and then complement	*R.A.; SLE; Hep B viral prodrome; serum sickness*
IV **Delayed hypersensitivity** (*cell-mediated*)	Specific T-cells that release lymphokines	*Contact Dermatitis GVHD Response to TB/fungal/ viral infections PPD testing*

✪ COMMON EXAMPLES OF CONTACT DERMATITIS	
ALLERGEN	**IMPORTANT EXAMPLES**
☞ Ethylenediamine (part of aminophylline)	✓ Dyes, fungicides
☞ K+ Dichromate	✓ Cement, leather, household cleaners, bleaches
☞ Nickel sulfate	✓ Earrings, zippers, hairpins, door handles, silverwork, hair dyes & bleaches, insecticides, fungicides
☞ Paraphenylenediamine	✓ Hair dyes, fur dyes, chemicals used in photographic work
☞ Thiuram	✓ Rubber products, fungicides, insecticides
☞ Rhus	✓ Poison ivy/poison oak
☞ Latex	✓ Gloves, elastic, condoms
☞ Nail polish	✓ E.g. eyelid dermatitis from scratching
☞ Neomycin	

ATOPIC DERMATITIS
1. High IgE associated
2. Depressed cell-mediated immunity
3. Patients tend to have a significant family history of allergic-type conditions, including allergic rhinitis, asthma, and eczema.

IN ORDER TO HAVE ASTHMA, YOU NEED 3 THINGS:
1. Reversible airway obstruction (as measured by PEFR or FEV1)
2. Airway inflammation
3. Airway hyperresponsiveness

✪ USUAL ALLERGENS IN ALLERGIC RHINITIS BY TIME OF YEAR		
Seasonal	**Springtime**	Tree and grass pollen
	Fall	Ragweed
Perennial		Dustmites; animal dander; molds

KEY INDOOR ALLERGENS → Dust mites, cockroaches, cats, dogs, and mold

KEY OUTDOOR ALLERGENS → Trees, grass, ragweed, and molds

✪ RAST TESTING

1. Measures specific IgE to various Ag

2. More specific, but less sensitive than skin testing, therefore RAST is indicated in those individuals who are so exquisitely sensitive to an Ag that skin testing may yield a systemic reaction.

3. RAST is also appropriate in patients who are unable to discontinue certain medications that would otherwise affect skin testing results.

HEREDITARY ANGIOEDEMA (HANE)

➤ Autosomal dominant deficiency or malfunction of C_1 esterase inhibitor (C_1INH)

➤ Recurrent attacks of nonpruritic angioedema involving the skin and mucosa of the upper respiratory and GI tracts.

➤ Death from laryngeal edema may occur in as many as a quarter of the patients

➤ Not associated with urticaria

➤ Family history is positive in 80% of patients

➤ Treatment: attenuated androgens (danazol or stanozolol)

IMMUNODEFICIENCY DISEASES ☉

DEFECT OR DEFICIENCY	CLINICAL EXAMPLES
B CELLS	➢ Recurrent infections with extracellular, encapsulated bacteria
	➢ *IgA deficiency* [most patients asymp; if symptomatic, may see GI or Pulm infections; remember also to take great care with transfusions since IgA-deficient patients are at increased risk of anaphylaxis from immunoglobulin infusions as well as blood transfusions (washed packed cells should be given if transfusion is needed)].
	➢ X-linked agammaglobulinemia
T CELLS	➢ TB, fungal, pneumocystis, toxoplasmosis infections; DiGeorge syndrome (deficient thyroid and parathyroids)
NEUTROPHILS	➢ Chronic granulomatous disease; ➢ Chediak Higashi disease
COMPLEMENT *Terminal components* *C3* *C6,7* *C1esterase inhibitor*	 ➢ Recurrent neisseria infections ➢ Pyogenic infections ➢ Raynauds phenomena ➢ Hereditary angioedema

MEDICATIONS THAT CAN INTERACT WITH GRAPEFRUIT JUICE:
(shared CYP3A4 metabolism)
- ❖ Antihistamines (ebastine, terfenadine)
- ❖ Calcium channel blockers (felodipine, nimodipine, nisolodipine, nitrendipine, pranidipine)
- ❖ Amiodarone
- ❖ Immunosuppressants (cyclosporine, tacrolimus)
- ❖ HMG-CoA reductase inhibitors
- ❖ Methadone
- ❖ Psychiatric meds (buspirone, carbamazepine, triazolam, midazolam, diazepam)
- ❖ Sildenafil
- ❖ Saquinavir (protease inhibitor)

9.   CARDIOLOGY PART I:
ELECTROCARDIOGRAPHY PEARLS PLUS!

HERE'S THE _EASY_ WAY TO FIGURE THE AXIS!

Look at the direction of the R-wave in leads I and aVF:

	I	aVF
Normal axis ("2 thumbs up")	↑	↑
LAD	↑	↓
RAD	↓	↑
Extreme RAD	↓	↓

CAUSES OF TALL R-WAVE (R>S) IN V1 OR V2:
1. Dextrocardia
2. Hypertrophic cardiomyopathy
3. Posterior wall MI
4. RBBB
5. RVH
6. WPW→√ for delta wave
7. RAD (right axis deviation)→check the axis!
8. Rotation of heart (5% of population)
9. Normal variant among young females

DDX OF ↑QTc (differential dx of increased calculated QT interval):
1. Ischemia: #1 cause
2. ↓Mg, ↓K+, ↓Ca; ↓thyroid
3. Pentamidine
4. Tricyclic antidepressants; Pheonothiazines
5. IA Antiarrhythmics (e.g. PDQ: procainamide; disopyramide; quinidine)
6. Amiodarone
7. Any combination of Seldane with erythromycin/azoles (e.g. ketoconazole)/lovastatin

---

PEARL: **QTc:** Even though the 'c' stands for <u>c</u>alculated, you should really think of it as '<u>c</u>orrected' for the heart rate—because imagine the heart rate was at 300: the QT would be very short indeed! The QTc therefore takes the heartrate into account.

⇒ **THEREFORE,** remember the **RULE OF THUMB to recognize ↑ QTc:** If the QT interval (whatever the rate) is more than half the R-R interval, then the QT is prolonged.

PEARLS:

➤ A **true 'pause'** is defined as ≥ 3s between 2 adjacent R-waves in symptomatic patients; >5s if asymptomatic

➤ The QT interval is inversely proportional to the serum calcium: ie hypercalcemia → short QT; hypocalcemia → long QT. QT is important because it **can progress to Torsades** (de Pointes) which can in turn progress to VT.

➤ **Digoxin** can: ↑PR, and ↓QTc; but **Quinidine** can ↑ all the intervals. **K+ can:** 1) flatten the PR; 2) broaden the QRS; and 3) peak the 'T'-waves. In severe cases, you may see a 'sign-wave' that can progress to asystole.

➤ Generally speaking, **rhythm** is best read by √ing V1, except if Afib or Aflutter, when rhythm is best made out in the inferior leads, and **intervals** are best read at lead II.

➤ **You can't read ST-T wave changes in AFib or Aflutter.**

➤ The only time *aVR* helps is in *pericarditis* where ST depression (*"bent knee" sign*) may sometimes be found. *Beware too*: the disappearance of pain may sometimes signal a new pericardial effusion.

NON-Q-WAVE MI

➤ Formerly 'subendocardial' infarction
➤ Due to a critical lesion that forms a thrombus which is effectively lysed by the patient's own fibrinolytic cascade, but is present long enough to cause necrosis that is primarily subendocardial and does not involve the full thickness of the myocardial wall.
➤ EKG: ST ↓ (don't confuse for ischemia!); no Q-waves

CORRELATING KEY INFORMATION IN ACUTE M.I.		
M.I.	**KEY LEADS**	**USUAL CULPRIT ARTERY**
Anteroseptal	V1-V3	LAD
Anterolateral	V4-V6, I, L	Circumflex
Inferior	II, III, F	RCA
RV infarction	Right sided precordial leads V4R to V6R,esp. ST elevation, in V4R	RCA
Posterior	Reciprocal ST↓ in V1-V3; tall R waves V1, V2	RCA or circumflex

- **PEARL**: Remember, you always have to repeat the EKG in chest pain syndromes to check for motion up or down of the ST segment (this is true also for T-wave inversion). Any movement is *usually* indicative of <u>ischemia</u>. On the other hand, *no* movement/resolution of an ST segment elevation or a T-wave inversion, given the proper scenario, may be indicative of <u>infarction</u> (could also be pericarditis, LV aneurysm, among others).

CHIEF CAUSES OF ST DEPRESSION
1. **Non-Q-wave M.I. (formerly 'subendocardial')—usually flat ST depression**
2. **Positive Stress Test (ischemia)**
3. Digoxin (concave or 'scooped-out' appearance)

EKG in POSTERIOR WALL MI
1. Tall R-waves V1-V2 (clinically defined as R>S)
2. Upsloping ST depression in V1-V2
3. Usually associated with signs of inferior MI

GENERAL PROGRESSION OF EKG FINDINGS IN ACUTE M.I.
1. First, hyperacute **T**-waves
2. Then, see **ST** elevations
3. Finally, **Q**-waves form

HYPERACUTE T-WAVES
1. M.I.
2. ↑K+
3. Normal Variant
4. LBBB

U-WAVES
1. Follows the T wave and is inverted just like the letter "U".
2. May be a normal variant; or
3. 2° to electrolyte imbalance

CAUSES OF AN ELEVATED ST SEGMENT
1. Pericarditis (diffuse, concave ST ↑; PR depression often noted)
2. Coronary spasm (Prinztmetal's angina, aka 'variant' angina)
3. Ventricular aneurysm
4. ↑K+
5. Ischemia
6. LVH
7. LBBB
8. Early repolarization
9. CHF

SOME CAUSES OF PATHOLOGICAL 'Q' WAVES
(≥1mm wide or ≥one-third of the entire QRS amplitude)
1. Cardiac contusion; myocarditis
2. Hyperkalemia
3. Hypertrophic CMP
4. LBBB
5. Poor lead placement
6. Transmural MI
7. WPW ('pseudoinfarction')

POOR R-WAVE PROGRESSION
1. In general, the height of the R-wave should ↑ as one moves across the precordium from V1→V6.
2. Normally, you should see an R-wave height of 3mm by V3, or 4mm by V4
3. If V3R>V4R, that's called "regression", and that's usually evidence of infarct.
4. Beware, however, that an EKG taken during a prolonged inspiration (heart moves away from chest wall leads) can simulate this, so should repeat on normal breathing.

ABSENT 'P' WAVES
1. A Fib
2. Sino-atrial block
3. Severe ↑K+

CAUSES OF LOW-VOLTAGE EKG
1. Calibration off
2. Obesity→other tissue
3. Tamponade→pericardial space
4. Pericardial effusion→pericardial space
5. Cardiomyopathy / Myocarditis →heart
6. Global ischemia→heart
7. Breast tissue (lead placement)→other tissue

ANTIARRHYTHMIC CLASSIFICATION (Vaughn-Williams)

Ia	PDQ (Procainamide, Quinidine, Disopyramide)
Ib	Lidocaine
Ic	Encainide
II	Amiodarone
III	β-blockers (eg Propranolol)
IV	CCBs (ev Verapamil)

> **PEARL:** PACs *(Premature atrial contractions) have longer PR intervals than sinus beats and can be an early sign of occult CHF.*

ASHMAN'S PHENOMENON ("SHORT-LONG-SHORT")

- Refers to *the 3 R-R interval immediately preceding a PAC to help identify the complex as a PAC* (as opposed to a PVC), particularly in AFib or A Flutter. Remember too that a PAC has a longer PR interval than the sinus beat (2° to conduction delay).

✓ **Criteria for LAE**: Width **> 3 boxes** (.12 s) or notched P wave in the inferior leads or V1, V2; a biphasic P wave in V1 should also make you think of LAE.

✓ **Criteria for RAE**: Height **> 2.5 boxes** (0.25 mV; 2 ½ small boxes), esp in lead II

Can remember, "LEFT → LENGTH; RIGHT → HEIGHT"

CRITERIA FOR LVH:
1. R-wave in lead I ≥ 11mm
2. R-wave in aVL ≥ 12
3. *S in V1/2 + R in V5/6 ≥ 35* (really any 2 precordial leads)
4. S in V2 ≥ 25
5. R in I + S in III ≥ 25

FOR RVH, LOOK FOR:
1. *Look for R>S in V1/2*
2. *Look for S>R in V5/6*

But you must first rule out...
1. RBBB (below)
2. LPHB (below)
3. Anterolateral or inferior wall MI

MORE PEARLS YOU HAVE TO KNOW...

- **PEARL:** If you see true **angina + ST↑ ≥1mm in ≥ 2 anatomiclly contiguous limb leads** AND **ST↑ ≥1mm in ≥ 2 contiguous precordial leads** AND **t <12h** from symptom onset, or if you **see angina + new BBB→ THROMBOLYTICS** are justified in the ER setting
- **Absolute contraindications** include:
1. Prior intracranial bleed or CNS tumor;
2. Recent prolonged CPR;
3. Active internal bleeding;
4. CVA or head trauma within the previous 6 months;

> **Relative contraindications** include:
> 1. GIB within 1 month
> 2. Surgery or trauma in the past 2 weeks
> 3. Pregnancy
> 4. BP >200/110

- **PEARL:** Remember that *any* Q-waves—even so-called 'baby' Q-waves, in leads **V1 or V2 are significant**.

- **PEARL:** **Routine/prophylactic use of Lidocaine peri-MI** should not be practiced as it can actually ↑ mortality, if used indiscriminately, and should only be used in patients who show evidence of VT.

- **PEARL:** When see **akinesia or severe hypokinesia** on echo, you must consider **coumadin to prevent thrombus formation/emboli**.

- **PEARL:** You cannot include a **'lateral' component to an inferior wall MI** if there are only T-wave inversions laterally (must have either ST↑ or Q-waves).

- **PEARL:** *Because* **RV infarction can complicate inferior wall MI**, *right-sided EKG should always be checked in cases of IWMI*, looking for ST ↑ in leads RV3 or RV4.

- **Suspect Right Ventricular Infarction when you see hypotension in the setting of an IWMI** (especially when preload-reducing agents like nitrates and diuretics have been given); additional signs include elevated JVD, distended liver, and clear lungs.

- **PEARL:** For a **posterior component** to the inferior wall MI, look at V1-2 for R>S &/or ST↓ ≥ 2mm. If IWMI + RBBB→can't use this; must do right-sided leads to R/O posterior wall MI.

- ☞ **TREATMENT FOR RV INFARCTION and posterior wall MI IS IV FLUIDS**
  → *usually 2 liters normal saline.*

  - ⇒ ***Do not give*** *Nitroprusside* (Nipride) to patients with RVI: it can markedly reduce the RV and therefore LV preload (primarily due to venodilatation) causing BP to drop dramatically. Efforts must be made to increase preload.

  - ⇒ The same goes for **Hypertrophic Cardiomyopathy** by the way. Diuretics, nitrates, and other vasodilators should be avoided since in HCM they will *increase* the obstruction.

PEARL: Remember to look for **T-wave inversions** ± **ST↓** (and never ST↑) in **UNSTABLE ANGINA**.

PEARL: Remember, **Digoxin** doesn't INVERT T-WAVES. **Ischemia** and infarction do.

PEARL: <u>**TO DIFFERENTIATE SVT WITH ABERRANCY versus VT**</u>,

- One can apply the principal of 'concordance' and 'discordance' fairly easily.

- *<u>Concordance</u>* is where all the main forces in the precordial leads (V1→V6) point in the same direction, i.e. all the R-waves point up or all point down. Concordance suggest *<u>VTach</u>*.

- *<u>Discordance</u>*, on the other hand, is where the main forces in those leads are not in agreement and do not all point in the same direction. Discordance is evidence of *<u>SVT with aberrancy</u>*.

- Another trick is to look for the start of the arrhythmia and see if you find a **PAC or PVC**. A PAC often precedes SVT with aberrancy, while a PVC often precedes VT.

PEARL: **DIGOXIN TOXICITY** can cause nearly every type of block. However, **<u>there are 2 that are the Sine Qua Non of Dig toxicity, namely:</u>**

   1)   **SA exit block;**

   2)   **PAT with 2:1 block**

However, there are 2 blocks that digoxin <u>never</u> causes:

   1)   **Mobitz II;**

   2)   **AFib**

PEARL: If you have a **<u>new BBB</u>** with an M.I., besides ASA and angioplasty/lytics/ etc., patient needs a **pacemaker**!

PEARL: **Pacemaker syndrome** is sometimes seen in patients with VVI pacemakers who, paradoxically, are short of breath at rest but relieved with exertion. EKG reveals retrograde P-waves.

BUNDLE BRANCH BLOCKS:

LAFB (Left Anterior Fascicular Block) (aka Left Anterior *Hemi*block)
1. QRS between .10-.12s
2. LAD > - 45°
3. *Small Q in I and L*
4. *Deep S inferiorly*
5. Small R inferiorly

LPFB (Left Posterior Fascicular Block; aka LAHB)
1. QRS between .10-.12s
2. RAD > +110°
3. *Small Q inferiorly*
4. *Deep S in I and L*
5. Small R in I and L

RBBB—see also next box
1. S wave in I
2. RSR′, T-wave inversion, and ST segment ↓ in V1-V3 (suspect ischemia or infarction is see T-wave inversion or ST↓ laterally)
3. S wave in V5,6
4. *May see ST ↑ inferiorly*.

LBBB-see also next box
1. RSR′, T-wave inversion, and ST segment↓ in I , L, and V4-6 (suspect ischemia or infarction is see T-wave inversion or ST↓ in V1-3)
2. S-waves inferiorly and V1-3
3. *ST↑ in V1-3*

Quickly! Is it a RBBB or LBBB? If the QRS is >0.12s, there is a BBB. You can tell if the BBB is a RBBB or LBBB by finding the location of the RSR′. Very simply, if it is at the right precordium, it is a RBBB. If it is to the left precordium, it is a LBBB.

⇒ Another perhaps even easier way is, once you've determined that the QRS is indeed >.12s and there appears to be a BBB, check the T-wave in V1. If the T-wave is upright, it's a LBBB. If the T-wave is inverted (down), you have a RBBB. A simple **mnemonic** to help you remember this is:
   "When you get RIGHT DOWN to it, it's LEFT UP to you!"

Complete Heart Block (CHB) **and AV Dissociation** (AVD):
♦ When the Atrial rate is faster than the Ventricular rate→that's **CHB**.
♦ When the Ventricular rate is faster than the Atrial rate→that's **AVD**.
♦ It's really semantics, though, because **BOTH NEED A PACEMAKER**.

AFIB AND CONVERTING TO NSR

- **If atria <5cm & AFib≤ 2 weeks**→may attempt to chemically convert without anticoagulation.
- **If atria < 5cm & Afib present for > 2 weeks**→must give anticoagulation x 3weeks before and after converting
- **If atria > 5cm & AFib present > 2 weeks**→patient is less likely to convert successfully; therefore the goal is to control the ventricular response with, e.g. Digoxin.

IMPORTANT CAUSES OF CARDIOGENIC SHOCK FOLLOWING ACUTE MI:

1. **RV infarct**→give IV fluids
2. **VSD** (*holosystolic murmur* with parasternal *thrill* typical)→IABP (intra-aortic balloon pump)
3. **Papillary muscle rupture** (*apical holosystolic murmur; often associated with a thrill; bedside echo a simple way to differentiate this from VSD)*→IABP
4. **LV Wipeout** (Massive MI with 2° loss of ≥ 40% of LV)→IABP
5. **LV aneurysm**—seen in anterior MIs, another reason for warfarin x 3-6 mo post-MI; surgery for clinically significant decreases in cardiac output
6. **Free wall rupture** → nearly always fatal
7. **Tamponade** (free wall rupture can lead also lead to tamponade) → pericardiocentesis

INDICATIONS FOR IABP (Intra-Aortic Balloon Pump):

1. Cardiogenic Shock
2. VSD
3. Papillary Muscle Rupture
4. Refractory Unstable Angina
5. VTach presumed 2° to ischemia

UNSTABLE ANGINA

➢ The syndrome of unstable angina includes new onset or crescendo effort angina, rest angina, early post-myocardial infarction (MI) angina, variant angina, and angina occurring soon after percutaneous transluminal coronary angioplasty (PTCA) or coronary artery bypass graft surgery (CABG). The pathogenesis of this syndrome is thought to involve plaque rupture followed by thrombus formation.

➢ **INITIAL MEDICAL THERAPY:**

✓ Both **intravenous nitroglycerin** (5 to 10 μg/min, increasing as needed to 40 to 400 μg/min) and an **intravenous beta blocker** are given as antiischemic therapy for symptom control:
- 5 mg of metoprolol
- 1 mg of propranolol
- Esmolol infusion [50 μg/kg per min increasing to a maximum of 200 to 300 μg/kg per min]) with the goal being a decrease in heart rate to 60 beats/min.

✓ The combination of **aspirin and heparin** (given by intravenous infusion, not subcutaneous or intravenous bolus) reduces progression to MI and perhaps mortality . *Clopidogrel or ticlopidine* can be given to patients who cannot take aspirin because of gastrointestinal intolerance or hypersensitivity. *Low molecular weight heparin* is an alternative to heparin; it has at least equivalent efficacy, and is easier to administer and has a lower incidence of thrombocytopenia.

✓ The **glycoprotein IIb/IIIa inhibitors** abciximab, tirofiban, and eptifibatide are approved for use in patients with unstable angina. The ACC/AHA Task Force and the Sixth American College of Chest Physicians (ACCP) Consensus Conference on Antithrombotic Therapy recommend that these agents be administered, in addition to aspirin and unfractionated heparin, **to patients with unstable angina who**: 1) manifest continuing ischemia or 2) have other high-risk features; and 3) to patients in whom a percutaneous coronary intervention is planned. Generally speaking, though, glycoprotein IIb/IIIa inhibitors are not given to low risk UA patients (no ↑ in cardiac enzymes; no ST↓, chest pain resolved) or patients with no prior angina; no ergional or global LVD; and no perfusion defects.

✓ In post-infarct (within a few days) and post-PTCA (within 48h) angina, the patient should also be reevaluated at the cath lab.

➢ **SUBSEQUENT MANAGEMENT**:

The 2 general approaches, still in contention, are conservative and invasive:.

✓ The conservative approach advocates that patients who become asymptomatic on the above medical regimen be given several days to "cool off," intravenous medications are discontinued within 48 hours, and, if the patient is still symptom free, exercise testing is performed, most often with some form of myocardial imaging, like nuclear or echo. Persistence of symptoms, symptom recurrence, or a positive stress test usually leads to prompt cardiac catheterization.

✓ The invasive approach advocates that all unstable angina undergo cath after initiating medical therapy and within 24 to 36 hours of admission.

✓ Generally, however, the *ACC/AHA recommends the following*:

  o All patients with unstable angina should be treated initially with a maximal medical regimen (including heparin, aspirin, and intravenous nitroglycerin).

  o Emergent catheterization is performed for prolonged episodes of angina unresponsive to medical therapy or for frequent recurrent episodes of ischemic chest pain.

  o All other patients who are candidates for revascularization should be considered for early angiography within the first 24 to 36 hours. Up to 15 percent of such patients have no significant coronary stenosis on angiography. Some of these patients may have coronary microvascular disease.

o As with stable angina, CABG is preferred over PTCA for the treatment of patients with left main coronary disease, severe three vessel disease, or severe two vessel disease involving the left anterior descending artery with left ventricular dysfunction

➢ In most cases, the in-hospital antiischemic medical regimen used to control symptoms, with the exception of intravenous nitroglycerin, should be continued after discharge to prevent recurrent ischemia. Sublingual or spray nitroglycerin should be given. And aspirin, of course, should be added. Lipid lowering is indicated even if there are only borderline high serum total or LDL-cholesterol concentrations. The goal serum LDL-cholesterol is less than 100 mg/dL.

VENTRICULAR BIGEMINY (i.e. PVC every other beat)—DDX
1. Hypoxia
2. Thyrotoxicosis
3. Electrolyte imbalance
4. pH ↑or ↑ (alkalosis/acidosis)
5. Ischemia

MAT (Multifocal Atrial Tachycardia)
1. *Heart rate usually >105*
2. *3 different P-wave morphologies*
3. *Seen in COPD classically and commonly*
4. Treatment is Verapamil and, of course, treating the underlying COPD (usually 2° to hypoxia)
5. *Don't give Digoxin (unless MAT progresses to Afib) because you can aggravate the arrhythmia.*

Wandering Atrial Pacemaker can look like MAT in that one can also see at least 3 P-wave morphologies. The key difference is in the rate. WAP rate is usually <95. Essentially, WAP is 'physiologic'; MAT is 'pathologic'.

Approach to the 'Skipped Beat': First, R/O blocked PAC. You'll identify the **blocked PAC** by noting that the P wave falls right in time/in sync with the other P-waves. Remember the Ashman's phenomenon. Once you've ruled out blocked PAC, you must R/O **Mobitz I** (Type I, 2° Heart Block, or "Wenckebach") by checking for ↑ing PR intervals (and ↓ing R-R intervals) just before the blocked beat.

COMMON CAUSES OF MOBITZ I (WENCKEBACK):
1. Digoxin toxicity

2. IWMI

MALIGNANT EFFUSIONS/TAMPONADE
- **In men→R/O** lung ca.
- **In women → R/O** breast ca.
- *Note also, melanoma and lymphoma also metastasize to the pericardium*

COMMON CAUSES OF BLOODY PERICARDIAL EFFUSIONS:
- Metastases
- Uremia
- TB

ADVANTAGES OF BETA-BLOCKERS IN CHRONIC CAD
1. Good control of stable angina, particularly exercise-related
2. Anti-HTN
3. Antiarrhythmic effects
4. Possible benefit in preventing sudden death, limiting MI size, or preventing the occurrence of MI should intense ischemia occur
5. Long-acting, reasonably cardioselective, reasonably inexpensive

INTERVENTIONS THAT HAVE BEEN SHOWN TO ↓ MORTALITY AFTER MI:
1. **ASA** →Aspirin should be administered at a dose of 160 to 325 mg as soon ASAP after onset of symptoms and continued at ≥75 mg/day indefinitely thereafter. Ticlopidine and clopidogrel are alternative anti-platelet options. Clopidogrel is generally preferred because of fewer side effects.
2. **Thrombolytics/angioplasty**
3. **Beta-blockers**→beware in those with severe asthma. Beta-blockers work by decreasing the myocardial wall stress and the cardiac work load. Remember to follow the PR interval (<.24), the HR (>45), the SBP (>100), and check for rales before each dose of IV Beta-blockade. (a 5-5-5mg IV metoprololol at >2 min intervals is commonly used). MI patients should be continued on Beta-blockers, advancing to 50mg PO q6h x1 day, and then to 100mg PO bid indefinitely as tolerated.
4. **ACE Inhibitor 3 days out** (only those with evidence of CHF or low EF% (≤40%) or cardiomegaly should remain on the ACEI)—these work to prevent so-called "remodeling" which can have an ill-effect following an MI.
5. **Statin** therapy initiated prior to discharge reduces 1-year mortality by 34% and reduce the risk of a recurrent MI up to 40% even in patients with average cholesterol levels.

- While *nitrates* relieve pain, i.e. ↓ morbidity, they *do not ↓ mortality*. Don't get fooled.
- *LV function* is the best prognosticator after MI.
- *Beta-blockers post-MI* have the greatest impact on survival in individuals with compensated CHF c/w those without CHF.

THE DIFFERENCE IN SURVIVAL AFTER M.I. ATTRIBUTABLE TO THESE INTERVENTIONS :
1. ASA→23%↑
2. Lytic therapy→20%↑
3. B-Blocker→ 9%↑
4. ACE Inhibitor 3 days out→7%↑

CARDIOLOGY II

COMMONLY ASKED MATERIAL ☺…

1. Recognize **Erythromycin** can ↑ digoxin levels as well as anticoagulant levels if used concomitantly; also ↑ risk of rhabodmyolysis when used in conjunction with lovastatin.

2. Usually several questions on **ASD**.

    a) Recognize that it gives a fixed split S2

    b) Biatrial enlargement on EKG

    c) Elevated pulmonary pressure

    d) 2 types: *secundum* (no endocarditis prophylaxis necessary; RAD) and *primum* (prophylaxis necessary; LAD); for primum (& VSD too), no prophylaxis is needed if ≥6 mo post-surgical repair.

3. Recognize the need for **Calcium Gluconate** in hyperkalemia with EKG changes. Severe hyperkalemia requires emergent treatment directed at minimizing membrane depolarization, shifting K^+ into cells, and promoting K^+ loss. In addition, exogenous K^+ intake and antikaliuretic drugs should be held. Administration of calcium gluconate decreases membrane excitability. The usual dose is 10 mL of a 10% solution infused over 2 to 3 min. The effect begins within minutes but is short-lived (30 to 60 min), and the dose can be repeated if no change in the electrocardiogram is seen after 5 to 10 min.

4. Know the treatment of **Unstable Angina**: ASA (preferred anti-platelet agent) + heparin (LMWH is ideal), beta-blockers, G 2b/3a inhibitor (high and intermediate risk U.A.), nitroglycerin, and oxygen. Generally speaking, if angina at rest and/or EKG evidence of ischemia persist despite 24 to 48 h of the comprehensive treatment described above, then cardiac catheterization should be performed

5. Recognize that **thrombolytics** can in fact be used in the elderly, even 80 yo or older, but know the contraindications in general for lytics.

6. Know which **anti-HTN meds** would be potentially dangerous (**increase the block**) in patients with preexisting increased PR/ QRS/ QTc intervals (i.e. already have block), e.g. Calcium Channel Blockers and the IA antiarrhythmics, etc.

7. Know the indications for a **CABG**: 3-vessel CAD with LV dysfunction; 2-vessel CAD with a proximal LAD stenosis; left main disease; and palliation of symptoms (angina)

8. Know that **Beta Blockers** have been definitely shown to decrease mortality and recurrence after an M.I.

9. Know that RV infarct and AV block are major complications following **Inferior Wall M.I.**

10. Recognize the **hemodynamics of RV Infarct and Tamponade** (e.g. equalization of pressures in tamponade):

	RA	PCWP	CO
RVI	↑↑	↓	↓↓
Tamponade	↑↑	↑↑	↓↓

11. Know the clinical manifestations of **tamponade**: hypotension; JVD with rapid "x" descent and attenuated "y" descent on examination of jugular venous pulsations; ***Kussmaul's sign; pulsus paradoxus***; narrow pulse pressure, tachycardia, ***electrical alternans***, and "distant" heart sounds. In pulsus paradoxus, the decrease in systolic arterial pressure that normally accompanies the reduction in arterial pulse amplitude during inspiration is accentuated (> 10 mmHg). The differential diagnosis for pulsus paradoxus includes pericardial tamponade, constrictive pericarditis, restrictive cardiomyopathy, COPD (exacerbation), asthma (exacerbation), superior vena cava obstruction, pulmonary embolus, hypovolemic shock, pregnancy, and obesity.

12. Be able to recognize **free wall rupture** following acute Anterior Wall M.I.; recognize ***PEA*** (Pulseless Electrical Activity) in this setting. The clinical presentation typically is a sudden loss of pulse, blood pressure, and consciousness while the EKG continues to show sinus rhythm. The myocardium continues to contract, but forward flow is not maintained as blood escapes into the pericardium.

13. Know that you can treat **papillary muscle rupture** (with secondary mitral regurgitation) following acute M.I. with a balloon pump.

14. Know also that an **intraaortic balloon bump (IABP)** can also be used to treat refractory unstable angina; VSD; cardiogenic shock; and VT presumed secondary to ischemia.

15. Recognize **calcific pericarditis** on a CXR.

16. Recognize that severe **dilated (congestive) cardiomyopathy** on lisinopril (or other ACE inhibitor) and diuretics would benefit from addition of digoxin.

17. Know that *quinidine, verapamil, thiazides, erythro, & amiodarone* can **increase digoxin level**.

18. Potential **toxicities of amiodarone** include: pulmonary fibrosis; hepatitis; thyroid dysfunction (so ✓ PFTs, LFTs, and TFTs !); optic neuropathy and/or optic neuritis; corneal deposits; photosensitivity; potentiates coumadin and increases digoxin level; prolongs PR, QRS, and most importantly QT, esp in combination with IA antiarrhythmics (quinidine, procainamide, disopyramide). *Hypotension* is the most common adverse effect occurring with intravenous amiodarone therapy. *Neurotoxicity* is the most common adverse effect occurring with oral amiodarone therapy.

19. Recognize when **nitroprusside** (Nipride®) would be indicated (and contraindicated!)

20. Usually several questions on **WPW...**

    ☞ Be able to recognize the <u>delta waves</u> on EKG, e.g. in a young man/athlete with syncope.

    ☞ ***Procainamide*** for rate control ***when these patients go into Afib or Aflutter***. Digitalis and intravenous verapamil are contraindicated in patients who have WPW syndrome plus AF, since these drugs can shorten the refractory period of the accessory pathway and can increase the ventricular rate, thereby placing the patient at increased risk for VF.

    ☞ ***Radiofrequency catheter ablation*** of bypass tracts is the treatment of choice in patients with <u>symptomatic</u> arrhythmias (not just anyone with WPW!).

☞ ***EKG findings*** in WPW syndrome: Short PR interval ; wide QRS complex; and slurring on the upstroke of the QRS produced by early ventricular activation over the bypass tract yielding the delta wave. Inferiorly, delta waves may appear as Q-waves, mimicking myocardial infarction—hence the term "pseudoinfarction" pattern.

21. Know that of all the **Goldman criteria** (re: preoperative), the S3 is the most important risk factor or prognosticator.

22. Complete heart block (third degree heart block and Mobitz II second degree block) as well as some symptomatic bradycardia→**pacemaker**.

23. RBBB + LAHB after acute M.I.→pacemaker.

24. Know the differential of "**Cannon 'a' waves**":
    a) The term implies atria contracting vs. a closed A-V valve
    b) DDx for true cannon a waves includes: Complete Heart Block; Vtach; and AV nodal tachycardia

25. Know when and why to use **adenosine** (re: can be diagnostic and therapeutic in SVT)

26. Know that we don't use **lidocaine** "prophylactically" anymore peri-MI as it can actually ↑ mortality.

27. Know indications for **cardioversion** in an awake individual→ arrhythmia causing low BP *with symptoms.*

28. Be able to recognize a **Roth spot** (re: the retinal finding from endocarditis/septic emboli).

29. Know who needs (or doesn't need!) **endocarditis prophylaxis**.

30. Usually no congenital heart disease questions, other than ASD and VSD

31. Recognize the presentation of **Malignant HTN**, especially schistocytes and mental status changes; nitroprusside is the drug of choice.

32. **ACE inhibitors** *contraindicated* in **pregnancy**; so is sulfa (unless she is HIV+ and develops PCP)

33. Recognize a classic case of **cholesterol emboli** post cardiac cath to renal arteries (acute ↑ creatinine; oliguria/anuria) and distal extremities (esp. toes).

34. Know that the **Low Molecular Weight Heparins**, like Lovenox or Fragmin, as alternatives to heparin, can be used in combination with ASA, for the treatment of both unstable angina and non-Q-wave MI, per AHA. (Fragmin=dalteparin, Lovenox= enoxaparin)

35. Know that a **pregnant woman** would use **SQ Heparin** for her anticoagulation, dose-adjusted.

36. Know what to do for a **pulsating abdominal mass**, say 2, 4, and 6 cm (using cutoffs of 3 and 5.5 cm).
    3cm asymp AAA → U/S or CT q 6-12 mo. *Screening U/S for male smokers starting at 65yo.*

37. Should know how to adjust Heparin in **DVT management** based on PTT, when to start Coumadin (≤ PTT therapeutic but after initiating heparin of course), and when to stop Heparin (INR therapeutic).

38. Changes in **Cardiac Physiology during 3rd trimester** of Pregnancy:
    ↑: Blood *volume*, Cardiac *Output* (so easier to remember also ↑ stroke *volume* and heart rate)
    ↓: SVR (systemic vascular resistance)

CARDIOLOGY   NOTES

COMPLICATIONS BY SITE OF MI
✪ *Anterior MI*
1. Ventricular arrhythmias
2. LV aneurysm
3. Free wall rupture; VSD
4. Mobitz II

✪ *Inferior MI*
1. Bradycardias, CHB
2. Papillary muscle dysfunction (common) or rupture (rare)
3. Associated RV infarction
4. Mobitz I

✪ ANTICOAGULATION IN NONVALVULAR AFIB: CURRENT RECOMMENDATIONS

RISK STATUS	Age < 65	Age 65-75	Age >75
Risk factors for CVA	Warfarin	Warfarin	Warfarin
No risk factors	ASA	Warfarin *or* ASA	Warfarin

✪ DDx of AFIB: PIRATE SHIP :

P ericarditis   **S** ick Sinus Syndrome
I schemia   **H** TN (#1 cause)
R heumatic heart disease   **I** diopathic (eg Lone AFib)
A trial myxoma   **P** E
T hyrotoxicity
E thanol

NYHA (NY Heart Association) Criteria for Assessing Cardiorespiratory Capacity
1. NYHA I—Dyspneic only on severe exertion
2. NYHA II--Dyspneic walking up hills, stairs
3. NYHA III-Dyspneic walking on level ground
4. NYHA IV-Dyspneic at rest

EFFECTS OF CAROTID SINUS MASSAGE OR ADENOSINE (Diagnostic And Therapeutic)
1. **A tach/A flutter/A fib** → AV block (can slow down the rhythm temporarily so you can check for the presence and pattern of any P waves)
2. **PSVT** → Termination/NSR (Normal Sinus Rhythm)
   - Included in this group are typical AV nodal reentrant tachycardia (AVNRT), AV reciprocating tachycardia with a concealed bypass tract, and AV reciprocating tachycardia (AVRT) in WPW.
3. **Sinus Tach*** → Transient slowing; re: max heart rate in sinus tach = 220 - (patient's age)
4. **VT** → No effect

TYPES OF PULSES

1. **Alternans** (alternating weak and strong pulses)→ CHF, rapid respiratory rates, tamponade
2. **Bisferiens** (A pulse waveform with two upstrokes during systole)→ AI, combined AS and AI, hypertrophic cardiomyopathy, hyperkinetic circulation
3. **Dicrotic** (first peak in systole, second peak in diastole) → Hypotension, hypovolemic shock, fever with decreased SVR, severe CHF, tamponade,
4. **Collapsing**→AI, IHSS, exercise, fever, patent ductus arteriosus
5. **Jerky**→IHSS (hypertrophic cardiomyopathy)
6. **Paradoxus** ✪→Tamponade; constrictive pericarditis; asthma
7. **Plateau/tardis/brevis** → AS

DDx OF IRREGULARLY IRREGULAR PULSE (i.e. not just AFib!)

1. A Fib, A Tach or A Flutter with varying block
2. MAT; WAP (wandering atrial pacemaker)
3. PVCs
4. Sinus Arrhythmia

PRESSURE WAVE FORMS (or JVP) ON RIGHT HEART CATH ✪ :

1. **Normal**
   - ☞ 'a' wave→   Right **a**trial contraction
   - ☞ 'x' descent→   Atrial rela**x**ation
   - ☞ 'c' wave →   Tricuspid **c**losure
   - ☞ 'v' wave→   **V**entricular contraction
   - ☞ 'y' descent→   Fall in RA pressure (tricuspid opening)

2. **Abnormal 'a' wave**
   - Absent→A Fib
   - F waves (sawtooth waves) → A flutter
   - **Large 'a' waves** (RA contracting against an ↑ resistance)
     - i. TS
     - ii. ↑ Resistance to RV filling
       - (a) Pulm HTN
       - (b) PS
     - iii. **CANNON 'a' WAVES** ✪ (*giant a waves due to the simultaneous contraction of atrium and ventricle while the tricuspid valve is closed*)
       - (a) Regular→ AV nodal tachycardia
       - (b) Irregular→ **CHB; VT**

4. **Elevations in the 'v' wave**
   - a. TR classic; severe MR
   - b. Volume overload to LA, eg from VSD
5. **RAPID 'Y' DESCENT**→TR
6. **Slow/absent 'y' descent** (obstruction to RV filling)→ tamponade; TS
7. **RAPID 'X' DESCENT** ✪→ constrictive pericarditis classic; tamponade
8. **Fixed elevation**→SVC syndrome
9. **Absent Hepatojugular reflux**→IVC obstruction, or Budd Chiari Syndrome
10. **KUSSMAUL'S SIGN** ✪→Paradoxical rise in JVD with inspiration (eg **constrictive pericarditis or right ventricular infarction**, where the heart is unable to adequately accommodate the volume; rare in tamponade)

KEY HEMODYNAMIC FINDINGS ON SWAN-GANZ ✪

CONDITION	CVP (RAP)	PCWP	SVR	CO
Hypovolemia	↓	↓	↑	↓
R + LVF	↑	↑	↑	↓
Neurogenic Shock	↓	↓	↓	↓/NL
PE	↑/NL	NL	↑	↓
RVI	↑	↓	↑	↓
Sepsis	↓	↓	↓	↑
Tamponade*	↑	↓/NL	↑	↓

Remember equalization of pressures can also be seen in tamponade (as well as severe constrictive pericarditis.

➢ CVP (=Right Atrial Pressure; 0-6 mm Hg is normal)
  o **DDx of ↑ CVP (>6):**
    ✓ RV Failure
    ✓ LVF with concurrent RFV
    ✓ TR
    ✓ Tamponade
    ✓ Constrictive pericarditis

➢ **PULMONARY ARTERY PRESSURES** (PA Systolic and PA Diastolic; PAD is important one since it approximates the wedge if the pulmonary vasculature is normal)
  o **DDx of ↑ PAD (>12):**
    ✓ High pulmonary vascular resistance
      ▪ Pulm HTN ± cor pulmonale
      ▪ PE
    ✓ VSD
    ✓ LVF

➢ Generally, the LVEDP ≈ LAP ≈ PCWP ≈ PAD
  o **DDx of ↑ WEDGE (PCWP > 12) :**
    ✓ LVF
    ✓ Mitral stenosis; Mitral regurg (pronounced V wave on PAS/PAD tracing)
    ✓ Pericardial tamponade
    ✓ Poor LV compliance due to ischemia, infarction, or hypertrophy

➢ Cardiac Output (C.O.)
  o **DDx of ↓ C.O. (or ↓C.I.)**
    ✓ Ischemia, infarction
    ✓ MR, VSD

- o **DDx of ↑ C.O.** ("PASTA")
  - Paget's Disease
  - Anemia
  - Septicemia
  - Thyroid (hyper)
  - AVMs

NORMAL SWAN-GANZ VALUES
- Cardic Index   2.4-3.8 L/min/m^2
- CVP   0-6
- PAD   5-12
- PAS   15-30
- PCWP   5-12
- RVDP   7-14
- RVSP   30-35

DDX OF A SOFT S1
1. 1st degree AV block
2. Cardiomyopathy, LVF
3. Large pericardial effusion
4. MR
5. MS with rigid valve

DDX OF LOUD S1
1. Mitral stenosis with mobile valve
2. Sinus tach (e.g. thyrotoxicosis)
3. WPW

TYPES OF SPLIT S2
1. ***Fixed split→ASD*** ✪
2. Loud A2→systemic HTN
3. Narrow split with loud P2→Pulmonary HTN
4. ***Paradoxical (P2 precedes A2) → LBBB; AS*** ✪
5. Physiologic—normally A2 is heard before P2, and this widens on inspiration.
6. Single S2 (inaudible A2)→calcific AS
7. Wide split with soft P2→Pulmonary Stenosis
8. Widely split→RBBB

DDx of "S3" *(true <u>S3</u> may be physiologic or 2° to CHF and is due to ventricular volume overload)*
1. Fixed split S2 in ASD
2. MS opening snap
3. MVP with mid-systolic click

- ***S4, incidentally,*** may be seen in ***xclt physical conditioning/HTN/CAD*** and is ***<u>2°</u> to ↓ventricular compliance to filling***.

S3 → *Markedly* **diminished LV diastolic function**
S4→ *Moderately* **diminished LV diastolic function**

SYSTOLIC MURMUR FOLLOWING AN MI ☻

1. Misdiagnosis→**Dressler's syndrome** (fever + pericarditis/pericardial rub seen weeks to months after transmural infarctions; ✓anti-*myocardial* antibody which is not to be confused with *another* AMA, anti-mitochondrial antibody of primary biliary cirrhosis)
2. **MR 2° to cardiac incompetence**
3. **Papillary muscle** dysfunction (common) > rupture > rupture of chordae tendinae (uncommon)
4. Ruptured interventricular septum (**VSD**)→check for harsh murmur palpable thrill

KEY PHYSICAL FINDINGS IN MS ☻

1. A *diastolic rumble* that increases with exercise and is heard best in the left lateral decubitus position
2. *Presystolic augmentation* of the rumble
3. *Opening snap*
4. *Loud S1*
5. Elevated JVD
6. Malar flush
7. Peripheral cyanosis

SIGNS INDICATIVE OF SEVERE MS

1. Graham-Steel murmur (functional PI) or TI
2. Left atrial enlargement, RVH
3. *Length of diastolic murmur*
4. *Proximity of opening snap to S2* *(The closer the A2/OS interval, the tighter the valve)*
5. RV strain pattern, elevated RV pressures
6. Signs of pulmonary HTN/congestion

SIGNS INDICATING VALVE MOBILITY IN MS

1. Loud S1
2. Opening Snap

GENERAL PRINCIPLES IN MANAGEMENT OF MS ☻

1. *Endocarditis prophylaxis*
2. *Rate control for patients in AF*
3. *Anticoagulation* (if AF or have evidence of pulmonary or systemic embolization)
4. *Diuretics*
5. Percutaneous balloon mitral valve *commissurotomy*
   - Mitral **valvulotomy** is indicated in the symptomatic patient with pure MS whose effective orifice is < 1.0 cm^2. Over half of all patients undergoing mitral valvulotomy require reoperation by 10 years.
   - *Patients considered for **MVR** should have critical MS, i.e., an orifice < 0.6 cm^2/m^2 body surface area and be in the New York Heart Association class III, i.e., symptomatic with ordinary activity, despite optimal medical therapy.*

SEVERITY OF MS BY ECHO GRADING OF CROSS-SECTIONAL VALVE AREA
1. Valve area (in square cms) >2.5 →asymptomatic
2. Valve area 1.5-2.5→symptoms on exertion only
3. Valve area .5-1.5→symptoms at rest
4. Valve area < .5→"severe"

MANAGEMENT OF MITRAL STENOSIS IN PREGNANCY
> In the pregnant patient with MS, valvulotomy or valvuloplasty should be carried out if pulmonary congestion occurs despite intensive medical treatment. If severe mitral stenosis is identified *prior to pregnancy*, *valvulotomy should be carried out before conception*, if possible. Asymptomatic pregnant women with mitral stenosis simply require *close observation*. However, if symptoms of pulmonary congestion develop, *diuretics and restriction of activity* are indicated.

DDX OF THE MS DIASTOLIC MURMUR

1. *Austin-Flint murmur* ✪ (regurgitant jet in severe AI encroaches on the anterior leaflet of the mitral valve creating a relative mitral stenosis)

2. *Graham-Steel murmur* ✪ (severe **MS** + Pulm HTN→this PI murmur)

3. Flow murmurs in volume overload
   a) Severe MR
   b) VSD, PDA
   c) Renal failure

4. *LA myxoma* --see below.

LOCATIONS OF MURMURS

Valve	Usual Location of Murmur
Aortic	R. sternal border, 2nd ICS
Pulmonic	L. sternal border, 2nd ICS
Tricuspid	L. lower sternal border (LLSB)
Mitral	Apex and LLSB

LEFT ATRIAL MYXOMA
1. Loud or soft S1; *'tumor plop'*

2. *Pansystolic* murmur

3. Symptoms are postural, e.g. syncope

4. Mass seen on echo

5. DDx on echo…
   a) LA thrombus
   b) Large MV vegetation
   c) Thick or redundant MV leaflets

SYMPTOMS AS PROGNOSTICATORS IN AORTIC STENOSIS ✪

1. <u>A</u>ngina→death within 3-5years (if untreated)

2. <u>S</u>yncope→death within 2 years

3. Dyspnea→death within 1 year

4. Overt cardiac failure→death within 6mo.

PEARL: *The later the peak* of the systolic murmur→the <u>worse</u> the AS. Similarly, *the loss of S2* connotes a <u>worse</u> AS

PEARL: In AS, valve areas ≤ 0.7 cm^2 are considered "critical".

CLINICAL CORRELATES OF MVP ✪
1. ASD
2. IHSS
3. Ischemic or rheumatic heart disease
4. Marfan's syndrome; Ehlers-Danlos syndrome
5. PAN
6. PCO
7. WPW

INDICATIONS FOR VALVE REPLACEMENT IN AI
1. Symptoms
2. Declining exercise tolerance on stress testing
3. ↑ heart size on CXR
4. Development of LV strain pattern*
5. LV end-systolic diameter>55mm in an asymp patient as seen by echo
6. ↓ in EF% on echo or MUGA

   * A **strain pattern** is seen in LVH where there is a widening of the QRS with ST↓ and ⊥ (T-wave inversion) in leads V5 and V6.

CAUSES OF AI
1. Bicuspid AV
2. HTN
3. Valvulitis
    a) Rheumatic
    b) Infective
    c) Rheumatoid arthritis
4. Aortitis
    a) Syphilis
    b) Ankylosing Spondylitis

SOME INDICATIONS FOR *PERMANENT* PACING
1. Alternating RBBB and LBBB
2. Complete Heart Block
3. Drug-resistant tachyarrhythmias
4. Intermittent Mobitz II A-V block
5. Symptomatic bradyarrhythmias, e.g. SSS (Sick Sinus Syndrome)
6. Prolonged sinus pauses (> 3 seconds in symptomatic; > 5 seconds in asymptomatic),
7. Patients with a long QT interval, as a preventitive measure
8. Symptomatic patient with bi- or tri-fascicular block and prolonged H-V interval

INDICATIONS FOR *TRANSVENOUS* PACING IN ANTERIOR MI
1. 2° or 3° AVB
2. Alternating RBBB and LBBB
3. New bifascicular block in the setting of AMI
4. New LBBB with pre-existing 1°AVB
5. New RBBB with pre-existing 1° AVB/LAHB/LPHB

ACC/AHA Guidelines for Implantation of ICDs (Implantable Cardioverter-Defibrillator)
1. Cardiac arrest due to VF or VT not due to a transient or reversible cause
2. Spontaneous sustained VT
3. Syncope of undetermined origin with clinically relevant, hemodynamically significant sustained VT or VF induced at EPS when drug therapy is ineffective, not tolerated, or not preferred
4. Non-sustained VT with CAD, prior MI, LV dysfunction, and inducible VF or sustained VT at EPS that is not suppressible by a class I antiarrhythmic.

✪ **PEARL:** Following MI (esp in those with non-sustained VT), **EPS** (to study inducibility of VT) and checking for **late potentials** are excellent ***risk stratifiers for sudden death*** if they are negative. That is, they are valuable based on their ***negative predictive value***. This is the <u>same as D-dimers in DVT or PE when suspicion is low</u>, when normal D-dimers can help *rule out* disease.

ADVERSE PROGNOSTIC FINDINGS ON EXERCISE EKG STRESS TESTS ✪

1. ↑ in complex ventricular ectopy (along with ST-segment shifts)
2. Exercised-induced typical angina
3. Low peak heart rate (e.g. <120 bpm without pacemaker)
4. Low workload (e.g., <6.5 METs or 5-6min on Bruce protocol)
5. Marked ST segment depression (eg. **>2mm**)
6. Prolonged ST-segment depression (e.g. **>6min**) after exercise
7. SBP ↓ (e.g. >10mm Hg from baseline) or flat response (peak<130mm Hg)
8. ST-segment depression in multiple leads
9. ST-segment elevation without abnormal Q wave

CARDIAC SYNDROME X: MAIN CLINICAL FEATURES
(*Don't confuse with the other Syndrome X discussed in Endocrinology*)

- *Exercise-induced chest pain*, so + EST
- *Atypical features* of chest pain (e.g. prolonged episodes, poor response to sublingual nitrates)
- Negative stress echo
- *Normal coronary angiogram*
- Abnormal pain perception in many patients
- *Microvascular angina* in some patients
- Antianginals ineffective in ~ 50% of patients
- *Good prognosis* overall
- More common in women with estrogen deficiency than those without deficiency.
- Still somewhat ill-defined

FEATURES OF VALVULAR HEMOLYSIS
1. Signs of gross (para)valvular regurgitation
2. Normochromic normocytic anemia
3. Schistocytes on peripheral smear
4. ↓Haptoglobin with negative Coombs' test

INDICATIONS FOR TISSUE (PORCINE) VALVES
1. Any patient with absolute contraindication to anticoagulation
2. Elderly patient in NSR with normal size left atrium requiring MVR
3. Elderly patient requiring AVR
4. Young woman desiring pregnancy

- *Remember*, the key difference between tissue and prosthetic valves is that tissue valves don't require anticoagulation. While prosthetic valves require anticoagulation, these valves last much longer.

VERAPAMIL—ABSOLUTE CONTRAINDICATIONS:
1. Digoxin toxicity (re: dig ↑s the levels of quinidine or verapamil by 50%, and vice versa)
2. High degree AVB
3. Hypotension, heart failure
4. Sick Sinus Syndrome
5. Simultaneous IV Beta-blockers
6. WPW

CONTRAINDICATIONS TO DIGOXIN THERAPY
1. AVB
2. WPW; MAT
3. Prior to elective cardioversion
4. Constrictive pericarditis; acute myocarditis
5. Hypertrophic CMP in NSR

INDICATIONS FOR CHECKING SERUM DIGOXIN LEVEL
1. Suspected toxicity
2. Refractory Afib
3. Appearance of new arrhythmias
4. Change in renal function
5. Initiation of new treatment, esp. *quinidine/amiodarone/spironolactone/verapamil*.

ARRHYTHMIAS IN DIGOXIN TOXICITY
1. Most any bradycardia or block
2. **PAT with 2:1 block** ✪
3. Sino-atrial exit block

- *Never see*: Afib or Mobitz II from digoxin toxicity.

INDICATIONS FOR EPS ✪
1. Recurrent VT
2. To evaluate patients at high risk for VT
3. To evaluate the feasibility of catheter ablation
4. To determine response to antiarrhythmic medications
5. Recurrent SVT of unknown mechanism
6. Evaluation of unexplained syncope

DDX OF WIDE-COMPLEX TACHYCARDIA
1. SVT with aberrant conduction (see <u>discordance</u>)
2. VT (see <u>concordance</u>)
3. WPW with anterograde conduction (look for <u>delta waves</u>)

ASSOCIATIONS OF WPW
1. Male sex; familial
2. MVP
3. Thyrotoxicosis

✪ **Arrhythmias seen in WPW: PAT is by far the most common; Afib is #2. These account for the large majority. <u>Procainamide</u> is excellent at treating WPW with 2° Afib.**

EKG MANIFESTATIONS OF SSS ✪
1. <u>**Prolonged episodes of sinus bradycardia**</u>
2. Profound sinus arrhythmia with symptoms of tissue hypoperfusion
3. Periods of sinus arrest (>3s)
4. Junctional escape rhythms
5. <u>**'Tachy-brady' syndrome**</u> **(backround bradycardia punctuated by paroxysmal bursts of Afib or flutter)**
6. Chronic Afib (end-stage sinus node dysfunction)

NEW GUIDELINES FOR HEART FAILURE TREATMENT ✪

- **HIGH DOSAGES OF ACE I**
- **DIGOXIN**
  - ⇒ Patients who *should not* receive digoxin include those with advanced AV block or those with asymptomatic heart failure. In general, too, dig should be avoided in the acute phase after MI.
  - ⇒ Digoxin *may not* be effective in patients who have normal LV systolic function
  - ⇒ The benefits of dig are greatest in patients with severe CHF, an enlarged heart, and an S3.
- **DIURETICS** (*esp. spironolactone*—but beware of ↑K with concurrent use of ACE inhibitor
- **BETA-BLOCKERS** (e.g. <u>Bisoprostol, Carvedilol, Metoprolol</u>—all characterized in major clinical trials)
  - ⇒ ***<u>Now considered standard therapy</u>***
  - ⇒ Nearly all patients with heart failure are considered candidates for β-blockers
  - ⇒ Most patients with diabetes can safely use β-blockers
  - ⇒ PVD is not considered a contraindication to the use of β-blockers in these patients
  - ⇒ *Initiate β-blocker in <u>Stage II or III</u> NYHA <u>CHF only after patient is stable on an ACE I, digoxin, and a diuretic.</u>*
  - ⇒ Also recommended, of course, for use post-MI

✪ *Remember*: 1) The treatment for ***dilated, i.e. 'congestive' CMP*** is ***also*** ACE inhibitor/dig/diuretics; 2) When a patient presents in ***CHF with a normal EF%***, one should R/O CAD and valvular heart disease; and 3) When you see increasing azotemia with diuretics yet no improvement in symptoms of CHF, this suggest low EF% / forward failure, which necessitates ***positive inotropy treatment*** (e.g. dobutamine or milrinone).

SYSTOLIC VS. DIASTOLIC DYSFUNCTION: *Generally*:

- ➢ CHF with a low EF% = **systolic failure**
- ➢ CHF with a normal EF% = **diastolic failure**
  - ▪ Major treatment options for diastolic failure include → diuretics and β-blockers.

DIAGNOSES TO CONSIDER IN REFRACTORY CHF

1. PE
2. Silent MI
3. Silent valvular stenosis
4. Anemia
5. Cardiac tamponade; constrictive pericarditis
6. High-ouput failure in elderly (thyrotoxicosis; Paget's dz)
7. LV aneurysm
8. Myocarditis
9. Overvigorous hydration
10. Thiamine deficiency

INDICATIONS FOR RIGHT HEART CATHETERIZATION
1. Uncertainty about the patient's volume status
2. Comorbid conditions, including ongoing ischemia, sepsis, renal insufficiency, or severe lung disease.
3. Lack of response to empiric therapy.

✪ FEATURES DISTINGUISHING HYPERTROPHIC CARDIOMYOPATHY (HCM) FROM AS
1. +FH-- premature sudden death
2. Apex beat--double impulse in HCM
3. HCM murmur is late systolic (not ejection); inaudible in carotids
4. Maneuvers (Incidentally, the MR murmur of MVP behaves exactly as per HCM below)

   a) HCM **murmur** ↑ by valsalva/standing/nitrates (*all with decreased left ventricular volume which in turn ↑the outflow obstruction*)

   b) HCM **murmur** ↓ by squatting/isometric exercises (by *increasing LV volume*)

> ✪ Echocardiographic findings characteristic of IHSS: '**SAM ASH**'→ "**S**ystolic **A**nterior **M**otion of the anterior MV leaflet with **A**symmetric **S**eptal **H**ypertrophy"

✪ PEA (Pulseless Electrical Activity): REVERSIBLE CAUSES WITH ACUTE INTERVENTIONS :

- **H**ypovolemia → bolus IV fluids
- **H**ypoxia → hyperventilate
- **H**ydrogen ion excess—acidosis → hyperventilate
- **H**yperkalemia/**H**ypokalemia → as appropriate
- **H**ypothermia (eg if see Osborne waves) → rewarm

- **T**hrombosis (PE and coronary) → thrombolysis for PE
- **T**ension pneumothorax →chest tube
- **T**amponade → pericardiocentesis
- **T**ablets (drug overdose) → as appropriate

✪ BIOCHEMICAL MARKERS OF CARDIAC INJURY IN COMMON USE:

Marker	Onset	Peak	Duration of Elevati
Troponin I and T	**4-6 h**	18-24 h	**Up to 10 days**
CK-MB	6-12 h	18-24 h	**1 ½-2 days**

TROPONINS → The markers of choice in **acute MI** and should be used instead of CK-MB. Their longer duration of elevation allows for diagnoses to be made days after the acute event. In addition, their high specificity for cardiac injury makes it the marker of choice for the **retrospective diagnosis** of acute MI, effectively replacing LDH as such. For all the troponins, any elevation is considered abnormal. The prognostic value of elevated serum troponins has been demonstrated in patients with unstable angina and MI.

CK-MB → Since CK levels return to baseline one to two days after infarction, resampling can be to detect **infarct extension**. New elevations that occur after normalization are indicative of recurre injury.

THROMBOLYTICS ✪

If you see true **angina with <u>t<12h from symptom onset + ST↑ (≥1 mm in 2 consecutive leads</u>)** or if you see **angina + new BBB→ thrombolytics** (or PTCA) are justified in the ER setting (assuming no contraindications to thrombolytics) .

<u>**Absolute** contraindications include</u>: 1) prior intracranial bleed or CNS tumor; 2) recent prolonged CPR; 3) active internal bleeding; 4) CVA or head trauma within the previous 6 months; and 5) use of Streptokinase for the second time in a year (since patient builds up antibodies to it and tends to react poorly the second time if used so soon after.

<u>**Relative** contraindications include</u>: 1)GIB within 1 month; 2) surgery or trauma in the past 2 weeks; 3) pregnancy; and 4) BP >200/110.

✪ Following AWMI, approximately 1/3 patients will develop ***mural thrombi***, so *long-term* anti-coagulation is also important to prevent thromboembolic disease.

HYPERTENSION:

✪ **"TODAY'S TWO FOR ONE SPECIALS"—WHEN YOU CAN TREAT HTN *AND*...**

CONDITION	KEY DRUGS TO CONSIDER
AFib/ATach	B-blockers, CCBs
African-American heritage	Thiazide diuretic and dietary salt restriction
Angina	B-blockers, CCBs
CHF	ACE inhibitors, diuretics (esp. spironolactone), carvedilol, losartan
Diabetes ± proteinuria	ACE inhibitors, diuretics
Dislipidemia	Alpha-blockers
Essential tremors	Beta-blockers (non-cardioselective)
Hyperthyroidism	Beta-blockers
Isolated systolic HTN in elderly patients	Diuretics, long-acting CCBs
M.I.	Beta-blockers, ACE inhibitors (if CHF or↓EF%)
Migraine	Beta-blockers (non-cardioselective), CCBs
Osteoporosis	Thiazides
Preoperative HTN	Beta-blockers
Renal insufficiency	ACE Inhibitors

☞ The ***diagnosis of HTN*** requires *at least* 2 formal measurements on different days.
☞ ***Isolated systolic HTN*** affects mainly the elderly.
☞ In HTN patients, <u>***LVH***</u> is a strong negative prognosticator for sudden death and MI.

- Know the **JNC VI** (or most recent) clinical definitions for adult **BPs**:

Category	Systolic		Diastolic
Optimal	<120	and	<80
Normal	<130	and	<85
High-normal	130s	or	85-89
HTN			
Stage 1	140s-150s	or	90s
Stage 2	160s-170s	or	100-109
Stage 3	>=180	or	>=110

CARVEDILOL
1. Non-selective beta-blocker
2. *Also* an alpha-blocker
3. Peripheral vasodilator effect
4. Most importantly, carvedilol is used in severe CHF, helping to ↑ the EF%;
5. ↓*morbidity AND mortality*

CONSERVATIVE RECOMMENDATIONS (prior to or in combination with medication)
1. ↓ Weight;
2. ↓ Fat intake
3. ↓Smoking
4. ↓Alcohol to < 2oz/day
5. ↓ Na+
6. ↑Regular exercise

VERAPAMIL
1. Should be avoided in SSS (sick sinus syndrome) as well as 2nd or 3rd degree blocks.
2. Avoid using with CHF when EF<40%
3. **↑ risk of digoxin toxicity**
4. Most common side effect=constipation

FMD (FIBROMUSCULAR DYSPLASIA)
1. Classic string-of-beads appearance on renal angiography
2. #1 cause of renovascular HTN in younger persons, esp women< 25

ATHEROMATOUS RENOVASCULAR DISEASE
1. #1 cause of renovascular HTN in elderly
2. Frequently bilateral
3. Bruit heard 50% of the time
4. Onset after 50 yo
5. ↓K+ due to 2° aldosteronism

6. *Remember, the sudden ↓ in renal function with the use of an ACE I should make you think of Bilateral RAS (renal artery stenosis)*.

7. Remember too with RAS, captopril scan is the screening method of choice, as it is safe in pts with renal insufficiency or history of allergy to contrast media. Doppler Duplex U/S may also be considered but is very "operator dependent", meaning the results are only as good as the tech performing the study.

ATHEROEMBOLIC RENAL DISEASE ✪

1. History is key→e.g. Occurrence *after angiography or aortic surgery*
2. *Livedo reticularis and peripheral emboli* (manifest as gangrene toes, e.g.)
3. Rapid decline in renal function
4. Sudden worsening of HTN

RENAL PARENCHYMAL DISEASE
1. #1 cause of 2° HTN
2. HTN (in turn) and DM are the biggest causes of renal parenchymal disease.
3. Remember, other than peripheral cortical scarring (seen with HTN renal dz), *renal size* (using U/S) is probably the easiest way to differentiate CRF secondary to HTN (kidneys smaller) vs. Diabetes (an infiltrative dz, therefore, kidneys larger)

PRIMARY HYPERALDOSTERONISM
1. Excess aldo(from unilateral adenoma or B/L hyperplasia) *leads to* HTN and ↓ K+ and ↓ renin
2. Suspected in pts with spontaneous ↓*K+* or precipated by usual dose diuretic therapy.
3. Clinical: muscle *weakness;* cramps; H/A; palpitations.
4. *EKG* changes: ↑ ST; inverted Ts; U waves.
5. Dx: after a 3-day high salt diet, measure Na+, K+, creatinine, and aldo in a 24 h urine.
   - a *24 h urine aldo*>12 ng (if urine Na+>200meq) is diagnostic.
6. Tx: adenoma→*surgery*;
   hyperplasia (if no mass seen on adrenal CT) →*spironolactone*

PHEOCHROMOCYTOMA
1. Extra-adrenal tumors are only norepi-producing, whereas adrenal pheos may be epi- or norepi-producing tumors.
2. *"Rule of 10's"*:
   10% of pheos are extraadrenal
   10% are malignant
   10% are familial
      10% are bilateral (since familial tumors tend to be bilateral)
3. *Common presentation*: H/As; sweating; palpitations; HTN *and* orthostatic hypotension.
4. *Screen* with 24 h urine for metanephrines (VMA) and catecholamines (Epi, Norepi).
5. *Next* step: Abdom CT to locate the tumor (for surgery)
6. *Preop*: administer alpha blockers followed by beta-blockers.

COARCTATION OF THE AORTA
1. May go undetected beyond childhood
2. Key ➜ *Upper extremities* HTN, esp. relative to lower extremities (low BP/cold feet)
   ➜ Also may see *rib notching* on CXR.

PREGNANCY & HTN ✪

1. **TREATMENT GUIDELINES FOR CHRONIC HTN IN PREGNANCY (CHP)**
   - CHP is defined as HTN that is present **before the 20th week** of pregnancy <u>or</u> that <u>persists</u> after delivery
   - CHP is now classified as either <u>mild or severe</u> (no longer phase I, II, & III)
   - **MILD HTN** (≥140/90 to 179/109)
     - ➢ Usually doesn't require treatment because the risk of complications is low even at these relatively high BPs.
     - ➢ *In fact the new guidelines say that antihypertensive meds can be stopped or reduced in pregnant women as long as BP remains < 160/110.*

   - **SEVERE HTN** (≥180/110)
     - ➢ <u>Methyldopa and labetalol</u> should be used first
     - ➢ Diuretics are OK to use if needed, *except in* women with preeclampsia or other conditions resulting in reduced perfusion
     - ➢ <u>Don't use atenolol</u> 2° to potential fetal growth retardation
     - ➢ <u>D/C ACE I and ACE receptor blockers</u> as they are associated with renal failure and death in the fetus.
     - ➢ Women with CHP are at ↑ <u>risk for going on to develop preeclampsia</u> (worsening HTN + proteinuria) and controlling the BP *does not* ↓ that risk.

2. **PREECLAMPSIA** → *triad* of **HTN, edema, and proteinuria** developing **after the 20th week**.
   - Can see ↑ **uric acid**, which you would *not* see with chronic HTN in pregnancy.

3. **ECLAMPSIA** → preeclampsia *plus* **convulsions**
   - *Warning signs*→H/A, blurry vision, epigastric pain, hyperreflexia, or cerebral symptoms.
   - **Magnesium** sulfate for impending eclampsia; *calcium gluconate* for *mag* toxicity!

MALIGNANT HTN ✪
1. Sudden severe ↑ in BP associated with acute injury to target organs.
2. Retinal hemorrhages, exudates, *papilledema* frequently noted
3. H/A, confusion, GI distress, seizures (in fact, *HTN encephalopathy* is really the preferred for malignant HTN)
4. *Schistocytes* (fragmented rbcs) seen on blood smear.
5. HTN Emergency--*Nitroprusside* is the drug of choice.

   - May result in cyanotoxicity if thiocyanate levels are not checked Q48h
   - Na+Nitrate and Hydroxycobalamin (Methylene Blue) used to treat toxicity.
   - Side effects of Nitroprusside: N/V, agitation, flushing, fasciculations and tremor.

HYPERTENSIVE CRISES

EMERGENCIES
☞ *DBP>115 <u>with</u> evidence of end-organ dysfunction or damage*
☞ BP should be lowered *gradually* over 2-3 hours to SBP 140-160 and DBP 90-110. To avoid cerebral hypoperfusion, the BP should not be lowered by > 25% of the MAP (mean arterial pressure). Except for ecclampsia, *nitroprusside* can be used for almost all hypertensive emergencies.

URGENCIES
☞ *DBP>115 <u>without</u> end-organ dysfunction/damage*
☞ *Gradually reduce BP over 24-48h*

PREDOMINANT RENOVASCULAR DISEASE BY AGE:
1. Fibromuscular dysplasia→age usually < 30yo
2. Atherosclerosis→age usually >60yo

IMPORTANT CAUSES OF SECONDARY/ACQUIRED HYPERTRIGLYCERIDEMIA
(*"seen in 3D"*)…

- ❖ **D**ISEASES
  - ▪ Metabolic causes
    - ➢ DM
    - ➢ Hyperuricemia
    - ➢ Obesity
    - ➢ Chronic renal failure
    - ➢ Nephrotic syndrome
- ❖ **D**RUGS
    - ➢ β-blockers
    - ➢ Diuretics
    - ➢ Glucocorticoids
    - ➢ Hormonal
        - o Estrogen replacement
        - o Insulin
        - o Thyroxine
- ❖ **D**IET
    - ➢ Alcohol
    - ➢ High carbohydrate ingestion

ESTROGEN and MECHANISMS OF RISK REDUCTION in CHD mortality

➢ ↑HDL, ↓ LDL, ↓Lp (a), ↓ LDL oxidation
➢ ↑Insulin sensitivity
➢ ↑Vascular dilatation
➢ ↓Coagulation factors
➢ ↓Coronary artery LDL uptake

Chylomicrons → Transport of dietary fat
VLDL → Transport of endogenous TG
LDL → Transport of cholesterol to peripheral cells
HDL → Transport of cholesterol from peripheral cells

NEW CHOLESTEROL GUIDELINES *(NCEP May 2001)*

➢ Similar to the old guidelines, <u>beginning at age 20, patients need a lipid profile q5y</u>. The difference is that the new guidelines recommend this <u>*fasting* lipid profile to include TC, TG, LDL, and HDL</u>, where *prior* guidelines had recommended only nonfasting TC and HDL.
➢ LDL < 100 is now considered ideal.
➢ The low normal for HDL has been raised from < 35 to < 40 mg/dL.
➢ The low normal for TG has been lowered from < 200 mg/dL to < 150.
➢ The new guidelines recommend that the highest risk group (CAD, PVD, AAA, symp carotid disease, and DM) shoot for LDL < 100 mg/dL

  ○ If none of these risk factors are present, risk factors are then counted (HTN, cigarettes, HDL<40, age ≥40 (men) or ≥55 (women), +FH of early CAD):
    ▪ 0-1 risk factor → LDL goal <160
    ▪ *≥ 2 risk factors → Risk stratify estimating the 10-year risk of coronary event:*
      • If < 10% →LDL goal <130 (meds 190)
      • 10-20% → LDL goal < 130 (meds 160)
      • If > 20% →LDL goal <100 (meds 130)

MAJOR INDEPENDENT CHD RISK FACTORS

➢ Age (men ≥ 45; women ≥ 55)
➢ Family history of premature CHD (male 1st degree relative < 55; female 1st degree relative < 65)
➢ Cigarettes
➢ HTN (BP ≥ 140/90 or patient on anti-HTN therapy)
➢ Low HDL (< 40 mg/dL)
➢ Elevated LDL (per previous section)

SEE NEXT PAGE FOR HYPERLIPIDEMIAS...

HYPERLIPIDEMIAS ✪

	PROBLEM	PLASMA	PRESENTATIONS	TREATMENT
Type I	Deficiency of lipoprotein lipase	↑ TG ↑ chylomicrons Creamy layer of supernatant after overnight incubation	*Eruptive* xanthomas Pancreatitis Lipemia retinalis (milky retinal vessels)	Fat free diet Medium chain TG + Fat-soluble vitamins
Type IIA	Deficiency of LDL receptors or overproduction of Apo B	↑LDL ↑TC	*Tendinous* xanthomas Premature atherosclerosis and CAD	Statin + Bile acid binding resins
Type IIB	↓ LDL and VLDL receptors	↑LDL ↑VLDL	CAD	Statin or Nicotinic acid
Type III	Abnormal Apolipoprotein E	↑LDL ↑VLDL	*Palmar & tuberous* xanthomas; Premature atherosclerosis and CAD DM; hypothyroidism	Statin or Nicotinic acid
Type IV	Overproduction of Apo B and VLDL	↑ VLDL	Premature atherosclerosis and CAD	Gemfibrozil or Nicotinic acid
Type V	Mixed I + IV	↑Chylomicrons ↑VLDL Creamy supernatant after overnight incubation	*Eruptive* xanthomas Pancreatitis CAD Lipemia retinalis	Gemfibrozil and/or Nicotinic acid + Low fat diet

10. Pulmonary and Critical Care Medicine

TUBERCULOSIS

WHO GETS INH AGAIN? ✪

- ○ **≥ 5mm induration**
  - ■ HIV-seropositive persons
  - ■ Recent contacts of patients with active TB
  - ■ Patients with fibrotic changes on CXR consistent with healed TB
  - ■ Organ transplant recipients and other immunosuppressed persons (receiving the equivalent of ≥ 15 mg/d of prednisone for ≥ 1 month

- ○ **≥ 10 mm induration**
  - ■ Injection drug users (HIV-seronegative)
  - ■ Recent immigrants (within the last 5 years) from countries with high TB prevalence
  - ■ Residents and employees* in high-risk settings, such as prisons, long-term care facilities, hospitals, homeless shelters
  - ■ Mycobacterial laboratory personnel
  - ■ Persons with DM, CRF, leukemias, lymphomas, weight loss ≥ 10% of ideal body weight; carcinoma of the head & neck or lung; or silicosis
  - ■ Persons with a history of gastrectomy or jejunoileal bypass
  - ■ Children younger than 4 yo
  - ■ Children & adolescents exposed to adults at high risk

- ○ **≥15 mm induration**
  - ■ Persons with none of the above risk factors for TB

  For persons who are otherwise at low risk and are tested at the start of employment, a reaction ≥ 15 mm induration is considered positive.

✪ BCG Vaccine & Skin Testing
➤ The skin test reactivity associated with BCG vaccination in childhood usually diminishes in 5 years. Moreover, many of the patients who have received BCG vaccine are from countries with a high prevalence of TB, and the likelihood of infection is high. *Therefore*, a positive skin test (≥10mm) in a patient who has received BCG more than 5 years before skin testing should be considered as caused by MTB and not the vaccine.

TREATMENT OF PULMONARY TB ✪
1. <u>Suspect</u> Drug <u>Resistance</u>→ R.I.P.E. until sensitivities return
2. Then, if INH-<u>Sensitive</u> → R.I.P. x 2 mo→ R.I. x 4 more months.
3. If INH-<u>Resistant</u>,→ R.E. ± P x 18 months (or 12 months after sputum culture negative, whichever is longer)

MDR-TB (MULTI-DRUG RESISTANT TB) ✪

1. Implies resistance to at least 2 drugs, usually INH and Rifampin
2. Risk factors include

   a. Recent immigration from Latin America or Asia
   b. Living in area of ↑ resistance ($\geq 4\%$)
   c. Previous Rx without Rifampin
   d. Previous incomplete treatment
   e. Exposure to known MDR-TB

3. Associated with a high mortality
4. Requires treatment with **_at least_** 3 drugs from among the following, _e.g._

R ifampin +	**_OR_**	S treptomycin or Capreomycin or Kanamycin +
I NH +		A mikacin +
P ZA +		F loroquinolone
E thambutol		

   ### Generally, you want to…
   ✓ _Give ≥ 3 drugs until culture becomes negative, including any first-line agent to which the patient is partially sensitive, ≥ 1 injectable agent (streptomycin, capreomycin, or kanamycin), and, possibly, a quinolone._
   {Typical MDR-TB regimen: R.I.P., oflaxacin, cycloserine, and capreomycin}
   ✓ _Then give 2-drug regimen for ≥ 12 months after culture-negative._

5. Note, may consider Rifabutin, instead of Rifampin, as ~30% of Rifampin-resistant strains are Rifabutin-sensitive.

TWO-STAGE TST (TB SKIN TEST) ✪

1. Use in **individuals who are tested regularly** for TB, e.g. nursing home residents.

2. _The idea_ → Because the immune response may wane with time/age, elderly patients may require a second "booster" test dose 1 week later to see if the first neg test was a false negative. The second dose should "wake-up" the immune system and help to identify a h/o TB exposure. Remember this is the appropriate testing in nursing home patients.

3. Also, if the first stage is +, but < 10mm→repeat in 1 week, and if then≥ 10mm, you can safely say this is **_not a recent conversion_** to directly diagnose recent converters. In other words, **recent converters will not have a boostered response.**

Note: **Steroids** are absolutely contraindicated in **TB** _unless_ the patient is receiving maximal anti-TB therapy and there is acute hypoadrenalism (Addison's) due to TB infiltration/ablation of the adrenals. Other controversial exceptions include: TB Pericarditis; Acute Miliary TB with septic shock; and TB meningitis.

TOXICITY OF ANTI-TB MEDICATIONS:

1. **INH** (Isoniazid)
   a) Hepatitis
   b) SLE
   c) Pyridoxine deficiency (rare)→neuropathy
   d) Potentiation of phenytoin, coumadin

2. **Rifampin**
   Daily Administration
      a) Antagonism of OCPs, warfarin, steroids, digoxin, and short-acting sulfonylureas
      b) Asymp ↑ of AST, ALT
   Intermittent Administration
      a) Hepatitis
      b) Orange-red discoloration to urine, tears
      c) Flu-like illness
      d) Hemolysis, ITP, DVT, azotemia

3. **Streptomycin**
   a) Hypersensitivity reactions—rash, malaise, ↑eos
   b) Vestibular damage (esp if renal impairment)
   c) Teratogenicity

4. **Ethambutol**—optic neuritis, esp in renal impairment
5. **PZA** (Pyrazinamide)—hepatotoxicity in 10%

INFLUENZA
1. Type A most common
2. Those ≥65yo have by far the highest mortality
3. Strep and Staph can secondarily infect
4. **Amantadine** is only effective vs. Type A and can shorten the course of disease in influenza only if given **within 48 hours** of symptom onset (Amantadine as ***TREATMENT***)
5. Amantadine + Vaccine confers ± 95% protection (Amantadine as ***PROPHYLAXIS***)
6. Amantadine toxicity = restlessness, insomnia, dizziness, renal
7. The flu vaccine **may in fact be given along with Pneumovax**
8. The following **risk groups** should receive annual vaccine:
   a) ≥65
   b) > or < 65 with chronic medical problems, such as cardiopulmonary disorders and DM
   c) Health care personal
   d) Nursing home residents and residents of other long-term care facilities, as well as their staff
   e) House-hold members of high-risk groups
   f) Healthy pregnant women who will be in their 2nd or 3rd trimesters during the flu season.
   g) HIV and immunocompromised
   h) Anyone who wishes to reduce the likelihood of becoming ill with influenza
9. Be ready to recognize the value of **Relenza** (zanamivir; for inhalation) and **Tamiflu** (oseltamivir; supplied as capsules), both **neuraminidase inhibitors**, in uncomplicated acute illness due to influenza virus if symptomatic **for ≤ 2 days**.

DDX of WHEEZING + EOSINOPHILIA

1. **ABPA**
2. **Churg-Strauss**
3. **PAN**
4. **Strongyloides**

- **Löeffler's syndrome** is not included in this list since, while there are transient pulmonary infiltrates and peripheral blood eosinophilia, *there is no wheezing*.

WEGENER'S GRANULOMATOSIS

1. **Pulmonary-renal syndrome (others include** Goodpasture's; Churg-Strauss; SLE; Cryoglobulinemic vasculitis; Leukocytoclastic vasculitis, i.e. small vessel vasculitis)
2. **c-ANCA** (Remember, "Yes, <u>WE</u> <u>c-AN</u>")
3. Pulmonary manifestations include hemorrhage and thick-walled, centrally-**cavitating nodules**
4. Renal manifestation is **Focal Segmental** GN
5. The mnemonic "**ELKS**" summarizes the organs affected:
   - **E** NT ('saddle nose' deformity; nasal discharge; paranasal sinusalgia)
   - **L** ung
   - **K** idney (involvement usually follows E/L/S of ELKS)
   - **S** kin

- *Think Wegener's* if see **triad of <u>sinusitis + hemoptysis + large cavitary nodules</u>** on CXR

GOODPASTURE'S SYNDROME ✪

1. *Hemoptysis* is usually always the initial symptom
2. *Pulmonary* involvement typically *precedes* renal involvement; <u>P</u>-ANCA
3. Serum ELISA technique can detect *anti-basement membrane antibody*
4. *Plasmapheresis* is an important adjunct to immunosuppression in reducing this autoantibody.

> **Generally, lung biopsy is preferable in diagnosing Wegener's, while a renal biopsy is preferable in diagnosing Goodpasture's.**

BORDETELLA PERTUSSIS

1. Responsible for **whooping** cough
2. Should R/O in cases of **prolonged bronchitis** in older children and adults
3. May cause ↑↑Lymphocytes
4. Treatment with **Erythromycin**

CHLAMYDIA PSITTACOSIS

1. Asymptomatic avian carriers→poultry workers, e.g. cleaning out bird cages
2. F/C, H/A, dry cough, stiff neck; TCN is treatment.

LEGIONNAIRE'S DISEASE ✪

1. Clinical: weakness, malaise, **high fever**, **cough**, and **diarrhea**, relative bradycardia, **bilateral patchy infiltrates**
2. Labs: **↓Na, ↓ Phos**, ↑ WBC, **↑ LFTs**
3. **Diagnosis:**
   a) Urine Antigen-1
   b) √ Ab with **IFA** (Indirect fluorescent Ab) test; ≥ 1:256 or a 4-fold ↑ is pos.
4. Treatment: Erythro ± Rifampin; Fluoroquinolone; or Azithromax

MISCELLANEOUS PEARLS FOR THE BOARDS ✪

➢ In **massive hemoptysis**, the cause of death is usually asphyxiation, not exsanguination (bleeding out)

➢ **Hypertrophic Pulmonary Osteoarthropathy** is generally caused by *adeno ca and large cell* ca of the lung. It can be seen on bone scan.

➢ **Horner's syndrome** consists of the triad of ptosis, meiosis, and anhidrosis. It is 2° to superior sulcus tumors (Pancoast tumors) which is usually caused by SVC syndrome or Squamous Cell Ca of the lung.

➢ **HRCT** (High Resolution CT) is the investigational tool of choice for diagnosing **bronchiectasis**.

➢ *Bronchial artery embolotherapy* can lead to *spinal artery embolism* which in turn can present with **neurologic deficits, since the spinal artery is a branch of the bronchial artery.**

➢ An **↑ serum ACE level** does not establish the dx of sarcoidosis, since it is non-specific and may be elevated in a variety of other conditions such as mycoses and hyperparathyroidism.

➢ Remember, in **emphysema**, air trapping leads to hyperinflation, **a ↓ in elastic recoil, and an ↑ in compliance**. Remember from way back? → compliance & elasticity are *inversely proportional*. You might want to think of an old rubberband to understand this concept: the older it gets, the more you can stretch it (more compliance), but it won't shoot as far (less recoil).

➢ **In aspiration pneumonia** CXR shows involvement of dependent pulmonary segments which are favored in aspiration: the lower lobes when aspiration occurs in the upright position; or the *superior segments of the lower lobes or posterior segment of the upper lobes* when aspiration occurs in the recumbent position.

COMMON CAUSES OF A CHRONIC COUGH (> 3 wk) ✪

1. **Asthma**
2. **Chronic bronchitis**
3. **GERD**
4. **Post-nasal drip**
5. **ACE Inhibitor**

COMMON CAUSES OF COPD→ "ABCDE" ✪

A sthma—*reversible* airway obstruction
B ronchitis
C ystic Fibrosis
D ilatation of the bronchi (Bronchiectasis)—*irreversible* →look for "train-tracking" on the CXR
E mphysema

☞ In general, <u>bronchiectasis</u> is seen in the <u>lower lung fields</u>. Important <u>exceptions</u> include:

- ✓ Cystic Fibrosis
- ✓ ABPA
- ✓ Chronic Mycoses

CYSTIC FIBROSIS ✪

1. + Family History (more common among caucasians)
2. **Sweat Chloride ≥ 60** on pilocarpine iontopheresis

3. *Common Complications and Clinical Correlates:*

- ✓ **Pseudomonal** infection common
- ✓ **Aspergillus** (ABPA in 10% of CFers)
- ✓ **Candida** Albicans
- ✓ Asthma
- ✓ **Pancreatic insufficiency**
- ✓ **Azospermia**
- ✓ **Infertility (nearly all men and women with CF)**
- ✓ **Sinusitis**
- ✓ Purulent sputum
- ✓ COPD in 90% of adult survivors; **bronchiectasis**
- ✓ **Hemoptysis** (71%)
- ✓ Nasal polyps (48%)
- ✓ Anorexia, weight loss, clubbing

KARTAGENER'S SYNDROME ('Immotile Cilia Syndrome')

1. Half of these patients have situs inversus (i.e. dextrocardia)

2. Sinusitis is common

3. Males are commonly infertile*

- Note: The infertility in Kartagener's syndrome is 2° to **immotility** of the sperm, whereas in CF, it is 2° to **azospermia** (reflecting obliteration of the vas deferens)

HEMOPTYSIS—MOST COMMON CAUSES
1. **B** ronchiectasis; bronchitis
2. **L** ung carcinoma
3. **T** B

OBSTRUCTIVE SLEEP APNEA—CLINICAL FEATURES ✪
1. **Snoring**
2. **AM Headaches**
3. **Feeling poorly rested on awakening**
4. **Daytime drowsiness**
5. **Systemic / Pulmonary HTN**
6. **Ventricular arrythmias** (2° to prolonged periods of apnea at night)
7. Peripheral edema 2° to **Pulm HTN**/cor pulmonale
8. Obstructive sleep apnea **2° to obesity**, the disorder is referred to as **Pickwickian** Syndrome
9. ↓pO2
10. ↑pCO2
11. **Polycythemia** 2° to ↓pO2
12. RVF→LVF in late stages
13. **Nasal CPAP** an important tool in treatment

IDIOPATHIC PULMONARY FIBROSIS (IPF) ✪
1. PFTs show a <u>restrictive</u> pattern with ↓DLCO
2. Any end-stage diffuse lung disease can **mimic** IPF;
   a) BOOP (Bronchiolitis Obliterans with Organizing Pneumonia)
   b) DAD (Diffuse Alveolar Disease)
   c) LIP (Lymphocytic Interstitial Pneumonitis)
   d) etc.
3. Commonly see **<u>hypoxemia exacerbated by exercise</u>** (similar to PCP)
4. **<u>Lung biopsy</u>** is important in this disease, since the causes are multiple
5. **<u>Honeycombing</u>** on CXR, if seen, is significant, since it signifies **<u>advanced</u>** IPF or interstitial fibrosis from any cause.
6. Prognosis is poor without **<u>lung transplantation</u>**.

CLUES FROM THE BAL (Bronchoalveloar lavage): Lymphs & Neutrophils in Interstitial Lung Dz:
➢ Lymphocytes predominate → hypersensitivity pneumonitis, sarcoidosis, TB,
➢ Neutrophils predominate → cigarettes, eosinophilic granuloma, IPF

BOOP (Bronchiolitis Obliterans with Organizing Pneumonia)
1. Pathology→Seen when bronchiolitis (inflammation and fibrosis of the small airways) spreads to adjacent parenchymal tissue.
2. Etiologies →RA; viral infections; toxic inhalations.
3. CXR→ parenchymal infiltates
4. PFTs→ restrictive defect

SARCOIDOSIS ✪

1. A <u>**systemic disease**</u> of unknown etiology which causes <u>**non-caseating granulomas**</u> throughout the body.
2. Presence of non-caseating granulomas is ***not* diagnostic** as they can be seen in other diseases, which often also produce hilar lymphadenopathy!
3. Think of this disease if presented with a young black women (W>M, B>F) in her 20's-30's with bilateral hilar LN + E. nodosum.
4. **Staging**/Progression:

Stage I	Hilar *lymphadenopathy*
Stage II	I + pulmonary *parenchymal* disease
Stage III	Pulmonary parenchymal disease *without* hilar LN (*tricky*!)
Stage IV	Pulmonary *Fibrosis with bullae*

5. <u>**False-negative PPD**</u> (2° to suppressed T lymphocyte function)
6. Remember, **serum ACE** levels are non-specific and are **corroborative** *only*.
7. Other labs frequently seen in sarcoidosis:
   a) ↑ vitamin D
   b) Hypercalciuria

8. Know these important <u>**INDICATIONS FOR STEROIDS**</u> in <u>**SARCOIDOSIS**</u>:
   a) Ocular involvement
   b) Cardiac involvement
   c) Neuro involvement
   d) Progressive pulmonary disease
   e) Hypercalcemia
   f) Hypercalciuria with renal insufficiency
   g) Disfiguring cutaneous manifestations (e.g. Lupus Pernio—violacious nodules occurring over the nose and malar regions)

PULMONARY INFILTRATES WITH EOSINOPHILIA (PIE). Here's <u>your PIE</u> chart:
   (*DDx of pulm infiltrates and ↑serum eos*):

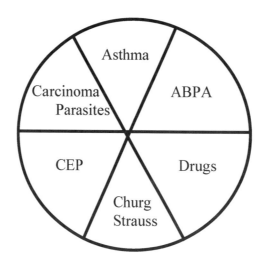

THE DIFFUSE INTERSTITIAL LUNG DISEASES (ILD) …
- ✓ Symptoms include dyspnea, decreased exercise tolerance, and usually a non-productive cough.
- ✓ ↓DLCO on PFTs
- ✓ Treatment options vary and include:
  - o Observation
  - o Addressing the primary cause of the ILD
  - o Prednisone; Cyclophosphamide; Azathioprine--check PFTs, CXR, and symptomatic improvement at 6 months on these.
  - o Transplantation (criteria include 1) limitation in activity; 2) room air Pa02 < 60; and 3) DLCO < 30%
- ✓ **Smokers** predisposes to 2 DLDs→ PEG (Pulmonary Eosinophilic Granuloma) and PAP (Pulmonary Alveolar Proteinosis)
- ✓ The other name for PEG is Histiocytosis X (might remember **"PEG is His X"**), because of the atypical histiocytes that are found in the tissue.

ILDs THAT CAN GIVE SPONTANEOUS PNEUMOTHORAX
1. **PEG**
2. **LAM** (Lymphangiomyomatosis) (*see next*)
3. Cystic Fibrosis

LAM
1. **Women** of childbearing age
2. Recurrent spontaneous **pneumothorax**
3. **Hemoptysis**
4. **COPD** picture on PFTs
5. Hyperinflation with reticulonodular infiltrates.

ILDs ASSOCIATED WITH HILAR/MEDIASTINAL ADENOPATHY
1. Lymphoma
2. Lymphagitic carcinomatosis
3. Sarcoidosis

ILDs ASSOCIATED WITH BOTH OBSTRUCTIVE & RESTRICTIVE DEFICITS:
1. LAM
2. PEG
3. Sarcoidosis

ASBESTOSIS:
1. **Pleural thickening (esp. apical) ± pleural plaques** best appreciated at the diaphragmatic border. Remember, though, sarcoid and TB also show pleural thickening.
2. Fibrosis usually predominates in the **lower** lung fields (as opposed to silicosis)
3. Due to the resulting fibrosis, PFTs reveal a *restrictive* pattern.

4. Mesothelioma usually follows asbestos exposure by an <u>average of 40years</u>.

5. <u>Another long-term complication of asbestosis is</u> **bronchogenic ca; smoking is markedly synergistic** in this regard. ✪

6. <u>Unlike bronchogenic ca, when</u> **smoking** is added to asbestos exposure, there is **no** additional ↑ risk of developing **mesothelioma**. ✪

SILICOSIS ✪

1. Associated with sandblasting, mining professions.
2. **No ↑ risk of lung ca**
3. **"Eggshell" calcifications** of hilar LNs (a term also used in sarcoidosis)
4. + RF and +ANA are common
5. **If you see fever** with silicosis (± weight loss)→ R/O Silicotuberculosis and **✓ a PPD**, as their is a significantly ↑ risk of developing TB in silicosis.

FARMER' LUNG ✪

1. **A form of HYPERSENSITIVITY PNEUMONITIS**
2. Caused by **fungal** precipitans (thermophilic actinomycetes) in modly hay, grain, or silage
3. Serum precipitins are almost always + for this fungus
4. ↑ Immunoglobulins, except Ig E
5. **+ RF** seen in most cases
6. Clinical presentation: **fever/chills/sweats/dry cough/ dyspnea**
7. These symptoms resolve faily rapidly (18-24 hours), and recur on reexposure to the antigens.
8. PFTs are **restrictive**
9. **No wheezing; no eosinophilia**
10. Treatment: "remove the patient from the source" (not too realistic if you're a farmer!); steroids

OCCUPATIONAL ASTHMA

1. Inciting agents are divided into <u>two broad categories</u>:

   a. *Low molecular weight chemicals* (eg, trimellitic anhydride, formaldehyde), which require combination of the chemical, which is an incomplete antigen (ie, a hapten), with a protein conjugate to produce a sensitizing neoantigen.

   b. *High molecular weight organic materials* (eg, grain dust, avian proteins) which may serve as complete antigens.

2. *Cigarette smoking* is a significant risk factor for occupational asthma.

3. *Peak flows*, i.e. peak expiratory flow rates, should be done to confirm the diagnosis *<u>at the end of the work period and during the period away from work</u>*. A *four-fold decrease* in

nonspecific bronchial hyperresponsiveness at the end of the work period confirms an association of disease with the work environment.

4. If you suspect a *high molecular weight compound*, *skin tests* to that extract can be done, and in the presence of nonspecific bronchial hyperresponsiveness, are highly suggestive of occupational asthma. There are no skin test reagents available for low molecular substances.

EXERCISE-INDUCED ASTHMA (EIA)

- Patients may complain of wheezing, cough, chest tightness, fatigue, or SOB during or after exercise.
- Of course, a resting physical exam may be completely normal.
- Dx usually supported when preexercise inhalation of a short-acting β-agonist causes symptom resolution.
- *Nonpharmacologic approaches* to EIA as well as advice to patients should include a pre-exercise warm-up, exercising in warm, humid air, and exercising in short bursts.
- Short-acting β-agonists are **1ˢᵗ-line drug therapy** for these patients.
- Cromolyn and nedocromil are considered **2ⁿᵈ-line therapy** and are effective in 70-85% of patients. They work by inhibiting mast cell degranulation and *should be taken 10-45 min prior to exercise*. Their duration is 1-2 h. They may be used alone or in conjunction with a β-agonist.
- Long-acting β-agonists, like salmeterol, may also help, although effects may wane over time.
- Leukotriene inhibitors also appear to be beneficial in a 75% of patients in a recent study.

PPH (Primary Pulmonary HTN) ✪

1. 2° to hyperreactivity of the pulmonary vasculature
2. F>M incidence

3. Clinical presentation:

   a) **Exertional dyspnea/syncope/presyncope 2° to…**
   b) Pulmonary HTN, which causes 2° cor pulmonale
   c) CXR: Cardiomegaly with prominent pulmonary artery and "pruning" of the pulmonary vessels
   d) ↑ Pulmonary pressures seen on right heart cath

4. **Management** includes:

   a) Supplemental oxygen for hypoxemia
   b) Diuretics for edema
   c) Digoxin for RV failure;
   d) Chronic anticoagulation for chronic thromboemboli and PPH
   e) Vasodilators (e.g., prostacyclin or nifedipine) for PPH, which should be initiated only in the setting of hemodynamic monitoring because they can cause profound hypotension and death
   f) Transplantation (lung or heart-lung)

5. **Criteria for transplant in pulmonary HTN**
   - ➢ Symptoms of right-sided heart failure
   - ➢ 2-year survival estimated < 50%
   - ➢ PA systolic pressure > 60 mm Hg

DRUG-INDUCED LUNG DISEASE ✪

DRUG	PULMONARY TOXICITY
Nitrofurantoin/phenytoin/hydralazine	SLE-like picture with pleural effusions (50%) and pulmonary infiltrates (30%); hydralazine→pleurisy.
Narcotics	ARDS; Non-cardiogenic Pulmonary Edema; Granulomas (e.g talc); pneumonia; Bronchiectasis; Endocarditis
'Crack' cocaine	Diffuse alveolar hemorrhage; BO ± OP; hypersensitiv pneumonitis
Busulfan/**B**leo*/**B**CNU*	All can lead to pulmonary <u>fibrosis</u> (Remember to "**B**.tough"). Bleo may also cause a pneumonitis.
Methotrexate	Hypereosinophilia; Hilar LN; pleural effusion
Steroids may predispose to	Nocardia; Mycoses (esp Aspergillus, Candida, Crypto) and may exacerbate TB
ASA overdose	Respiratory Alkalosis (following an anion gap metabolic acidosis)
Prolonged O2 at high FIO2	ARDS
Amiodarone*	Diffuse infiltrates (remember, patients on this amiodarone should have their *PFTs, TFTs, and LFTs* closely monitored.
Penicillamine	BOOP; SLE
Methylsergide	Fibrosis

* THE PULMONARY INJURY WITH THESE IS <u>DOSE-RELATED</u>.

- Remember, **High Altitude Pulmonary Edema** occurs among high-altitude natives on returning to altitude after being at sea level.several weeks.

SOLITARY PULMONARY NODULES ✪

1. Large majority are benign; remember the key always is _serial films_; an SPN that shows no growth over 6-9 months is usually benign.

<table>
<tr><td colspan="2" align="center">ETIOLOGIES OF SPN:</td></tr>
<tr><td>Malignant nodules</td><td>40%</td></tr>
<tr><td>Bronchogenic carcinoma</td><td>33%</td></tr>
<tr><td>Other 1° malignancies</td><td>2%</td></tr>
<tr><td>Solitary metastasis</td><td>5%</td></tr>
<tr><td>Benign nodules</td><td>60%</td></tr>
<tr><td>Infectious granulomas</td><td>50%</td></tr>
<tr><td>Benign tumors</td><td>5%</td></tr>
<tr><td>Other</td><td>5%</td></tr>
</table>

2. _**Benign**_ SPNs are usually $\leq$ **2.5-3cm** in diameter
3. _**Malignant**_ SPNs which tend to be **> 3cm**
4. Dx: For more proximal SPNs→can usually do a wedge biopsy. More distal SPNs usually require either a CT-guided or Fluoroscopy-guided transthoracic needle biopsy.
5. The following clinical features are quite useful in _**differentiating**_ benign and malignant SPNs:

	MORE LIKELY BENIGN	**MORE LIKELY MALIGNANT**
Age	Age <35	Age > 35
Gender	Female	Male
Smoker?	No	Yes
Size	< 2.5-3 cm	> 2.5-3 cm
Margins	Smooth margins	Irregular margins/spiculated edges
Calcification	Central/popcorn/ diffuse/ laminated pattern	Eccentric pattern
Growth (on CXR)	No	Yes
Satellite lesions	Yes	No
CT scan +C	Less likely to enhance	More likely to enhance
PET	No uptake (with fluorodeoxyglucose)	↑ uptake

DIAGNOSTIC VALUE OF GROSS SPUTUM EXAM
1. Rusty, mucoid→Pneumococcal pneumonia
2. Currant jelly sputum → Klebsiella
3. Rubbery brown plugs→ ABPA
4. Purulent, malodorous→ Lung abscess; bronchiectasis
5. Clear, watery, copious→Alveolar cell ca
6. Frank blood with simultaneous mucopurulent sputum→TB
7. Pink, frothy→CHF
8. 'Anchovy sauce'→ Amebic abscess
9. Black→coalworker's pneumoconiosis with progressive, severe fibrosis

DDx of ↑ A-a (Alveolar-arterial) Gradient→Remember, "<u>VSD</u>" ✪

V/Q mismatch
1. PE
2. Airway obstruction (asthma, COPD)
3. Interstitial lung disease
4. Alveolar disease

Shunt
1. Intracardiac (e.g. *VSD!*)
2. Intrapulmonary shunt (e.g. ARDS or intrapulmonary AVM) and "intraalveolar filling" (pus=pneumonia; water=CHF; protein (AP); blood)
3. Alveolar collapse (atelectasis)

Diffusion defect, e.g.
1. IPF
2. Emphysema

DETECTION OF LEFT TO RIGHT SHUNTS
➤ Arterial blood sampling from the RA, RV, and PA provides helpful information when evaluating a suspected intracardiac (left to right) shunt. Detection of an <u>*oxygen saturation "step-up"*</u> allows confirmation of the shunt and determination of its location.
  ○ If a left-to-right shunt is suspected, the oxygen saturation of the above chambers as well as the SVC and IVC should be measured while inserting the catheter under fluoroscopic guidance to ensure proper sampling sites.
  ○ *A step-up is defined as a <u>greater than 10 percent rise in oxygen saturation</u> when comparing the calculated saturation of mixed venous blood to the saturation of blood in the RA, RV or PA.*

INTERPRETING PFT'S "Quick & Dirty" ✪

1. **First**, ✓ the relative **<u>FLOWS</u>** (FEV_1/FVC): *(normal FEV1% is 75-80%)* — If ↓, then patient usually has **obstructive** disease, so f/u with a <u>bronchodilator</u> challenge to ✓ for improvement in FEV1 (asthma); <u>if no change, ✓ DLCO</u> (↓in emphysema; nl/↑ in asthma; nl in bronchitis).

2. **Next**, look at the **VOLUMES** (e.g. FVC): If ↓, then patient has **restrictive** lung disease, and a f/u <u>DLCO</u> will differentiate interstitial lung disease (↓DLCO) vs. chest wall lesions (normal DLCO; essentially pleural disease or weakness of the diaphragm)

3. **Finally**, if FEV_1/FVC and FVC are normal: Consider a **methacholine challenge to R/O asthma** (checking for reversible lung disease, mostly FEV1)

RESTRICTIVE LUNG DISEASE

➤ **These disorders cause reduction of lung volumes (restriction; eg VC)**

➤ **Can be divided into three groups:**
1. Intrinsic lung diseases, which cause inflammation or scarring of the lung tissue (interstitial lung disease) or fill the airspaces with exudate or debris (acute pneumonitis).
2. Extrinsic disorders, such as disorders of the chest wall or the pleura, which mechanically compress the lungs or limit their expansion.
3. Neuromuscular disorders, which decrease the ability of the respiratory muscles to inflate and deflate the lungs.

DDx of ↑ DLCO ✪

1. **Asthma**
2. Alveolar hemorrhage
   a) Mitral Stenosis
   b) Goodpasture's syndrome
   c) Trauma, etc.
3. Polycythemia

DDx of ↓ DLCO ✪ (↓surface area available for gas exchange)

1. **Emphysema**
2. **IPF** (Idiopathic Pulmonary Fibrosis)
3. **PE**
4. **PPH** (Primary Pulmonary HTN)
5. Sarcoidosis
6. Anemia

✪ To diagnose **REVERSIBLE** obstructive lung disease (e.g. asthma), the following parameters should ↑ **in response to bronchodilators: FEV1 (or VC) ≥12%** or >0.2L or FEF_{25-75} ≥ 50%; **additional criteria include** ≥ 15% increase in FEV1 over time with anti-inflammatory-bronchodilator therapy ; **≥ 20% variability in peak flow** measurements over time; and hyperreactivity on **methacholine** testing, as evidenced by a ↓ **in FEV1 by ≥ 20%**

✪ Remember also, <u>FEF $_{25-75}$</u> is one of the best measures of <u>**SMALL AIRWAY disease.**</u>

✪ A sudden <u>↓ in the FEV 1 by ≥ 20% is an indication for hospitalization</u>.

• In patients with COPD, *exercise tolerance correlates more with FEV 1*, in general, than with their pO2. In fact, low FEV1 and chronic mucus hypersecretion are predictors of hospitalization due to COPD.

✪ <u>**Home O2 is indicated**</u> for patients with pO2 <55 or O2 sat% <88.

PREOPERATIVE EVALUATION For Candidates Undergoing Lobectomy Or Pneumonectomy ✪

☞ Studies evaluating patients undergoing *pneumonectomy* have found that those patients with a <u>preoperative FEV1 in excess of 2 L tolerate the resection well</u>. (In contrast, the suggested threshold value for preoperative FEV1 in patients undergoing lobectomy has generally been 1.0 to 1.5 L).

☞ For pneumonectomy candidates who fall below the 2L threshold, a <u>predicted *postpneumonectomy* FEV1 greater than 0.8 L</u> is used; this is achieved through a quantative V/Q scan. A more accurate way, however, is to use % predicted postop FEV1 (% relative to normal expected) rather than in absolute units; a cutoff of 40% (ie ≥40% of the predicted normal value for that patient) is frequently used as the predicted postoperative FEV1.

✪ PLEURAL FLUID HINTS	
WHEN YOU SEE...	**THINK OF THESE FIRST**
↓ Glucose	➢ Empyema ➢ Esophageal rupture (esp with ↓pH and ↑amylase) ➢ RA (esp. if also find ↓pH and ↑LDH) ➢ TB (don't forget pleural biopsy if suspect)
↑Amylase	➢ Esophageal rupture ➢ Pancreatitis
pH < 7.2	➢ Empyema ➢ Esophageal rupture
Bloody fluid	➢ Pulmonary infarction ➢ Pleural carcinomatosis ➢ TB
Lymphs predominate	➢ TB ➢ Fungal infection ➢ Malignancy

| SPECIALIZED TESTS FOR DETECTING CAUSES OF PLEURAL EFFUSION ||
TEST	DIAGNOSIS
TG> 110 mg/dl	Chylothorax
Amylase >200 U/dl	Esophageal perf; malignancy; pancreatic dz; ruptured ectopic pregnancy
RF ≥ 1:320 and ≥ serum titre	Rheumatoid effusion
ANA ≥1:160 and ≥ serum titre	Lupus pleuritis
CEA >10ng/dl	Malignancy
Adenosine deaminase >43U/L	TB pleuritis

COMMON DDX OF <u>TRANSUDATIVE</u> PLEURAL EFFUSIONS
1. ↓Albumin
2. CHF (#1 cause)/cirrhosis (ascites)/nephrosis
3. Constrictive pericarditis; SVC syndrome
4. Iatrogenic
5. PE

COMMON DDX OF <u>EXUDATIVE</u> PLEURAL EFFUSIONS: *(mostly 1° pulmonary processes)*
1. Pulmonary / pleural malignancy
2. Pneumonia; empyema (below); other pulmonary infections
3. PE (yes, here too!)

CRITERIA FOR AN EXUDATIVE PLEURAL EFFUSION (≥ 1 OF THE FOLLOWING)
1. Pleural fluid/serum **total protein ratio > .5**
2. "   "   "   **LDH**   ratio   **> .6**
3. Pleural fluid LDH > 2/3 of the upper limit of normal serum LDH (traditionally)
4. Pleural fluid pH > 7.3

EMPYEMA ✪
➢ Essentially pus in the pleural space with the following typical pleural fluid findings:
    ✓ Glucose < 40 mg/dl
    ✓ LDH > 600 mg/dl
    ✓ pH < 7.0
    ✓ Protein > 3g/dl
    ✓ WBC > 5000 cells/mm^3

✪ **Pleural biopsy** is valuable in cases of unexplained exudative effusions and suspected cases of TB and malignancy.

AGE-RELATED CHANGES IN PULMONARY FUNCTION ✪
1. ↓FEV
2. ↓ VC
3. ↑FRC (Functional Residual Capacity) and ↑ in RV
4. ↓ in pO2
5. There is no ↑ in pCO2 with aging

IMPORTANT DIAGNOSTIC LINKS

- Recurrent sinusitis + infertile young adult male
- Chronic productive cough + DM in young adult
- Obstructive lung dz + lower lung bullae + hepatic inflammation
- Productive cough on most days ≥ 3mo ≥ 2 consecutive years

DIAGNOSIS TO LOOK FOR
Kartagener's syndrome
Cystic Fibrosis
Alpha-1 antitrypsin deficiency
   (see below)
Chronic bronchitis

ALPHA-1 ANTITRYPSIN DEFICIENCY
1. An inherited disorder which leads to accumulation of the destructive enzyme elastase in the lung. AAT, remember, is an effective inhibitor of the proteolytic enzyme elastase. The structural integrity, therefore, of lung elastin depends on this antienzyme.
2. May lead to liver disease, *emphysema* or both in some individuals
3. The emphysema is more severe at the *lung bases*
4. *Management*
   - ✓ Population studies suggest a minimum plasma threshold of 11 μmol/L (corresponding to 80 mg/dL), below which there is insufficient AAT to protect the lung, leading to a risk of developing emphysema. The normal plasma levels of AAT are 20 to 53 μmol/L (150 to 350 mg/dL).
   - ✓ Exogenous intravenous augmentation therapy via the infusion of pooled human AAT is currently the most direct and efficient means of elevating AAT levels in the plasma and in the lung interstitium.
   - ✓ The current goal in the treatment of AAT deficiency is to raise the plasma AAT level (and therefore the concentration of AAT in the lung interstitium) above the protective threshold.
   - ✓ Currently, weekly infusions are the only Food and Drug Administration-approved regimen, although monthly infusions have similar clinical efficacy and safety and are widely used.
   - ✓ Liver transplantation has been reserved for patients with end-stage hepatic disease. It has the additional advantage of correcting the AAT deficiency, because the healthy donor <u>liver</u> produces, secretes, and thereby restores the normal levels of AAT.

HRCT ESPECIALLY USEFUL IN:
1. Bronchiectasis
2. LAM
3. Lung mets
4. PEG
5. Patient with diffuse interstitial infiltrates of unclear cause

MODERN APPROACH TO THE DIAGNOSIS OF PULMONARY EMBOLUS:

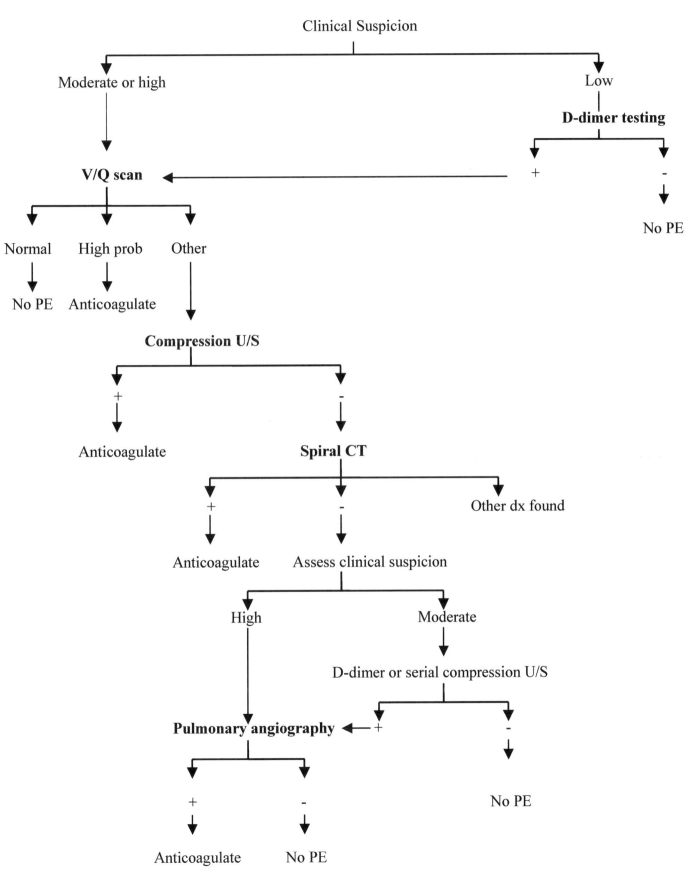

✪ *Remember*, in V/Q scanning, a normal scan essentially rules out PE, and an angiogram should follow an indeterminate scan if your clinical suspicion is high.

TESTING FOR PE WITH A D-DIMER ASSAY:

✪ *A D-dimer assay can help rule out PE in patients with nondiagnostic lung scans or a low pretest probability of disease:*

- For those patients with a **low pretest probability** of disease and a normal D-dimer result, the D-dimer assay has been shown to yield a <u>negative predictive value of 99%.</u>
- For those with a **nondiagnostic lung scan** and a normal assay, the D-dimer assay has been shown to have a <u>negative predictive value of 97%.</u>

PULMONARY INVOLVEMENT IN RA

1. *Caplan syndrome* (pneumoconiosis + rheumatoid nodules in the lungs)
2. Crycoaretenoid joints affected→upper airway obstruction may be seen.
3. Interstitial fibrosis
4. Obliterative bronchiolitis
5. Pleural effusions (re: low glucose)
6. Restrictive picture to PFTs and/or ↓DLCO
7. Subpleural rheumatoid nodules (usually only seen with high titres RF or when additional features are present)

THEOPHYLLINE dose should be monitored especially closely when used in:
(all of the following slow the rate of elimination of theo ✪)

1. CHF; COPD

2. Obesity

3. OCPs

4. Severe liver disease

5. Simultaneous use of cimetidine, erythromycin, fluoroquinolones (e.g. cipro), digoxin, verapamil, propranolol, allopurinol, and OCPs.

✪ <u>*Smoking*, on the other hand, causes theophylline to be more rapidly cleared; hence theophylline dose should be adjusted upwards as appropriate.</u>

THEOPHYLLINE TOXICITY—PRIMARILY 3 SYSTEMS ✪

1. **Neuro**→tremor/seizures; insomnia

2. **Cardiac**→arrythmias

3. **GI**→N/V

POOR PROGNOSTICATORS IN COPD
1. ↓FEV 1
2. Cor Pulmonale
3. Poor ABG findings
4. Tachycardia

A COMPARISON OF THE MAIN SMOKING-RELATED COPDs:

Emphysema	vs	**Chronic Bronchitis**
'Pink Puffers'		'Blue Bloaters'
Dyspnea		Coughing
Hyperventilation ("pink puffer")		No hyperventilation
No cyanosis		Cyanosis ("blue") Right heart failure→edema ("bloater")

SILO-FILLER DISEASE ✪
1. 2° to inhalation of **nitrous oxide**
2. Causes **non-cardiogenic pulmonary edema**
3. May see symptoms in 2 patterns, early (immediately after exposure) and weeks later.

CHRONIC EOSINOPHILIC PNEUMONIA (CEP) ✪
1. Diffuse interstitial infiltrates in the peripheral lung fields. When bilateral, this is referred to as the "**photonegative**" of pulmonary edema.

2. **Asthma and BOOP** are common associations

3. **Eosinophilia** in the blood and lung tissue
4. May also see ↑ platelets, ↑↑ESR, and an Fe def anemia
5. **Unlike PEG, it responds well to steroids**

DRUGS WHICH CAUSE NON-CARDIOGENIC PULMONARY EDEMA
1. Opiates (heroine; morphine; methadone)
2. ASA
3. Propoxyphene (Darvon®)

ARDS ✪
1. Remember, the **wedge (PCWP) is normal** (as opposed to CHF); compliance is decreased
2. **Hypoxemia** is the major clinical manifestation
3. **Sepsis is the #1 cause** (trauma, burns, pancreatitis are just some of the many other causes)

4. **PEEP** is an important resource to use <u>because</u>:
   a. It prevents alveolar collapse
   b. It plays an important role in recruiting collapsed alveolar units
   c. It allows you to dial down the FIO2 that might otherwise cause further damage that actually resemble ARDS. This usually occurs at levels ≥ 60% FIO2 for >24 hours.
   d. Beware, though, as PEEP can cause a drop in the cardiac output.
5. Another potential resource in ARDS is the use of a **reverse I:E ratio** in venting the patient. Normal ventilation has a shorter inspiratory time (I) than expiratory time (E), so a reverse I:E gives a longer inspiratory (I) time, which therefore allows for better oxygenation across the stiff lungs of these patients.
6. Carries a high mortality

VENTILATORS ✪

Ventilator SETTINGS:

> ☞ **To affect the pH or pCO2, you adjust the <u>RATE</u> and/or <u>TIDAL VOLUME</u>.**
>
> ☞ **The rate is usually altered first.To affect the pO2 or sat%, the <u>FIO2</u> and/or <u>PEEP</u> are usually adjusted, usually the FIO2 first.**
>
> ☞ [Recall that a **NORMAL** pH=7.<u>**40**</u>; a normal pCO2=<u>**40**</u>; a normal pO2 is about 100.]
>
> ☞ The only other ventilator setting is the **MODE**. The most common modes are IMV, SIMV, CPAP, and Assist Control. It is important to know how each of these modes work.

✪ **Intermittent Mandatory Ventilation (<u>IMV</u>).** <u>IMV</u>: The patient can breath his or her own spontaneous breaths at his own rate and volume, AND the machine will coordinate the dialed-in number of breaths to be delivered in synchrony.

✪ **Continuous Positive Airway Pressure (<u>CPAP</u>).** The machine provides no breaths, but does provide air at a preset FIO2 with a constant airway pressureThe patient does all of the ventilation in this mode, but remains connected to the ventilator primarily for monitoring purposes. It is useful as a test before extubation. IMV is also used as a weaning or exercise mode. So is **"T-piece"**, which is often <u>likened to *breathing through a large straw*</u> to exercise the respiratory muscles before extubation. Patients usually rest at night on Assist Control mode (*see next*).

✪ **Assist Control (<u>AC</u>).** *This is the <u>usual preferred initial mode</u>.* The patient initiates a breath and the machine cycles on to deliver the preset tidal volume. Essentially the machine senses the negative inspiratory pressure exerted by the patient and **"assists"** the patient by helping with the remainder of the inspiratory effort. If the patient fails to make a breathing effort altogether OR if the patient's intrinsic respiratory rate is less than the ventilator rate you've dialed in the machine has a **"back-up rate"** or set number of breaths that is delivered anyways.

ADJUSTING THE SETTINGS: GENERAL RULES OF THUMB...

☞ **When the pO2 is high**, lower the FIO2. Use the **Rule of 7's** to guide your adjustment in FIO2: For every 1% decrease in FIO2, the pO2 will drop by 7. So, for example, if the pO2 is 310 on 80% FIO2, take 310-100 (goal)=210, which is the amount of decrease we will need to make in the pO2. Dividing 210 by 7, we see we need to lower the FIO2 by 30. So 80%-30% leaves 50%, which is where we should order the new FIO2 in order to bring down the pO2 to 100.

☞ If the pO2 is high and your FIO2 is already low, then the PEEP can be lowered (usually in increments of 2 with follow-up blood gases). Because of oxygen toxicity, patients with a high pO2 should have their FIO2 lowered first, then the PEEP.

☞ *Conversely*, **for low pO2s**, one should similarly first adjust the FIO2 up before adjusting the PEEP. Let's briefly reiterate several important points about PEEP:
> **PEEP** is an important resource to use <u>because</u>:
> a. It prevents alveolar collapse
> b. It plays an important role in recruiting collapsed alveolar units
> c. It allows you to dial down the FIO2 that might otherwise cause further damage that actually resemble ARDS. This usually occurs at levels $\geq$ 60% FIO2 for >24 hours.
> d. Beware, though, as PEEP can cause a drop in the cardiac output.

☞ **When the pCO2 is high**, this typically indicates hypoventilation, so, assuming our tidal volume is set at 10-15cc/kg, simply dial up the rate first.

☞ *Conversely*, **when the pCO2 is low**, this usually indicates hyperventilation (for whatever reason) and either the rate should be lowered, or, if it is noted the patient's spontaneous breaths (not machine-delivered breaths) are tachypneic, then sedation or even paralysis with further evaluation may be necessary.

COMPLIANCE: 2 Types: Static vs. Dynamic:

$$\textbf{STATIC Compliance} \atop \textit{(indicates airway resistance)} \quad = \quad \frac{\text{Tidal Volume}}{(\textbf{\textit{Plateau}} \text{ pressure-PEEP})}$$

$$\textbf{DYNAMIC Compliance} \atop \textit{(reflects parenchymal disease)} \quad = \quad \frac{\text{Tidal Volume}}{(\textbf{\textit{Peak}} \text{ pressure-PEEP})}$$

RECOGNIZING COMMON VENTILATOR PROBLEMS:

Problem	→	**Usual Answer**
High peak pressure		Mucus plugging *
Low pressure (peak) alarm		Cuff leak/cuff rupture **
High peak and plateau pressures		Pneumothorax, CHF common
Low compliance		ARDS

*   Also ✓:   ETT down right mainstem bronchus; pneumothorax; kinked tube; bronchospasm; and patient bucking the vent

**   Also ✓:   ETT dislodged into oropharynx; disconnected tubing

---

☞ Because of the frequent observation that high airway pressures often result from attempts to normalize pCO_2, causing microstructural lung damage, propagating lung injury, and ultimately **barotrauma, PERMISSIVE HYPERCAPNIA** is a technique commonly employed in combination with the preferred Pressure-Control Ventilation mode (as opposed to the other Volume-Control modes of ventilation, discussed earlier) to *purposely* allow pCO_2 to increase in order to limit peak airway pressure. Barotrauma can present with interstitial emphysema, pneumomediastinum, subcutaneous emphysema, or pneumothorax. Although these signs may resolve simply by decreasing airway pressures, clinically significant pneumothorax, (eg noting hypoxemia, decreased lung compliance, or hemodynamic compromise) requires tube thoracostomy.

WEANING

WEANING CRITERIA:

Before starting to wean the patient from the machine, these parameters should be met:
1. FIO_2 <40%
2. PEEP<5
3. PaO_2>60
4. Patient alert and stable

The patient must have adequate ventilation on their own; therefore:
5. MIF (maximum inspiratory force) must be ≥ -25 (more negative); and
6. TV (tidal volume) >400cc in a normal sized adult;
7. Vital Capacity > 10cc/kg
8. Minute volume (resp rate x TV) *of the ventilator* ≤ 10 L/min

☞ For all *ventilator emergencies*, remember to *first disconnect* the patient from the ventilator *and bag* the patient with 100% oxygen until an adequate solution is found and problem is resolved.

IMPORTANT WEANING MODES

1. T-piece

2. CPAP

3. SIMV

CHOICE OF WEANING MODE

⇒ _T-piece and CPAP_ weaning are good options for patients who have undergone mechanical ventilation for short periods and therefore do not require much in the way of respiratory muscle reconditioning. _SIMV_ is better for patients who have been intubated for prolonged periods and therefore require gradual respiratory muscle reconditioning.

DOING THE ACTUAL WEAN

✪ **T-piece weaning** involves brief spontaneous breathing exercises or trials with supplemental oxygen. Trials are usually initiated for 5 min/h and are typically followed by a 1-h rest interval (on AC mode, or "resting mode"). T-piece trials are gradually increased in 5- to 10-min increments until the patient demonstrates that s/he can remain off the vent for several hours at a time. Extubation can then be tried.

✪ **CPAP weaning** is similar to weaning on the T-piece except that trials of spontaneous breathing are done while the patient is physically on the ventilator in CPAP mode. This is usually applied _with pressure support_ (PS), which one can liken to another PS, "Power Steering", since it helps to "drive" the breath in (pardon the pun), making it easier for the patient to pull the entire breath. In addition, pressure support is also useful in weaning patients (CPAP _or_ IMV modes), since it helps prevent any microatelectasis, thereby decreasing shunting and easing any weaning attempts.

✪ **IMV weaning** entails gradually lowering the mandatory backupor machine rate in increments of 2-4 breaths per minute while monitoring the patient's blood gases and respiratory rates. Respiratory rates > 25 usually indicate respiratory muscle fatigue and the need to combine such trials with periods of rest. Exercise periods are progressively increased until the patient can tolerate this mode all the way down to 4 breaths per minute. T-piece or CPAP trials can then be attempted before considering extubation.

11. __ENDOCRINOLOGY__

✪ HIRSUTISM

- Diagnosis--The idea is to figure out if _the androgens are coming from the ovary_ (✓ _testosterone_) or from the **_adrenals_** (✓ _DHEAS_; congenital adrenal hyperplasia; adrenal tumor).

- **DHEAS levels**: _DHEAS is an adrenal androgen_

  >7 ng/dl→DDx includes **adrenal tumor or CAH**
  <7 ng/dl→ excludes adrenal tumor or CAH → then check Testost.

- **TESTOSTERONE**: >200 →Suspect **ovarian tumor**.
  <200 →PCO

- ↑ T + ↑ DHEAS → adrenal cause
- ↑ T only → ovarian cause

- _Other hyperandrogenic signs_ that may be appreciated...
  1. Acne
  2. Abnormal menses
  3. Clitorimegaly
  4. Masculinization
  5. Defeminization

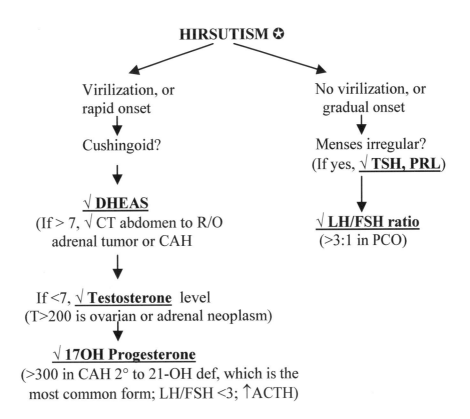

HIRSUTISM ✪

Virilization, or rapid onset

Cushingoid?

√ DHEAS
(If > 7, √ CT abdomen to R/O adrenal tumor or CAH

If <7, √ **Testosterone** level
(T>200 is ovarian or adrenal neoplasm)

√ 17OH Progesterone
(>300 in CAH 2° to 21-OH def, which is the most common form; LH/FSH <3; ↑ACTH)

No virilization, or gradual onset

Menses irregular?
(If yes, √ **TSH, PRL**)

√ LH/FSH ratio
(>3:1 in PCO)

✪ THE RELATIONSHIP BETWEEN THE CORTISOL AND ANDROGEN SYNTHESIS PATHWAYS
<u>GONADAL & ADRENAL</u> SOURCES OF ANDROGENS :

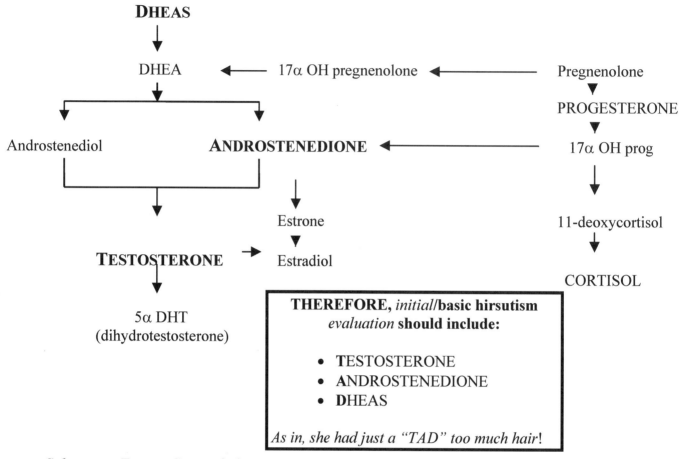

THEREFORE, *initial*/**basic hirsutism** *evaluation* **should include:**

- **T**ESTOSTERONE
- **A**NDROSTENEDIONE
- **D**HEAS

As in, she had just a "TAD" too much hair!

Subsequent Testing Can Include…
1. LH, FSH, SHBG (Sex hormone-binding globulin)
2. Free testosterone
3. DHT
4. Estradiol
5. Prolactin
6. ACTH
7. Cortisol
8. Dexamethosone Suppression Testing
9. Transvaginal U/S

✪ CAH (CONGENITAL ADRENAL HYPERPLASIA)
☞ *Must <u>know these clinical associations</u>…*

✪ <u>**17 α hydroxylase** deficiency</u> ⟶ <u>**HTN**</u> *[think of a "<u>hyper</u>" teenager (17)]*
✪ <u>**21-hydroxylase** deficiency</u> ⟶ <u>**VIRILIZATION**</u>; 21-hydroxylase deficiency is the most common (95%) form of CAH. (*<u>SEE also FIG. 3 APPENDIX</u>*)

AMENORRHEA WORKUP:

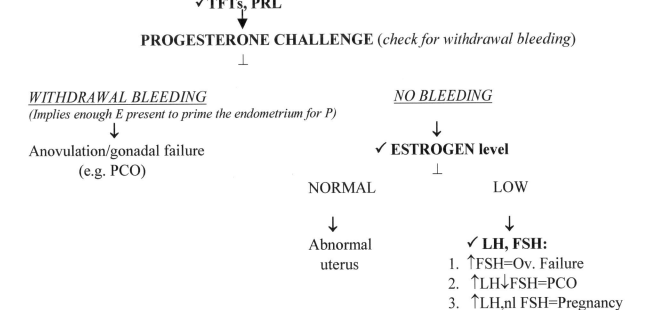

AMENORRHEA ✪
↓
✓β-HCG
↓
✓TFTs, PRL
↓
PROGESTERONE CHALLENGE (*check for withdrawal bleeding*)
⊥

WITHDRAWAL BLEEDING
(*Implies enough E present to prime the endometrium for P*)
↓
Anovulation/gonadal failure
(e.g. PCO)

NO BLEEDING
↓
✓ **ESTROGEN level**
⊥

NORMAL   LOW
↓   ↓
Abnormal   ✓ **LH, FSH:**
uterus   1. ↑FSH=Ov. Failure
                2. ↑LH↓FSH=PCO
                3. ↑LH,nl FSH=Pregnancy
                4. ↓LH↓FSH=Hypopit.

- Remember that the #1 cause of amenorrhea and ↑PRL is *pregnancy*!

- *Ovarian disorders* are common causes of 2° amenorrhea; **PCO** (*Polycystic Ovary Syndrome* is the most common of these).
  - ✓ The diagnosis is often made by recognizing an *obese, hirsute* patient with complaints of abnormal menses. An ↑LH/FSH ratio (>3:1) is common in this disorder. ↑PRL in $^1/_2$-$^1/_3$ of these pts.

- *"Postpill" amenorrhea* accounts for 30% of 2° amenorrhea; it occurs in 2% of women taking BCPs; 30% of *those* have *hyperprolactinemia*; remember, psychotropic drugs (**phenothiazines), haloperidol, and metoclopramide** can ↑ PRL levels→2° amenorrhea.

- HyperPRL accounts for 25-40% of all 2° amenorrhea;

- *1° hypothyroidism* is also a common cause

- If adult female sex characteristics are present and neg βHCG→R/O *structural causes* of amenorrhea as well as *TFM*.

- If patient is sexually infantile, R/O 1° amenorrhea, checking *hormone levels*.

ORAL CONTRACEPTIVES

> ➢ Can be either a combination of estrogen + progestin, *or* progestin only.

> ➢ Inhibit GnRH secretion and the mid-cycle LH surge so that ovulation does not occur.

> ➢ *Potential complications*...
>   1. Migraine
>   2. HTN
>   3. Hepatic adenoma
>   4. ↑ risk of thromboembolism, CAD, CVA

> ➢ *Precautions*...(use carefully in these individuals)
>   1. Obese
>   2. Smokers
>   3. Varicose veins
>   4. History of hypercoaguability

CONTRAINDICATIONS TO ERT FOR OSTEOPOROSIS
Absolute
- ✓ Estrogen-dependent neoplasm
- ✓ H/o breast cancer
- ✓ H/o or active thromboembolic disorder
- ✓ Undiagnosed or abnormal vaginal bleeding

Relative
- ✓ + FH for ↑TG
- ✓ Chronic hepatic dysfunction
- ✓ Endometriosis
- ✓ Gall bladder disease
- ✓ H/o thromboembolism
- ✓ Migraine
- ✓ Strong FH of breast cancer
- ✓ Uterine cancer
- ✓ Uterine leiomyomas

HYPOGONADISM

> ➢ Semen analysis almost always abnormal

> ➢ ↓ SHBG (Serum Hormone Binding Globulin); ↓ serum Testosterone is not specific for hypogonadism.

> ➢ Primary gonadal failure→see ↑ LH, FSH
> ➢ Secondary gonadal failure ("hypogonado**trop**ism")→ see ↓ LH, FSH; one should therefore also evaluate the rest of the pituitary functions.

- These pairs should be analyzed together…
  a)   FSH level↔semen analysis
  b)   LH level ↔Testosterone level

➢ If patient presents with delayed puberty + ***anosmia/hyposmia*** (abnormal development of olfactory lobes)→***Kallmann's Syndrome***.

➢ MANAGEMENT:

  ✓ *Testosterone replacement* therapy is the treatment of choice for men with hypogonadism

  ✓ Testosterone should be administered only to a man who is hypogonadal, as evidenced by a distinctly *subnormal serum testosterone* concentration. In comparison, increasing the serum testosterone concentration in a man whose testosterone concentration is already normal will have no beneficial effect *even if* the man has symptoms suggestive of hypogonadism.

  ✓ Testosterone can be replaced satisfactorily whether the testosterone deficiency is due to *primary or secondary hypogonadism*.

  ✓ Native testosterone is absorbed well from the intestine, but it is metabolized so rapidly by the liver that it is virtually *impossible to maintain a normal serum testosterone* concentration in a hypogonadal man *with oral testosterone*. Transdermal patches and IM injections of testosterone are the most common forms of treatment. The principal goal of testosterone therapy is to restore the serum testosterone concentration to the normal range.

  ✓ In *Klinefelter's Syndrome (next), remember to delay testosterone supplementation as long as possible to allow for closure of the epiphyses to allow appropriate growth.*

KLINEFELTER'S SYNDROME

  ▪ 47 XXY
  ▪ *Clinical*
    1. Small, firm testes
    2. Azospermia; infertility
    3. Testosterone ↓
    4. LH, FSH ↓
    5. Gynecomastia (incidentally, unilateral gynecomastia should make one think of carcinoma)
    6. Eunuchoidism
    7. Positive buccal smear (for karyotyping)

MALE INFERTILITY

Common causes

1. Abnormal sperm count/quality
2. Ductal obstruction (e.g. 2° to varicocele—90% are left-sided)
3. Ejaculatory disorders

Azospermia—physician must differentiate #1 from #2; FSH levels and sometimes testicular biopsy (ouch!) can settle.

IMPOTENCE (1° vs. 2°)

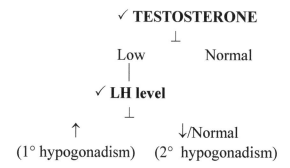

✪ TFM (TESTICULAR FEMINIZATION)

1. Genetic males affected with ambiguous genitalia (thus aka "*Male Pseudohermaphroditism*")
2. Lack the enzyme *5 alpha-reductase* for *peripheral conversion of testosterone to its active form, DHT* (dihydrotestosterone), in the tissues.
3. At adolescence, normal breast and female 2° sex characteristics seen; however, no pubic hair and no menarche
4. Managed with *gonadectomy after puberty completed*

TURNER'S SYNDROME

- Female phenotype
- 45XO
- **Clinical**—may see…

    1. Short stature
    2. Webbed neck
    3. Low-set ears
    4. Small jaw (micrognathia)
    5. Short metacarpals/metatarsals
    6. Epicanthal folds
    7. Shield-like chest
    8. ↑ carrying angle at the elbows
    9. Coarctation + Aortic Stenosis
    10. Amenorrhea—in fact this is the #1 cause of 1° amenorrhea

- *Turner mosaics may have none of these stigmata and may present with either 1° or 2° amenorrhea.*

☞ In treating patients with both ACTH and TSH deficiencies, eg in hypopituitarism from any cause, remember to ***give the glucocorticoid first***, since supplementing the thyroxine first may exacerbate the need for cortisol and precipate an acute adrenocortical crisis.

✪ PROLACTINOMAS

- *Manifest as…*
    1. *Amenorrhea/galactorrhea in women*
    2. *Decreased libido and potency in men*
        - ☞ These symptoms are often dismissed/passed off as psychiatric factors, thus delaying the diagnosis in men.
    3. Delayed sexual maturation in adolescents

- *Diagnosis*
    1. In women, always R/O pregnancy first
    2. Check serum PRL (prolactin) level. Serum prolactin values between 20 and 200 ng/mL are often due to functional causes, like those listed below. On the other hand, serum prolactin values above 200 ng/mL usually indicate the presence of prolactinoma. *Important functional causes of hyperprolactinemia to know:*

        a. *Drugs*
            (1) Several drugs are known dopamine D2 receptor antagonists, and raise serum prolactin by that mechanism. These include *phenothiazines, haloperidol, butyrophenones, metoclopramide, sulpiride, domperidone , and risperidone*
            (2) *Methyldopa* decreases dopamine synthesis—remember, this is a preferred drug for HTN in pregnancy
            (3) *Estrogen*-- estrogen to the estrogen receptor, which then binds to an estrogen response element on the prolactin gene, in the lactotroph cell of the pituitary

        b. *1° hypothyroidism*
        c. *CRF*
        d. *Chest wall trauma/lesions*
        e. *Pregnancy*
        f. *Ovarian disorders, esp PCO*

- ✪ **TREATMENT**-- Patients who have **MICROPROLACTINOMAS** (<u><10mm</u>)and who have any degree of *hypogonadism* (or infertility, galactorrhea, or hirsutism felt to be attributable to the lesion) should be treated first with a **dopamine agonist**.

Important dopamine agonists to consider are ...

> ➤ *Cabergoline*— Cabergoline is a nonergot dopamine agonist that is administered *once or twice a week*, and has much less tendency to cause nausea than bromocriptine and pergolide. It may be effective in patients resistant to bromocriptine.
> ➤ *Bromocriptine* — Bromocriptine is an ergot derivative that has been used for approximately two decades for treatment of hyperprolactinemia. It *must be given at least twice a day* to have maximal therapeutic effect.
> ➤ *Pergolide* — Pergolide is also an ergot derivative and has been approved by the FDA for the treatment of Parkinson's disease but not for hyperprolactinemia. Its *advantage over bromocriptine is that it can be given once a day, and its advantage over cabergoline is that it costs about one-sixth as much.*

- ✓ *serum PRL level at ONE MONTH* and evaluate for side effects. Subsequent treatment depends upon the response:

  - PRL now ↓ to normal/Pt tolerates → continue dose → gonadal function expected to return in a few months

    - The drug should be continued unless the patient becomes *pregnant*. After approximately one year, the dose can often be decreased. Complete cessation of the the drug, however, usually leads to recurrent hyperprolactinemia.
    - *After menopause, the drug can be discontinued* and the serum prolactin concentration can be allowed to rise. *Imaging should be performed if the value rises above 200 ng/mL* to determine if the adenoma has increased to a clinically important size. If so, drug therapy should be resumed.

  - If PRL level NOT down to normal, titrate your dopamine agonist up until a normal level is achieved
    - If no effect titrating up or if the patient can't tolerate any one, try switching dopamine agonists

MACROPROLACTINOMAS (>10mm)—Management is similar to microprolactinoma. *In addition*:

- ✓ Treatment of patients with prolactin macroadenomas, no matter how large or how severe the neurologic sequelae, *should also be initiated with a dopamine agonist*.
- ✓ *If vision was abnormal before therapy*, it should be reassessed within one month, although improvement may occur within a few days. An *MRI should be repeated in 6 to 12 months* to determine if the size of the adenoma has decreased.
- ✓ The size of the adenoma *decreases to approximately the same degree as the serum prolactin* concentration.

- ✓ *The decrease in size usually cannot be demonstrated until weeks or months after the prolactin secretion has decreased.*
- ✓ If the serum prolactin concentration has been normal for *at least one year* and the adenoma has decreased markedly in size, the dose of the dopamine agonist can be decreased gradually, as long as the serum prolactin remains normal.
- ✓ *Unlike microprolactinomas, the agonist should NOT be discontinued entirely, even after menopause, because hyperprolactinemia will probably recur and the adenoma may increase in size.*
- ✓ If the patient cannot tolerate, or the adenoma does not respond to agonist therapy, *transsphenoidal surgery* should be performed and, if a significant amount of adenoma tissue remains after surgery, *radiation therapy* should be administered.

✪ ACROMEGALY

Clinical Presentation (2° to GH/IGF-1 excess):

1. Acromegalic features
2. ***Carbohydrate intolerance*** in 20%
3. ↑ Sweating and oily Skin; skin tags
4. ↓ Heat tolerance
5. Acroparesthesias
6. ***Carpal tunnel*** dz and other **N**erve entrapment syndromes
7. Prolactinemia (in up to half the cases), causing amenorrhea/↓libido/galactorrhea
8. ***Proximal myopathy***
9. Acanthosis Nigricans (other causes of A.N. are obesity; DM; gastric ca)
10. Sleep apnea
11. Cardiomyopathy or HTN

> ✪ ***Remember*** → ***"PM SNAC"*** (**P**rolactinemia/**P**roximal **M**yalgia; **S**weating/oily **S**kin/**S**kin tags; **S**leep apnea; **N**europathies (entrapment);**A**cromegalic features/ **A**croparesthesias; **A**canthosis Nigricans; **C**arbohydrate intolerance/**C**ardiomyopathy)

DIAGNOSIS is either by:
1. ↑ *Serum IGF-1 (somatomedin); or*
2. OGTT (*oral glucose tolerance test), checking for non-suppressible GH,* i.e. GH that remains ↑ after administering ↑glucose load(this is the standard reference test). If GH does not suppress to < 10ug/L, the test is positive for GH excess.

MORTALITY is ↑ SECONDARY TO:
1. HTN
2. DM
3. Cardiovascular effects

DIABETES INSIPIDUS ✪

1. Causes polyuria and polydipsia (often with preference for ice-cold water); nocturia common.
2. May result from…
   a. <u>Production</u> of AVP→central DI→e.g. breast/lung ca mets, with ***abrupt*** onset of symptoms.
   b. <u>Sensitivity</u> of the kidneys to AVP→nephrogenic DI→e.g. ***Lithium*** toxicity
   c. Functional suppression of AVP →primary <u>polydipsia (compulsive water drinking)</u>→e.g. a ***psych***iatric patient.

3. **WATER DEPRIVATION TEST ✪**

   Deprive the patient of water and measure the subsequent urine and plasma osmolality q2h until plasma osm > 295 mosm/kg H20 is reached OR a 5% weight loss occurs. <u>Normally</u>, this would cause an individual to secrete ADH to conserve their water, causing <u>elevations in subsequent measurements of serum and urine concentration</u>. But in DI, there is either not enough ADH released from the brain or a lack of responsiveness to ADH at the level of the kidneys, so concentrations will not ↑ as expected to. If the plasma osm > 295, but the urine osm does not exceed 500, the test is positive (for DI) and the patient should be further evaluated with a vasopressin challenge.

   Overview ✪

Water deprivation	Response to AVP	DIAGNOSIS
Normal	Absent	1° Polydipsia
+	**Present**	Central DI
+	**Absent**	Nephrogenic DI

   More specifically…

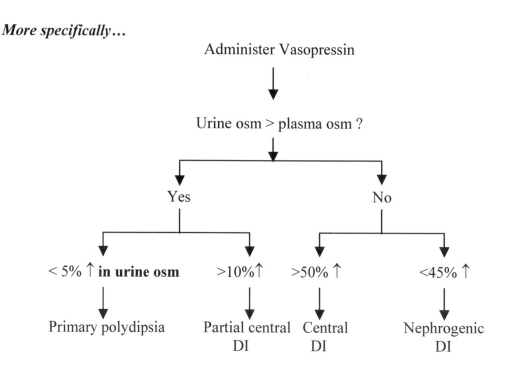

4. *Treatment depends on the cause...*
   a. Central DI→intranasal dDAVP (ADH analog)
   b. Partial central DI→Chlorpropamide (AVP agonist)
   c. Nephrogenic DI→Thiazides (diuresis causes ablation of medullary gradient which, in turn, decreases urine volume output), but patients must be on a Na^+ restricted diet to work

SIADH (Syndrome of Inappropriate ADH Secretion)

1. SIADH *should be suspected in patients who have hyponatremia and a concentrated urine (osmolality >300 mmol/kg) in the absence of* edema, orthostatic hypotension, and features of dehydration.

2. *Urine osmolality inappropriately > serum osm*

3. **Spot urine Na^+ >30**

4. ↓ serum Na+ ; a ↓ serum uric acid is also a frequent concomitant.

5. To make this diagnosis, you *must first rule out* the following conditions...
   a. ↑ or ↓ volume (SIADH is a euvolemic state)
   b. Effect of diuretics
   c. Thyroid deficiency (✓TSH)
   d. Adrenal deficiency (✓ACTH)

6. IMPORTANT CAUSES to know:
   a. Medications (eg carbamazepine, cyclophosphamide, TCAs, narcotics, phenothiazenes, vincristine & vinblastine)
   b. Pneumonia, COPD, pulmonary abscess, TB
   c. Meningitis
   d. Nausea
   e. Pain
   f. Postsurgical
   g. Small cell lung ca

7. TREATMENT

   a. **Fluid restrict** to 1-1.5 L/day is the mainstay of treatment.

   b. If the patient has **symptomatic** ↓Na+ with neurologic sequelae, then **hypertonic saline** is the tx.

   c. It is said that overly rapid correction of the serum Na+ with hypertonic saline can lead to CPM (Central Pontine Myelinolysis).

   d. *Demeclocycline* (an *antibiotic that inhibits the effects of ADH at the collecting ducts*)

THYROID DISORDERS

> ❂ **THE RELATIONSHIP BETWEEN GOITERS AND THYROIDITIS :**
> *(EITHER can be thyrotoxic or underactive) :*

GOITERS

⊥

GRAVES' Disease
(thyrotoxic)

THYROIDITIS

⊥

Silent
and Subacute
(these may be either
thyrotoxic **OR** hypothyroid)

HASHIMOTO'S
(hypothyroid)

☞ **THYROID SCANNING** (24 hour **Iodine** [131] **uptake**)

- Useful in the DDx of **THYROTOXICOSIS WITH DIFFUSE GOITER :**

> ❂ ↑UPTAKE→**Graves' Disease**
> ❂ ↓UPTAKE→**Subacute and silent thyroiditis**

❂ **SUBACUTE & SILENT THYROIDITIS** (can be ↑ or ↓ thyroid)

➢ Inflamed/damaged thyroid tissue causes release of stored hormones→a few weeks of mild **thyrotoxicosis that may be followed by** a short period of **hypothyroidism** while the thyroid recovers.

➢ **2 TYPES (BOTH SELF-LIMITING) …**

1. **SUBACUTE**
   a) Uncommon
   b) Painful, *tender* goiter
   c) Causative agent felt to be <u>viral</u>
   d) ↑ *thyroglobulin;* ↑ *temp;* ↑ *ESR*; ↓ I uptake
   e) Self-limiting
   f) For moderate disease→may treat with NSAIDs
   g) For more severe disease→may treat with prednisone

2. **Painless lymphocytic; so-called "<u>SILENT</u>"**
   a) Common
   b) Acute (often postpartum), transient thyrotoxicosis usual
   c) Self-limiting disease, but a tendency to recur ; beta-blockers prn
   d) Normal ESR

DIFFERENTIATING THYROIDITIS:

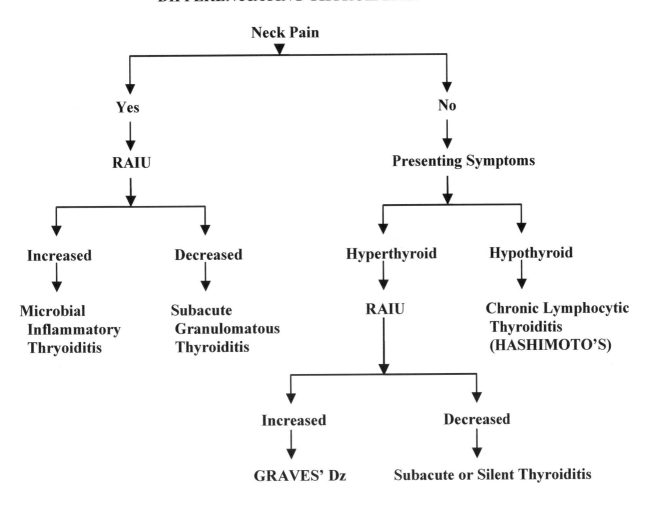

THYROIDITIS TERMS/SYNONYMS:

Chronic Lymphocytic Thyroiditis	aka **Hashimoto's** thyroiditis
Subacute Thyroiditis	Re: tender, *painful*; usually *viral* etiology
Silent Thyroiditis	Re: *painless*; lymphocytic; *postpartum*
Granulomatous	aka Subacute granulomatous thyroiditis; de Quervain's
Microbial inflammatory	Suppurative thyroiditis; acute thyroiditis
Invasive fibrous	Riedel's struma; Riedel's thyroiditis.

✪ ***REMEMBER***, the #1 cause of <u>Hyperthyroidism</u> is *Graves'* Disease, and the #1 cause of <u>hy</u>pothyroidism is *Hashimoto's* thyroiditis. <u>**Therefore**</u>, the #1 cause of both is an ***<u>autoimmune</u>*** disorder.

✪ The ACP now recommends screening *TSH in asymp women q5y beginning at age 50.* By contrast the American Thyroid Assn recommends screening asymp *adults q5y from age 35.*

HYPOTHYROIDISM (Hashimoto's Thyroiditis)

1. Also the most common form of thyroiditis
2. **<u>Anti-microsomal Ab</u>** is usually present; **<u>Antithyroglobulin Ab</u>** present over ½ the time.
3. Clinical
    a) Bradycardia
    b) Constipation
    c) Carpal tunnel syndrome
    d) Pericardial/pleural effusions
    e) Associated autoimmune disorders (e.g. DM)
    f) Hyperlipidemia
    g) HTN; cardiomyopathy

4. May present with ***<u>lymphocytic thyoiditis</u>*** (***<u>postpartum</u>*** transient hyperthyroidism followed by transient hypothyroidism as is seen within 6 months of delivery.) Antimicrosomal Ab is usually +.

5. May be goitrous or atrophic.

HYPERTHYROIDISM

1. ***Main causes include…***
    a) Nodular goiter—
    b) Single (Toxic Nodular Goiter, or TNG) *or*
    c) Multiple (Toxic Multinodular Goiter, or TMG—below)
    d) Thyroiditis—silent or subacute
    e) Graves' disease
    f) Tumors

2. **GRAVES' Disease**
    a) **<u>2 types of ocular findings</u>** ✪
        (1) *Infiltrative findings* (<u>only Graves'</u>):
            (a) Proptosis
            (b) Optic neuritis
            (c) Extraocular muscle dysfunction

        (2) *Noninfiltrative Findings* (<u>any thyrotoxicosis</u>)
            (a) Lid lag
            (b) Lid retraction
    b) Diffuse goiter (remember, *20% of patients, especially elderly, may not evince goiter*)
    c) Thyrotoxicosis 2° to ***thyroid-stimulating antibodies***

3. **Diffuse Goiter**
   a) *Graves''s Disease*
      (1)   ↓sTSH
      (2)   ↑Iodine uptake
   b) *Silent Thyroiditis*
      (1)   ↓TSH
      (2)   ↓ Iodine uptake

4. **TOXIC MULTINODULAR GOITER** (TMG)
   a) A disease of the elderly
   b) An **"APATHETIC" HYPERTHYROID** ✪ (note the oxymoron) (may mimic depression); picture dominates with…
      (1)   Weakness
      (2)   Loss of appetite
      (3)   Loss of energy
      (4)   Cardiovascular effects (arrhythmias;CHF)

5. **Toxic Nodular Goiter** (TNG)
   a)   Solitary nodule > 3cm
   b)   Isolated intense ↑ uptake on thyroid scan

6. **Thyroiditis**—previously discussed—*remember*: can be ↓ or↑ thyroid

7. **FACTITIOUS Thyrotoxicosis**
   a)   Ingested T3 or T4
   b)   Suspect it in thyrotoxic individuals with all of the following…
      (1)   High T4 or T3
      (2)   **No** goiter
      (3)   ↓ TSH
      (4)   ↓ serum thyroglobulin
      (5)   ↓ I-131 UPTAKE

8. **TREATMENT**…

   a) **BY DISEASE:**

      (1) *Graves'*→RAI (Radioactive Iodine)---If patient is pregnant, surgery (subtotal thyroidectomy) or antithyroid meds—see below—are appropriate treatment alternatives to RAI.

      (2) *TNG*→RAI or surgery

      (3) *TMG*→RAI or surgery

Remember, ***pregnancy*** *is the only absolute contraindication to RAI; the only major drawback of RAI is the development of hypothyroidism*

(4) ***Silent Thyroiditis***→symptomatic/supportive since self-remitting

(5) ***Subacute Thyroiditis***→as per silent thyroiditis + steroids/NSAIDs

(6) Tumor→surgery

b) **ANTITHYROID MEDICATION**

(1) **Methimazole**--↓ T4 production
(2) **Propylthiouracil (PTU)**--↓ T4 production & blocks T4→T3 conversion
Remember, **P**TU for **P**regnancy
Side effects of these agents...
  i. Agranulocytosis
  ii. Aplastic Anemia
  iii. Hepatitis
  iv. Vasculitis

(3) Beta-Blockers should be considered as adjunctive treatment only.

ALGORITHMIC WORKUP OF A THYROID NODULE...

FINE NEEDLE ASPIRATION:

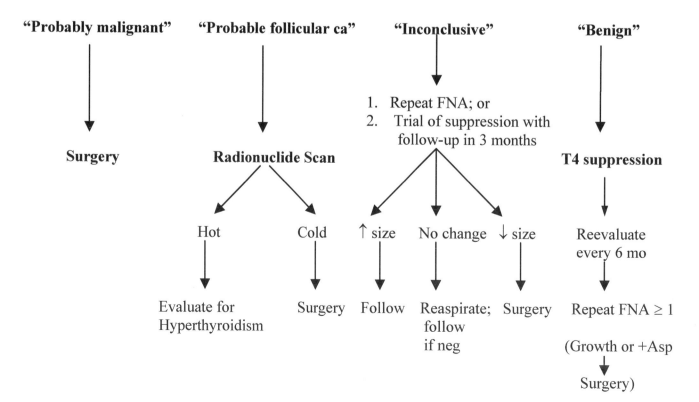

THRYOID NODULES--*90% rule of thumb*:

☞ 90% are benign
☞ 90% (!) are "cold" (Note: only 20% of these are actually malignant; 1% for hot nodules)
☞ 90% are solid

THYROID CA ✪

1. Nevertheless, remember, the classic link "**C** old" nodule↔**C** ancer.
2. "Hot" nodules→nearly always benign
3. **Papillary ca** is the most common and has the ***best prognosis***. It ***spreads via lymph***
4. *nodes*, and can present with thryoid mass and + cervical LNs.
5. **Follicular ca**—spreads ***hematogenously***
6. **Anaplastic ca**
   a. Seen mostly in the elderly
   b. ***Very aggressive***
   c. ***Worst prognosis***
7. **Medullary ca**
   a. *Calcitonin* is the tumor marker
   b. Amyloid deposits common
   c. May be isolated or part of MEN IIA or IIB, so *should therefore R/O pheo and hyperparathyroidism (IIA) if you see this on your exam (or given any 2, look for the third* !)

EUTHYROID SICK SYNDROME ✪

1. Aka "Adaptive hypothyroidism"
2. Seen in hospitalized patients (thus "euthyroid sick")
3. ↓T3 ↓T4 ↓sTSH (therefore **can look like Central Hypothyroidism**, except may also see ↑ *cortisol* levels from); *free T4 is normal*; ↑ reverse T3.
4. Because of the ↓sTSH, sTSH should not be used alone to screen for thyroid dz in hospitalized patients.
5. The condition is primarily a laboratory phenomenon, is only a reflection of the patient's generally ill condition, and warrants no additional treatment.

HYPERTHYROIDISM AND PREGNANCY

1. *In Graves' disease, surgery is considered a viable option in the second trimester*. ✪
2. During pregnancy, Graves' hyperthyroidism is typically treated with **PTU** (propylthiouracil).
3. TSH-receptor antibodies are IgG and can cross the placenta and cause *neonatal hyperthyroidism* as well.
4. *Postpartum thyroiditis* occurs in about 8-10% of women and *can be confused with Graves'*.
5. Women taking medication for Graves' *must not breast-feed*.
6. *Postpartum depression* may be exacerbated by postpartum thyroiditis.

Normal Pregnant State
1. ↑T3 and ↑T4 2° to estrogen-induced ↑ in TBG
2. FTI unchanged
3. *RAI should not be given.*

THYROTOXIC CRISIS:

1. Untreated or inadequately treated **HYPER**thyroid patients undergoing surgical treatment or who have another acute illness
2. Clinical:
   a. ↑ Temp; ↑ Pulse; ↓ BP
   b. Vomiting/diarrhea
   c. Irritability; delirium
   d. coma and even death if untreated
3. PTU, Na Iodide, and Propranolol are used to control the crisis
   - Remember, PTU blocks the synthesis of thyroxine, and Na Iodide blocks the release of thyroxine from the thyroid

MYXEDEMA CRISIS ✪

1. Occurs in severe **HYPO**thyroidism
2. While it may occur spontaneously, it can be brought on by severely inadequate dosing, noncompliance with one's levothyroxine, infection, cold, and other physiologic stressors. (these risk factors are not unlike those for DKA.)
3. 20-50% mortality
4. Clinical:
   a. ↓: Temp/BP/Resp/Na/Glucose
   b. Remember, myxedema is seen in severe hypothyroidism with deposition of mucopolysaccharides in the dermis, giving a doughy appearance to the skin (remember also that it can also occur in hypERthyroidism as pretibial myxedema)
   c. Gradual onset with lethargy→stupor→*coma*
5. TREATMENT:
   - ✪ **IV levothyroxine (T$_4$)**
   - ✪ **IV liothyronine (T$_3$,** due to these patients often having reduced ability to convert T$_4$ to
   - ✪ **IV steroids**-- Until the possibility of coexisting adrenal insufficiency has been excluded, the patient must be treated with glucocorticoids in stress doses (hydrocortisone given intravenously, 100 mg every 8 hours).
   - ✪ **Supportive measures as appropriate**-- These can include treatment in an ICU, mechanical ventilation if necessary, judicious administration of IV fluids including electrolytes and glucose, correction of hypothermia, and treatment of any underlying infection.

PARATHYROID DISEASE

Remember...

1. *Magnesium* is necessary for PTH secretion, so you certainly couldn't dx hypopara without first checking a magnesium.

2. Serum Ca is the key controlling factor for PTH secretion

3. The best PTH to order is an *__Intact PTH__*

4. Vit D comes from diet and from photogenesis of vit D precursors in the skin.

✪ **1° <u>HYPER</u>parathyroidism** [See Figure 1 (Appendix): <u>ALGORITHMIC APPROACH TO ↑ SERUM CA:</u>]

1. Usually from an *adenoma* (not hyperplasia); adenoma is solitary 80% of the time

2. Hyperplasia only 15% of the time (e.g. in MEN I, IIA)

3. Carcinoma only 2% of the time

4. May be part of *MEN I or IIA; these types are hyperplastic* lesions.

5. Usually asymptomatic; however, if you see a hypercalcemic patient with *HTN and renal stones* or chondrocalcinosis/pseudogout→ think hyperparathyroidism→ ✓ an *intact PTH*

6. Additional skeletal lesions that can be found include…

   a. Periosteal bone resorption e.g. at the distal phalanges
   b. Salt and pepper lesions seen on skull plain film

7. The key differential diagnosis is FHH (Familial Hypocalciuric Hypercalcemia), another cause of ↑ serum Ca. The way to DDx these is by ✓ *Urine Ca. It's low in FHH*; normal to ↑ in 1° hyperpara.

8. ↑ PTH. If the PTH is ↓, must consider parathyroid-independent hyperCa (tumors; sarcoid; vit D intox; etc).

9. Treatment is surgery when clinically significant.

FAMILIAL HYPOCALCIURIC HYPERCALCEMIA (FHH)

1. Autosomal dominant hypercalcemia in a relatively young patient

2. PTH is ↔ to slightly ↑, and therefore, cannot be used to DDx with 1° hyperpara, so *check the Urine Ca.*

3. *Important in the differential of hyperpara since diagnosis precludes parathyroidectomy*!!

4. A benign condition; no treatment necessary

☞ **Thiazides → Cause mild ↑serum Ca; and ↓ Urine Ca (unlike other diuretics).**
☞ **Lithium → Causes ↑ serum Ca in 10% since it ↑'s the setpoint of PTH secretion.**

☞ *Remember* → **FHH, THIAZIDES, AND LITHIUM** are common causes of "normal" or "minimally elevated" PTH.

✪ HYPERCALCEMIA OF MALIGNANCY

1. *Statistically is the #1 cause of ↑Ca in hospitalized patients.*

2. *Many mechanisms depending on the tumor...*

   ✪ *Multiple Myeloma, Breast, Prostate→↑__OAF__ (Osteoclast Activating Factor)→bone resorption*
   ✪ *Lymphoma (also sarcoidosis)→ __ectopic production of 1,25 Vit D__*
   ✪ __PTH-rP__ *(PTH-related Protein)*—humoral hyperCa of malignancy
      (i) Squamous cell ca of lung, head, and neck; and
      (ii) Ca of breast/kidney/GU tract.

✪ TREATMENT OF HYPERCALCEMIC DISORDERS:

1. Volume repletion first →THEN forced "saline diuresis"

2. Inhibitors of osteoclastic activity (i.e. of bone resorption; *Remember*: Osteo**B**lasts **B**uild; Osteo**C**lasts **C**hew up bone):

   a) Calcitonin—can see Tachyphylaxis
   b) Bisphosphonates (e.g. Etidronate; Palmidronate)
   c) Gallium Nitrate

   ■ *Remember→   ↑ Ca^{2+} in Addison's, vit D intoxication, and sarcoidosis are all __steroid-responsive__.*

__HYPO__parathyroidism

1. ↓ serum Ca
2. Clinical:
   a) Cardiovascular--↑ QTc; CHF
   b) GI—Abdominal pain; N/V
   c) Neuromuscular—paresthesias; muscle spasms; Chvostek's and Trousseau's signs.
   d) Neurologic—basal ganglia calcification; benign intracranial HTN

3. *Remember to first RULE OUT...*

   a) ↓ **Mg**: *a common cause of hypopara, since Mg needed for PTH secretion and action.*

   b) Low serum Albumin. If albumin, calculate the corrected Ca or order an ionized Ca. Re: **Corrected Ca**= measured Ca + [(4-measured albumin)x0.8]; *must memorize*

   c) Renal insufficiency

4. REMEMBER, JUST AS HYPERpara can be 1°, 2°, and 3°, so HYPO para can be…

    a) **HYPOPARA-- ↓ PTH**

    b) **"PSEUDO" hypopara—↑PTH** (r/o ↓ vit D and renal failure); genetic; 2° to **end-organ resistance to PTH; urinary cAMP is ↓**

    Clinical—may see…
    - (i)   Short stature/short neck/short metacarpals
    - (ii)   Rounded face/obesity/mild mental retardation
    - (iii) SQ Calcification

    c) **"PSEUDOPSEUDO"** hypopara—same as (b) **but without the biochemical markers**.

5. **Treatment**
    Correct any readily identifiable cause:
    - If life-threatening, give Ca supplementation intravenously
    - Oral phosphate binders may be useful as well as thiazides to ↓ urinary Ca excretion.

✪ **MEN I Syndrome** (Multiple Endocrine Neoplasia)—aka Wermer Syndrome

1. Pituitary tumors
2. Parathyroid tumor
3. Pancreatic ca

✪ **MEN IIA Syndrome**—aka Sipple Syndrome

1. Pheo—remember, you have "**II**" adrenals (and in fact, the pheo in Sipple's in usually bilateral)
2. Parathyroid tumor
3. Medullary thyroid ca

INSULINOMAS

1. Not unlike pheo (!), there is a rule of 10's…

    a)   10% are multiple

    b)   10% are malignant

    c)   10% are MEN I - related

2. Rare islet-cell tumor

3. Important in the DDx of hypoglycemia

[See APPENDIX, FIGURE 2: LABORATORY EVALUATION OF HYPOGLYCEMIA]

DIABETES

<table>
<tr><td colspan="6">CRITERIA FOR DIAGNOSING DIABETES</td></tr>
<tr><td rowspan="2"><u>TEST</u></td><td colspan="4"><u>RESULTS</u></td></tr>
<tr><td>Normal</td><td>IFG[1]</td><td>IGT[2]</td><td>Diabetes</td></tr>
<tr><td>Fasting glucose</td><td><110</td><td>110-125</td><td></td><td>126</td></tr>
<tr><td>Glucose intolerance (2h after 75g glucose load)</td><td><140</td><td></td><td>140-199</td><td>200</td></tr>
<tr><td>Random glucose</td><td></td><td></td><td></td><td>200 with symptoms</td></tr>
</table>

[1] IFG, impaired fasting glucose
[2] IGT, impaired glucose intolerance

✪ *The new cutoff for diagnosis is FBS ≥ 126.*

• *Ideally, FBS should be <115*

• *A1C% (Normal is < 6%); Goal is < 7%; >8% is certainly an indication for action.*

• Note, 70-85% of **NIDDM** patients are usually **obese**

<table>
<tr><td colspan="4">IMPORTANT THRESHOLDS IN TYPE 2 DIABETICS</td></tr>
<tr><td>INDEX</td><td>IDEAL</td><td>GOAL</td><td>UNACCEPTABLE</td></tr>
<tr><td>Fasting/preprandial</td><td>< 110 mg/dL</td><td><120 mg/dL</td><td>< 80 or > 140</td></tr>
<tr><td>Postprandial</td><td><140</td><td>180</td><td>>200</td></tr>
<tr><td>Bedtime</td><td><140</td><td>100-140</td><td><100 or > 160</td></tr>
<tr><td>HbA1C</td><td><6%</td><td><7%</td><td>>8%</td></tr>
</table>

SOMOGYI EFFECT vs. DAWN PHENOMENON !

✪ *SOMOGYI effect= rebound hyperglycemia <u>2° to release of counter-regulatory hormones</u>* that follow a hypoglycemic episode (these hypoglycemic episodes are often accompanied by vivid nightmares)

Treatment → 1) Take the NPH or lente insulin before bed instead of before dinner; or 2) switch to a longer-acting insulin preparation (such as ultralente insulin).

✪ *DAWN phenomenon*=↑ early AM glusoses **2° to insulin resistance** (there is an increased need for insulin in the early morning due to the early morning release of growth hormone which antagonizes the action of insulin.)

Treatment → increase the patient's insulin.

NOTE: *Both of these early AM phenomona are hyperglycemic in nature, yet the treatments are exact opposites. Usually, the dawn phenomenon can be differentiated from posthypoglycemic hyperglycemia (Somogyi) by measuring the blood glucose at 3 AM (↓ in Somogyi)*

TARGETS FOR LIPIDS, BLOOD PRESSURE, AND MICROALBUMIN IN **DIABETICS**

Lipids (mg/dL)	LDL	HDL	Total Cholesterol	Triglycerides
	≤ 100	> 35-45	< 200	< 200
BP	< 130/80 mm Hg			
Microalbumin	< 30 mg/24 h OR			
	< 20 µg/min on a timed specimen OR			
	< 30 mg/g creatinine on a random sample			

ADA. Diabetes Care, 2001; 24 (supp 1): S33-43
ADA. Clinical Practice Recommendations. Diabetes Care. 2001; 23: S32-42

CLASSES OF ORAL ANTIDIABETIC AGENTS & HOW THEY WORK:

AGENT	PRIMARY ACTION
Thiazolidinediones [e.g. rosiglitazone (Avandia®); pioglitazone (Actos®)]	Bind to peroxisome-proliferator-activated receptor-gamma (PPAR-gamma) in muscle, fat, and liver to ↓ insulin resistance
Miglitinides [e.g. *sulfonylureas* (gliburide, glipizide), *repaglinide* (Prandin®); *nateglinide* (Starlix®)]	Stimulate pancreatic beta cells to ↑ insulin output.
Biguanides (e.g. metformin)	Liver: ↓ glucose production Muscle: ↑ glucose uptake
Alpha-glucosidase inhibitors [e.g. acarbose (Precose®); miglitol (Glyset®)]	Inhibit intestinal enzymes that break down carbohydrates, thus delaying carbohydrate absorption
Sulfonylureas (2nd generation) [e.g. glipizide (Glucotrol®); glyburide (Diabeta®, Micronase®, Glynase®--micronized); glimepiride Amaryl®)]	

DIABETIC EYE DISEASE *(see Opthalmology)*

DIABETIC RENAL DISEASE

1. *Microalbumin*, defined as 30-250mg/24h, precedes overt proteinuria and identifies patients at risk for nephropathy; therefore it is an important screening test in diabetics.
2. If microalbumin is detected, an ACE inhibitor can be started to slow down/halt the progression of proteinuria and decrease one's risk of developing nephropathy
3. *ACE inhibitors* are also 1st line therapy in HTN + DM with normal renal function.
4. Contrast dyes may precipitate renal failure, depending on other risk factors, including old age, dehydration, liver disease, and preexisting renal dz.
5. *Kimmelstiel-Wilson* kidneys seen on pathology and represent progression of renal disease.
✪ **Hypo**reninemic **hypo**aldosteronism is the type 4 RTA of DM.

DIABETIC NEUROPATHY

1. **Peripheral polyneuropathy** is most commonly seen
   a) Usually bilateral, symmetric—so-called "stocking-glove" distribution
   b) Paresthesias, numbness, hyperesthesia, or deep pain worse at night

2. **Mononeuropathy**
   a) Etiology most likely vascular
   b) Commonly spontaneously remit
   c) Clinically may see…
      (1) Footdrop (*isolated peroneal neuropathy*)
      (2) Sudden wristdrop
      (3) Painful diplopia 2° to dysfunction of cranial nerves 3/4/6
3. **Autonomic** Neuropathy
   a) Constipation most common, but can also see diarrhea
   b) Diabetic *gastroparesis*—important 2° to potential unpredictable swings in plasma glucose.

DIABETIC AMYOTROPHY

1. Progressive *weakness, pain, atrophy* of the pelvic girdle and anterior thigh muscles.
2. Spontaneously abates after 6-12 months

DKA (Diabetic Ketoacidosis)

1. *Seen in Type I diabetes only (Type II diabetes can have Hyperosmolar Nonketotic Coma, HONC)*
   - *In general, blood glucose and volume deficits are much higher in HONC than in DKA. Patients with DKA are usually 4-6L behind (versus 8-10L in HONC).*

2. When replacing fluid losses in **DKA (**and HONC), the Na+ may be deceptively low (*pseudohyponatremia*) as a result of the dilution secondary to the hyperglycemia.

✪ **CALCULATING THE <u>CORRECTED</u> Na+** is also important since results can guide whether you replete with NS or ½ NS. The **2 rules of thumb** here are that:

☞ **For every 100 mg/dl that the glucose is > 100 mg/dl ("normal"), the Na+ will drop approximately 1.5**. As an example, let's say that the measured Na+ = 131 and the glucose is 500. That means the true Na, ie the corrected Na would be 500-100=400/100=4, so you'd add 4 x 1.5 = 6 to the measured Na of 131, giving you a corrected Na of 137.

☞ The other rule of thumb is that **if the Na ≤ 142, you can replete with NS; > 142 gets ½ NS** (normal saline would only contribute to persistent hyperosmolality). So, in this case the patient with a corrected Na of 137 would receive NS.

---

3. *Characterized by…*

    a) Insulin deficiency
    b) ↑Glucose
    c) Dehydration 2° osmotic diuresis
    d) Ketonemia
    e) Metabolic acidosis
    f) Pseudohyponatremia

4. Common *SYMPTOMS*

    a) Abdominal pain
    b) Anorexia
    c) Change in vision
    d) Fatigue
    e) Nausea and vomiting
    f) Thirst and polyuria
    g) Weakness

5. Common *SIGNS*

    a) Dehydration
    b) Hyperventilation
    c) Hypotension
    d) Impaired consciousness and/or coma
    e) Tachycardia
    f) Warm, dry skin
    g) Weight loss

6. *Typical Laboratories*

    a) Arterial pH <7.2 (also the level below which supplemental bicarbonate is indicated)
    b) Plasma bicarbonate ≤15meq/L
    c) Blood glucose ≥250mg/dl
    d) Ketones + in the blood and urine

7. *Precipitating factors* for DKA include most any major physiologic stressor, e.g....

    a)   CVA

    b)   Emotional stress

    c)   Infection

    d)   MI (thereofore an EKG is indicated in all adult patients)

    e)   Noncompliance with insulin regimen

✪ As you correct the metabolic acidosis and hyperglycemia, __*serum K+*__ ↓, so remember to add KCl to your IVF when K+ drops. Remember the *inverse correlation* between serum K+ and pH. That's why __*Bicarbonate*__ is given with ↑ serum K+. Speaking of Bicarb, it should only be added if pH <7.2

✪ Remember, DKA patients are *deficient in total body K+* regardless of their plasma K+ concentration.

✪ __*Remember to switch*__ from IV insulin to SQ when serum glucose ↓s to 200-250

✪ The best way to monitor a patient with DKA for improvement is *serial Anion Gaps*, and *not* urine ketones.

HONC (HYPEROSMOLAR NONKETOTIC COMA)

1. Very high glucoses with significant osmotic (thus HONC) diuresis.

2. Patients are typically 8-10 L behind! Consequently, these patients need even more *aggressive IV Fluid resuscitation*. Start with Normal Saline to correct the volume deficit→then switch to ½ NS to correct the hyperosmolarity.

    ✪ The __FLUID DEFICIT__ (in Liters) may be __CALCULATED__ AS FOLLOWS:

$$(0.6 \times \text{weight in kg}) \times \frac{(\text{current } S_{Na} - 140)}{140}$$

> ☞ *One half of the fluid deficit is replaced with normal saline over the first 6-8 hours. The remaining deficit should be replaced over the next 24 hours as ½ NS.*

3. *No ketoacidosis* (thus HONC) since enough insulin is available to inhibit ketone production.

4. Seen only in *Type II DM*

CHARACTERISTICS OF THE METABOLIC SYNDROME

- The constellation of **abdominal obesity, hypertension, diabetes, and dyslipidemia** — has been called "syndrome X", the "deadly quartet", the insulin resistance syndrome, the metabolic syndrome, and the obesity dyslipidemia syndrome, dysmetabolic syndrome, multiple metabolic syndrome.

- *More specifically, features may include*:
  - ➢ Hypertriglyceridemia
  - ➢ Low HDL
  - ➢ Small, dense, easily oxidized LDL cholesterol particles
  - ➢ Insulin resistance and hyperinsulinemia
  - ➢ Hyperglycemia and relative insulin deficiency
  - ➢ HTN
  - ➢ Central obesity
  - ➢ Procoagulant state

- Recent guidelines from National Cholesterol Education Program (Adult Treatment Panel III) suggest that the clinical identification of the insulin resistance syndrome be based upon the presence of *any three of the following*:

  1. Abdominal obesity, defined as a waist circumference in men >102 cm (40 in) and in women >88 cm (35 in)
  2. Triglycerides ≥150 mg/dL
  3. HDL cholesterol <40 mg/dL in men and <50 mg/dL in women
  4. Blood pressure ≥130/≥85 mmHg
  5. Fasting glucose ≥110 mg/dL

- The associated hyperinsulinemia can lead to HTN and an abnormal lipid profile, both of which promote the development of *atherosclerosis*.

- Individuals with syndrome X have a *markedly increased risk of coronary artery disease*.

- The insulin resistance syndrome *should not be confused with another disorder called syndrome X* in which angina pectoris occurs in patients with normal coronary arteries. Regardless of the mechanisms, avoidance of obesity, particularly abdominal obesity, should reduce the potential for the development of the various features of the insulin resistance syndrome.

- When all is said and done, however, management is still exercise & diet.

PREGNANCY AND DIABETES

1. *Tight control* of sugars in preexisting diabetic during pregnancy is important

   a) If poor control in *first trimester*→ ↑ risk of congenital malformations
   b) If poor control in *2ⁿᵈ/3ʳᵈ trimesters*→ ↑ risk of …

      (1)   Macrosomia
      (2)   Neonatal ↓glu, ↓Ca, ↑RBCs, ↑bili,
      (3)   Resp distress

2. As sulfonylureas are contraindicated, ***insulin*** therapy is the treatment.

3. Advanced maternal age is a risk factor for gestational DM.

4. Gestational DM is itself a risk factor for ***future development of Type II DM*** (50-60% risk over the ensuing 15 years)

ADRENOCORTICAL FAILURE [See Figure 3 for <u>Synthesis Pathways of Cortisol,Testosterone, & Aldosterone</u>]

1. ↓ ***Aldosterone and*** ↓ ***cortisol*** which lead to the following clinical picture:

    a) Weakness; fatigue
    b) ↓Appetite
    c) ↓BP
    d) ↓ Glucose
    e) ↓Na+
    f) ↑Pigment (e.g. at the palmar creases)
    g) ↑K+

2. Causes of ↓ aldo for the boards…

1° FAILURE (ADDISON'S Disease)—*these patients have <u>hyperreninemic</u> <u>hypoaldosteronism.</u>*

    a) *Autoimmune is the <u>#1 cause</u>* ✪
    b) TB; fungal disorders;
    c) Malignancy

    ✪ *Waterhouse-Friederickson Syndrome (bilateral adrenal hemorrhage) 2° to sepsis (e.g. meningococcal)*, trauma, anticoagulants--#2 cause in the US.

2° FAILURE (MOST PATIENTS)

    a) *Prolonged steroid use* (suppresses ACTH)--<u>#1 cause</u> of 2° failure ✪
    b) Following removal of adrenal tumor—may take up to 1 year for the HPA axis to recover.
    c) NSAIDs
    d) ACE inhibitors

3. Frequent association of antithyroid antibodies in autoimmune Addison's.

✪ Diagnosis: ***Cosyntropin test***. This test checks the cortisol response after infusing Cosyntropin (an ACTH analogue). A subnormal cortisol response indicates adrenocortical failure (although it doesn't differentiate 1° vs. 2° causes—*ACTH levels* do that). A normal response excludes it.

4. **THE TREATMENT DIFFERS FOR 1° VS 2° ADRENOCORTICAL FAILURE**. ✪

    ☞ 1°→Glucocorticoid (hydrocortisone) + Mineralcorticoid therapy (fludrocortisone)

    ☞ 2°→Glucocorticoid only

5. **DISTINGUISHING FACTORS** in Primary vs. Secondary/Tertiary adrenal insufficiency:

PRIMARY	SECONDARY/TERTIARY
Associated with **hyperpigmentation**	No hyperpigmentation
Mineralcorticoid and liberal salt intake important in management	Mineralcorticoid secretion intact
↑**ACTH**	↓ACTH

POLYGLANDULAR AUTOIMMUNE SYNDROMES

Type I: *essential components*:   **"IPAC"** *(remember the Sony IPAC? 1000 mnemonics in your pocket!)*
   1. Hypo**p**arathyroidism
   2. **A**drenal insufficiency
   3. Mucocutaneous **c**andidiasis

Type II: *typical presentation*:   **"2D TAG"**
   ☞ Lymphocytic infiltration of *the adrenal and thyroid* glands along *with type 1 diabetes* mellitus and *hypogonadism*

Type III: **"T + (A or D) = III"**
   ☞ **D**iabetes and autoimmune **t**hyroid disease OR **a**drenal insufficiency and autoimmune **t**hyroid disease in the absence of other autoimmune disorders.

CUSHING'S DISEASE (generally speaking)

- 2° to steroid excess (↑cortisol; opposite of adrenocortical failure!)
- Actually, the *terminology* goes…
   a) Cushing's **Disease**=2° disease at the level of the pituitary; caused by ACTH-producing tumor or hyperplasia.
   b) Cushing's **Syndrome**=1° disease at the level of the adrenal.
- *Etiologies*
   - *65% Cushing's Disease per se*
   - *10% Adrenal adenoma*
   - *10% Adrenal carcinoma*
   - *15% Ectopic ACTH*
   - *1% Ectopic CRH*

- *Clinical* (these are also the potential side effects of long term exogenous steroid use!)
    - a) Obesity
    - b) HTN; DM
    - c) ↑Androgens
    - d) Cataracts
    - e) Easy bruising
    - f) Osteoporosis
    - g) Striae (stretch marks)
    - h) "Moon face" (rounded face)
    - i) "Buffalo hump" (fat pad)

✪ CUSHING'S DIFFERENTIAL AND DIAGNOSTICS

DIAGNOSIS:	ACTH:	Suppressible with High Dose (8mg) Dexamethasone (DST) ?
Disease (pituitary level)	↑	Y
Syndrome (adrenal level)	↓	N
Ectopic ACTH (e.g. tumors)	↑	N

The two screening tests for Cushing's includes 24-hour urine collection for free-cortisol and the overnight dexamethasone suppression test (1 mg by mouth at 11 p.m. with measurement of an 8 a.m. cortisol level). *__A 24 hour urine for free cortisol__ is the simplest screen for Cushing's syndrome.*

☞ *If results of your screening test are abnormal, then advance to low and high-dose DST for confirmation and etiology…*

✪ DEXAMETHASONE SUPPRESSON TEST (DST) ESSENTIALS:

a) **Overnight** DST is for *screening*; aka *(or can do a 24h urine for free cortisol)*

b) **Low-dose** DST is for *confirmation*, ie to R/O false positives, such as:

- (1) Estrogen or BCPs or pregnancy
- (2) Simple obesity
- (3) Depression
- (4) Alcoholism
- (5) Hospitalized patients

c) **High-dose** DST is for *pinpointing* the exact cause. high dose can pinpoint the dx:

☞ Do the high dose test if low dose fails to suppress cortisol

☞ If the cortisol **suppresses** to < 5 µg/dl → **Cushing's disease** (pituitary)

☞ If not → ectopic ACTH or adrenal tumor

HYPERALDOSTERONISM

- Clinical: **HTN** + **↓K⁺**
- **Primary causes** have ↓*renin*; similar to hyperparathyroidism, most (70%) are adenoma; 30% hyperplasia.; only imaging can differentiate these; *think primary hyperaldosteronism in a HTN patient with ↓K+ not on diuretics.*
- **Secondary causes** have ↑*renin* and include malignant HTN; renovascular HTN; renal artery stenosis; and renin-secreting tumor

- *Workup* for Hyperaldosteronism:

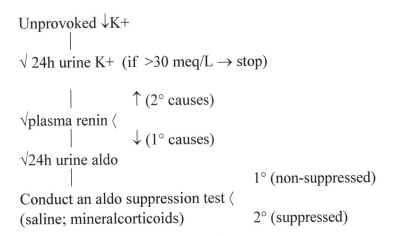

```
Unprovoked ↓K+
        |
√ 24h urine K+  (if >30 meq/L → stop)
        |                   ↑ (2° causes)
√plasma renin ⟨
        |                   ↓ (1° causes)
√24h urine aldo
        |                       1° (non-suppressed)
Conduct an aldo suppression test ⟨
(saline; mineralcorticoids)         2° (suppressed)
```

PHEOCHROMOCYTOMA

- **Rule of 10's** (*don't confuse with insulinoma's rule of 10's*):
  1. 10% are familial (MEN 2A, 2B)
  2. 10% are extraadrenal
  3. 10% are bilateral
  4. 10% are malignant

- **Clinical** (easy to recall since *all hyperadrenergic symptoms*)
  1. HTN
  2. Orthostatic Hypotension
  3. Headaches 2° to HTN
  4. Tachycardia/palpitations
  5. Sweating
  6. Weight loss

- **Diagnosis via 24 urine for:**
  1. Free catecholamines (Epi; Norepi);
  2. Metanephrines (the metabolites); and
  3. VMA (vanillylmandelic acid)

- **MANAGEMENT**

    1. Surgical excision is curative

    2. MIBG (meta-iodobenzylguanidine) nuclear scans are used to R/O metastatic disease as appropriate.

    3. **Preoperative medical management**:

        ✪ α *blockers, such as phentolamine or phenoxybenzamine, are most important, esp for treating the HTN;*

        ✪ β *blockers (only <u>after</u> adequate α blockade) for any tachyarrhythmias*

"INCIDENTALOMAS" (Incidentally discovered adrenal mass)

- Approx'ly 1 in 10 autopsies

- A little over ½% of all CT scans

- Ca is usually > 4cm; the more common adenomas usually < 6cm

---

✪ <u>If <4cm and non-hypersecreting, reimage (MRI, CT) in 3 months and periodically thereafter.</u>

✪ If, on the other hand, the <u>adrenal mass is > 4cm, has grown, or is hypersecreting</u>→ it should be excised.

- **MUST RULE OUT:**

    1. Pheo → ✓ <u>24 h urine</u> as above

    2. Cushing's syndrome → ✓<u>24 h urine for free cortisol</u>

    3. Primary hyperaldo→ ✓ <u>Serum K+</u> for starters; then as shown above

    4. Androgen producing tumors→ ✓ <u>serum DHEAS</u> levels

    5. TB/fungus/carcinoma→ ✓ <u>CXR</u>

APPENDIX

FIGURE 1.   <u>**ALGORITHMIC APPROACH TO ↑ SERUM CA:**</u>

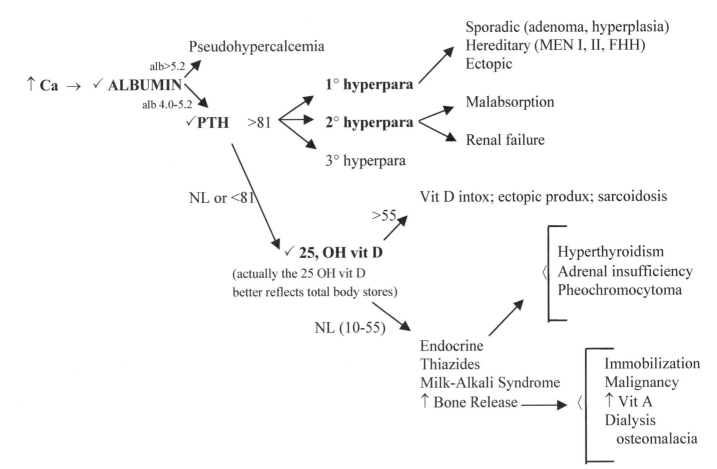

FIGURE 2.   <u>**LABORATORY EVALUATION OF HYPOGLYCEMIA**</u>

Diagnosis	Glucose	Insulin	C-peptide	Proinsulin
Sulfonylurea abuse	↓	↑	↑ *	↔
Surreptitious insulin	↓	↑↑	↓**	↓
Insulinoma	↓	↑	↑	↑

✪   *   <u>HIGH C-PEPTIDE</u> implies *endogenous* insulin secretion, which can result from either:
   a) Insulinoma; or
   b) Sulfonylurea abuse—this can be confirmed by simply checking sulfonylurea levels.
   • Consequently, in hyperinsulinemic patients, the exclusion of sulfonylurea abuse points to insulinoma. Remember, sulfonylureas ↑ insulin secretion.

✪   ** <u>LOW C-PEPTIDE</u>, on the other hand, implies *exogenous* source, such as surreptious insulin

FIGURE 3.   **SYNTHESIS PATHWAYS OF CORTISOL AND TESTOSTERONE :**

a thru c = enzymes, from which you should *know for your exam*,

> **a = 17α-hydroxylase**
> **b = 21-hydroxylase**
> **c = 11β-hydroxylase**

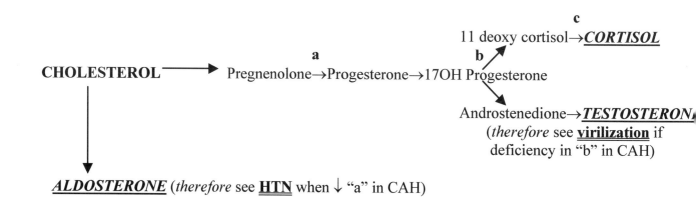

c

11 deoxy cortisol→***CORTISOL***

a   **b**

CHOLESTEROL ⟶ Pregnenolone→Progesterone→17OH Progesterone

Androstenedione→***TESTOSTERONE***
(*therefore* see **virilization** if
deficiency in "b" in CAH)

ALDOSTERONE (*therefore* see **HTN** when ↓ "a" in CAH)

12. I. NEPHROLOGY
II. CLINICAL TOXICOLOGY

I. NEPHROLOGY

Commonly Asked Material:

1. Know your RTAs:

RENAL TUBULAR ACIDOSES (RTAs) ✪			
	TYPE I	**TYPE II**	**TYPE IV**
Location	Distal	Proximal	Distal
Problem	Impaired distal acidification	Reduced proximal bicarb reabsorption	↓ aldo secretion/effect
Serum K+	↓	↓	↑
Urinary pH (5.3 cutoff)	↑	↓	↓
Important examples	Ampho, Sickle cell dz, RA, SLE, Cirrhosis, Lithium	Fanconi's, Amyloidosis, Myeloma, Carbonic anhydrase inhibitors	DM, BPH, NSAIDs, ACEI, Heparin, primary adrenal insuff., CAH, HIV, K+-sparing diuretics, Pentamidine
Management	K+, bicarb	K+, bicarb	Mineralcorticoids, Low K+ diets
Normal Anion Gap Acidosis & postive Urine Anion Gap	✓	✓	✓

> ✪ **Knowing the urinary pH and the K+** can clinch the diagnosis:
> ✓ **First** look at the serum K+. If the K+ is ↑, it's Type IV. If not, **then look at the urinary pH**…
> ✓ If the urinary pH is ↑, it's Type I; ↓ is Type II.

2. Know that _microalbuminuria_ in a diabetic (with or without e.g. borderline HTN) is an indication for ACE Inhibitors (e.g. lisinopril and enalapril)

3. Usually by the time a diabetic has developed microalbuminuria, s/he has developed signs of retinopathy.

4. In slowing the rate of progression of diabetic nephropathy, achieve good BP control (an ACE I would also accomplish this) and shoot for good glucose control.

5. Nephrotic syndrome
   - See ≥3.5g protein/24h urine; proteinuria→↓albumin→edema; ↑chol
   - Proteinuria→Antithrombin III deficiency (a protein important in anticoag)→renal vein thrombosis (RVT)→thrombemboli can be seen→pulmonary emboli.

6. Know how to calculate the corrected calcium, given the measured calcium and the albumin, and that if the corrected calcium is low, you obviously have to replete.

$$\textit{Corrected Ca} = \text{serum Ca} + [(4\text{-measured alb}) \times 0.8]$$

If the corrected calcium or ionized calcium is low (normal **ionized calcium** value is 4.5-5.0 mg/dl), check the magnesium, phosphorus, BUN, and creatinine to rule out ARF or CRF. <u>Symptomatic</u> cases of **hypocalcemia** should receive calcium gluconate as IV bolus (100-200 mg over 10 minutes) followed by infusion at 0.3-2 mg/kg/hr until ionize calcium normalizes.

7. Know the management for severe **hypercalcemia**:
   - a **Normal saline** hydration (volume repletion and enhances calcium excretion) ⎫ *Saline*
   - b **Loop diuretic** further promotes calciuresis ⎬ *Diuresis*
   - c **Bisphosphonates** (e.g. <u>pamidronate</u>) to bind to hydroxyapatite and inhibit dissolution of crystals

   but also...
   - d **Plicamycin** to inhibit RNA synthesis in osteoclasts
   - e **Calcitonin** to inhibit bone resorption,

8. You must learn the *formula for* glomerular filtration rate:

$$\text{GFR} = \frac{(140\text{-age}) \times \text{Kg patient}}{72 \times \text{creat}}$$

9. Know that in **Metabolic Alkalosis**,

   ✪ a <u>Urine Chloride<10</u> points to <u>surreptious vomiting (loss of HCl yields a met alk)</u>

   ✪ a <u>Urine Chloride>10</u> points to <u>Bartter's syndrome</u> and <u>diuretics.</u>

   <u>Don't confuse</u>: <u>Laxative abuse</u>, while it will give you a Urine Cl<10, is metabolic *acidosis* 2° to loss of bicarb!

✪ Remember, in **<u>Bartter's Syndrome</u>**, because of pathology at the tubules, Na+ is lost, leading to volume loss, which in turn causes ↑renin →↑ aldo→↓K. *The Blood Pressure is low/normal* despite the ↑ renin and ↑ aldo.

---

10. It might help you to remember one if you know the other since they are practically *opposites* in these regards:

	TYPE 4 RTA	BARTTER'S Syndrome
Renin	↓	↑
Aldo	↓	↑
K+	↑	↓
BP	↑	↓/normal
Acid-base	Met. **acidosis** (nonAG)	Met. **Alkalosis** (Chloride resistant)

11. Know the electrolyte picture **NSAIDs** can give→↑K+, ↓Na+.

12. Crusty facial lesion followed by nephritis→*Post-Streptococcal Glomerulonephritis*.

13. Know what medicines can *increase your Uric Acid*, such as thiazides and ethanol.

14. ✪ Recognize a case of *E. Coli 0157H7-induced HUS* (Hemolytic Uremic Syndrome) with Anemia; Thrombocytopenia; Renal failure following, e.g., ingested of tainted beef (ATR, which is the middle part of "F**AT R**N" (**F**ever-**A**nemia-**T**hrombocytopenia-**R**enal **F**ailure-**N**eurologic signs), used to help remember the clinical signs of TTP (Thrombotic Thrombocytopenic Purpura)

15. *Acyclovir*→renal intratubular obstruction with crystals.

16. 2 Q's on *Multiple Myeloma*;

   - Know that a *UPEP* (urine protein electropheresis) will do just that and will show any light chains and/or monoclonal IgM spikes.
   - Know that a *dipstick* does not detect light chains, so e.g. you might see only 1+ protein on the dipstick but, say, 5 grams of protein on a 24 hour collection!
   - Know that a *low Anion Gap* is consistent with the diagnosis.

17. Remember, in *symptomatic hypovolemic hypoNa+*→the first step is NS (normal saline) even before hypertonic saline, and that the danger of restoring the Na+ too fast is CPM (Central Pontine Myelinolysis).

18. **Fluid replacement in postobstructive diuresis** (typical scenario = after a foley has been placed with resultant severe volume depletion)→ Replacement of no more than two-thirds of urinary volume losses per day and use ½ NS (NS will worsen the Na overload that results from the diuresis)

19. Know the mechanism of **NSAID-induced renal toxicity**:

   a) Renal *prostaglandin inhibition*→↓renal blood flow→prerenal azotemia. This is a *vascular* phenomenon and is the main mechanism of injury for the exam.
   b) ↓Renin→↓aldo→↑K+; =Type 4 RTA

20. Autosomal Dominant Polycystic Kidney Disease (**ADPKD**) is often associated with:

    a) *Cerebral aneurysms* (MRI/MRA not necessary for all ADPKD unless + FH of aneurysm)
    b) *MVP*
    c) Hepatic cysts
    d) Elevated Hct

21. Struvite stones ↔ staghorn calculi ↔ urease-splitting bacteria (e.g. proteus; u.urealyticum).

22. Of all the types of renal stones, Calcium Oxalate stones are the most common, and can result from any of the following aberrations in the urine: ↑Ca (remember to r/o hyperpara); ↑Oxalate, ↑U.A.; or ↓ citrate (usually a protective factor)

23. Uric Acid stones are radiolucent.

24. Remember, a workup for causes of nephrolithiasis or renal stones is indicated for:

    a) Recurrent stones (≥2 stones)
    b) Significant + FH of stones
    c) Young (<25) or older (>60) patients

25.

OVERVIEW OF MANAGEMENT OPTIONS IN NEPHROLITHIASIS	
Treatment Option	**Indications**
Extracorporeal shock wave lithotripsy (ESWL)	Radiolucent stones Renal stones < 2cm Ureteral stones < 1cm
Ureteroscopy	Ureteral stones
Ureterorenoscopy	Renal stones < 2cm
Percutaneous nephrolithotomy	Renal stones > 2cm Proximal ureteral stones > 1cm

> ➢ Referral to a urologist is appropriate for patients with a ureteral stone > 5 mm in greatest diameter or a stone that has not passed after 2-4 weeks.

26. **Commonly Seen Examples of Mixed acid-base disturbances:**

    Combined Acidoses (Resp—1st example + Metabolic-2nd example)
    a) Resp failure + Circulatory failure (lactic acidosis)
    b) Sedatives + ASA
    c) COPD + Renal failure (or sepsis)

    Combined Alkalosis (Resp--1st + Metabolic—2nd)
    • [(Pregnancy or cirrhosis)—hyperventilation] + (diuretics or vomiting)

    Resp Acidosis—1st + Metabolic Alkalosis—2nd
    • COPD + (diuretics or steroids)

Metabolic Acidosis + *Resp Alkalosis*
   a) ASA (Resp Alk first then Met Acidosis)
   b) Sepsis (lactic acidosis with secondary resp alk)
   c) Cirrhosis

Metabolic Acidosis—1ˢᵗ + *Metabolic Alkalosis—2ⁿᵈ*
   • (Diabetic or alcoholic ketoacidosis) + vomiting

Triple Disorder **(combination of the previous 2 categories)**
   • (Diabetic or alcoholic ketoacidosis) + (sepsis or cirrhosis)

27. Muddy brown casts → ATN (Acute tubular necrosis)

28. Overview of **Management of Renal Stones by Size**:

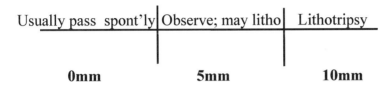

| Usually pass spont'ly | Observe; may litho | Lithotripsy |

0mm   5mm   10mm

29. **Acute Interstitial nephritis** 2° to drug hypersensitivity →check Hansel's stain for ***urine eosinophils***. Common **medications** that can cause AIN include: β-lactam antibiotics NSAIDs sulfa antibiotics thiazide diuretics

30. **LUPUS NEPHRITIS:**

W.H.O. CLASSIFICATION	IMPORTANT POINTS	TREATMENT
Class I (normal)	✓Usually no clinical renal dz	Observe
Class II (mesangial)	✓Microscopic hematuria is common with this lesion, and 25 to 50 percent of patients have moderate proteinuria.	Observe
Class III (focal proliferative)	✓Up to 1/3 have nephrosis	Observe or prednisone
Class IV (diffuse proliferative)	✓Nephrotic syndrome and renal insufficiency are present in at least 50 percent of patients ✓Most common type at biopsy; ✓Most aggressive lesion	Cyclophosphamide + prednisone
Class V (membranous)	✓Nephrotic presentation in 90%, but significant impairment of GFR is relatively unusual (10 percent).	Observe or prednisone

31. SLE flair up during pregnancy→25% fetal mortality.

32. The #1 cause of **Glomerulonephritis** (GN) and the #1 cause of incidental microscopic
    a. hematuria is IgA Nephropathy (Berger's Disease); there is no proven treatment for IgA nephropathy.

33. In differentiating **GN following URI**, remember the timing is important: Poststreptococcal GN averages 10 days after pharyngitis and 21 days after impetigo. This is in contrast to IgA Nephropathy, which typically occurs 3-5 days after URI or GI infection.

34. *Rhabdomyolysis*: labs: ↑CPK,↑K+, ↑U.A., ↑Phos→↓Ca, and ↑creat may be seen if myoglobinuria develops; if urine dipstick + for heme (Hgb or Mgb) and yet few or no RBCs→suspect myoglobinuric renal failure.

35. *Phosphate levels* <1 mg/dl are truly critical, since life-threatening muscle weakness (cardiac and diaphragmatic) may lead to CHF/ respiratory failure. Hemolysis/rhabdo/ARF may also develop.

36. If you see **RBC casts**   → Think *glomerular* nephritis
    "   "   "   **WBC/ WBC casts**→ Think inflammation *(e.g interstitial* nephritis) or infection (e.g. pyelonephritis); the term "pyuria" means > 5 leukocytes per high power field

37. Pregnant women with asymptomatic bacteriuria are at increased risk of pyelonephritis if bacteria are ≥ 10,000.

38. The **FENa+** (fractional excretion of Na+) is the most helpful urinary index to differentiate prerenal from intrinsic renal failure (<1% vs. >1-3%):

$$FENa= \frac{\text{clearance of Na+}}{\text{clearance of Creat}} = \frac{Urine_{Na}/Plasma_{Na}}{Urine_{Cr}/Plasma_{Cr}} = \frac{Urine_{Na}}{Plasma_{Na}} \times \frac{Plasma_{Cr}}{Urine_{Cr}}$$

39. **Contrast nephropathy** classically presents as an acute rise in BUN and creatinine with onset within 24 to 28 h, peaks 3 to 5 days, and resolves within a week.

40. Risk factors for **radiocontrast-induced ARF**:

    a) All the above factors for NSAID-induced ARF;
    b) DM with azotemia
    c) Large contrast load or multiple exposures
    d) MM (multiple myeloma) with dehydration

41. These are the risk factors for developing **NSAID-induced ARF**:
    a) Preexisting renal insufficiency
    b) Diuretics/volume depletion/hypotension
    c) States of relative intravascular volume depletion (cirrhosis; nephrosis; CHF)
    d) Advanced age

42. Know the difference between nephrotic and nephritic presentations:

> **Nephritis/nephritic syndrome** usually requires RBC casts, hematuria (microscopic or macroscopic), and proteinuria, whereas **nephrotic syndrome** encompasses the constellation of proteinuria (>3.5g/24h)→ hypoalbuminemia → edema; and hyperlipidemia.

> Renal syndromes can be divided into ARF, RTAs, nephritic syndrome, and nephrotic syndrome. Just as ARF is classified in terms of prerenal/renal/postrenal and RTAs are classified into types 1,2, & 4, so nephritic and nephrotic syndromes have their subclassifications. **Nephrotic** syndromes are divided into **renal vs. systemic.** **Nephritic** syndromes are subclassified into **normal vs. low serum complement (C3).**

43. Don't forget the big picture! In nearly all cases: ↑ serum Na+ is 2° to dehydration, and serum Na+ is 2° to fluid overload

44. Therefore, the treatment of *Hyponatremia* 98% of the time is *fluid restriction* (isovolemic—also called euvolemic—and hypervolemic branches of the hyponatremia algorithm). The other 2% is the hypovolemic branch and the treatment of that is either isotonic saline (.95NS) if patient is asymptomatic or hypertonic saline (3% NS) if symptomatic.

45. You must know *all* of the following key associations for the following glomerulopathies:

GN	IMPORTANT ASSOCIATIONS
MPGN	SLE, Sickle Cell, ↓C′
Minimal Change Disease	*Hodgkins* Dz, NSAIDs, 80% respond to
Focal Segmental Sclerosis	*HIV; heroine*
Membranous	*Solid organ neoplasms*(esp lung, colon). Membranous yields renal vein thrombosis in 25-50% of cases. It is also the #1 cause of idiopathic nephrosis in adults
Note: Both **Hep B and Hep C** can cause **membranous, membranoproliferative,** and **diffuse proliferative** (classic post-infectious) GNs.	

46. **Know these important causes of ↑K+: "RHABDO":**

R habdomyolysis
H emolysis
A ddison's Disease
B ad kidneys (ARF, CRF)
D rugs (ACE I, K+ sparing diuretics)
O (hyporenin hypoaldo)

47. Know the DDx for ↓ Mg: "ABCDEFGH":

A TN, ↑ Aldo
B artter Syndrome
C yclosporin*, Cisplatinum*
D iuretics
E thanol
F at losses (malabsorption syndromes)
G astric losses (NG suction, vomiting)
H ypoparathyroidism

48. * CYCLOSPORIN, CISPLATINUM, AND NEPHROTOXICITY

> ✪ <u>Cisplatin</u> can damage the <u>tubules</u> thru either ATN or a Type IV RTA; don't confuse with **Cyclophosphamide → hemorrhagic cystitis**
>
> {Streptozocin (an alkylating agent) can also cause renal tubular damage.}

49. SUPPLEMENTS TO CONSIDER IN CRF: "<u>BCDE</u>"

B icarbonate
C alcium (e.g. phosphate binders such as calcium carbonate and calcium acetate)
D vitamin
E rythropoietin

50. INDICATIONS FOR ACUTE DIALYSIS ("AEIOU")

A cidosis
E lectrolyte abnormalities (↑K, ↑Mg)
I ntoxication (eg ethylene glycol, salicylates)
O verload (fluid)
U remia

TYPES OF CASTS ON URINARY SEDIMENT	
TYPE	**KEY CULPRITS**
RBC casts	*Acute GN* Malignant HTN
WBC casts	Pyelonephritis *Interstitial nephritis* (re: also WBCs and urine eos)
Hyaline	*Prerenal azotemia;* HTN; often just normal
Pigmented granular casts, aka **"muddy brown"** casts	*ATN*
Fatty casts	*Nephrotic* syndrome
Waxy casts	*Chronic renal failure*

IMPORTANT FIGURES TO LEARN:

ACUTE RENAL FAILURE: *The Big Picture*

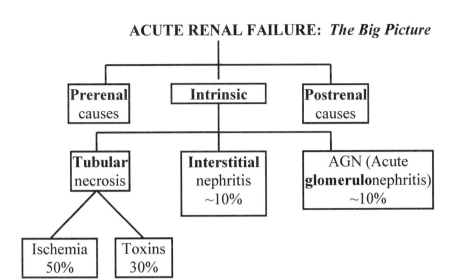

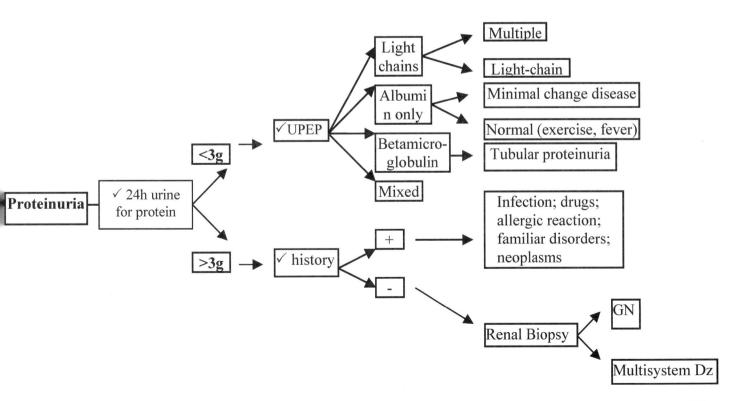

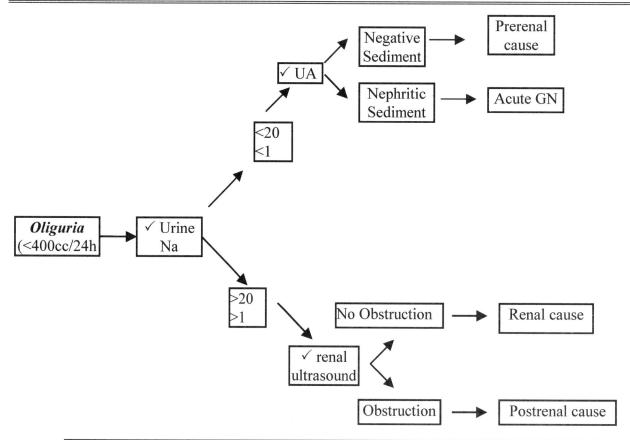

DISORDER		KEY IMPLICATED AGENTS
ARF		
Prerenal azotemia	→	NSAIDs; ACEI; radiocontrast
ATN	→	Aminoglycosides; Amphotericin
Intratubular obstruction	→	Acyclovir; Methotrexate
Rhabdomyolysis	→	Lovastatin; Gemfibrozil; heroin
Glomerulonephropathy		
Membranous GN	→	Gold; PCM (Penicillamine)
Focal segmental GN	→	Heroin
Obstructive Uropathy		
Urolithiasis	→	Allopurinol; Triamterene
Retroperitoneal fibrosis	→	Methylsergide
Vascular or Microvascular Disease		
HUS	→	Mitomycin; Cyclosporin
Tubulointerstitial nephritis		
AIN (Acute Interstitial Nephritis)	→	B-lactam Abx; NSAIDs; sulfonamides; diuretics; rifampin; cimetidine.
Chronic Renal Failure	→	ASA; Acetaminophen
Fluids & Electrolyte disorders		
RTA	→	Amphotericin; outdated TCN
Nephrogenic D.I.	→	Lithium
HyperK+	→	ACE I; NSAIDs; Cyclosporine
HypoNa+	→	NSAIDs; thiazides
HypoMg+	→	Amphotericin; Cisplatin; Aminoglycosides
Hypocalcemia	→	Cisplatin
HypoK+	→	Thiazides; Aminoglycosides

II. CLINICAL PHARMACOLOGY & TOXICOLOGY

Commonly Asked Material:

1. Know that *isopropyl alcohol* (rubbing alcohol) causes ketones, and an osmolar gap but NOT an anion gap.

2. *Anion Gap* = [Na - (HCO3 + Cl) = 8-12]

   ✪ *Causes of High Anion Gap* (>12) : **K-U-S-S-M-A-U-L** (Ketoacidosis; Uremia; Starvation; Salicylates; Methanol; Alkali loss; Unusual chemicals; Lactate) ; may use in combination with **C--M-U-D P-I-L-E-S** (Cyanide; Methanol; Uremia; DKA; Paraldehyde/Propylene glycol; INH/Iron; Lactate; Ethylene Glycol; Strychnine/Salicylates/Starvation.)

3. *Osmolar Gap* = 2[Na+] + [Glucose/18] + [BUN/2.8] . Greater than 10 is abnormal.

   ▪ Osmolar Gap= the measured osmolarity (lab) - your calculated osmolarity

   ✪ Main causes are alcohols (generally end in **-OLS**) ⇒ methan**OL**; ethan**OL**; ethylene glyc**OL**; isopropyl alcoh**OL**; mannit**OL**; and acetone.

   ✪ Know that *ethylene glycol* (antifreeze) gives calcium oxalate crystals.

4. Management of *theophylline toxicity*→ Charcoal lavage and hemodialysis are excellent.
   ▪ Presentation of theo toxicity→***Cardiac/GI/Neuro*** symptoms.

SPECIFIC OVERDOSE SYNDROMES with presentations/mnemonics/management:

ANTICHOLINERGIC SYNDROME (Atropine; TCA's; Antipsychotics; Anthistamines; some Parkinson's meds)

   Presentation—Dry skin and mucous membranes; hyperthermia; flushing;tachycardia; HTN; mydriasis; ↓ salivation and sweating; ileus; urinary retention; anxiety/confusion; seizures.

   ✪ *Mnemonic:* " **Dry as a bone; red as a beet; blind as a bat; mad as a hatter; hot as hades**".

CHOLINERGIC SYNDROME (Organophosphate poisoning)

   Presentation—Essentially the opposite of anticholinergic syndrome, with ↑sweating /salivation/ lacrimation; vomiting; diarrhea; miosis; bradycardia; wheezing; muscle cramps; fasciculations; altered mental status.

   ✪ *Mnemonic*--"**S-L-U-D-G-E**": **S**alivation/sweating; **L**acrimation; **U**rination; **D**efecation; **G**I upset; **E**mesis.

OPIATE OVERDOSE (e.g. morphine, codeine, heroine, methadone)

Presentation—Miosis; *respiratory depression*; drowsiness; N/V; Pulmonary edema; seizures.
❖ ***Classic Triad***---↓Mental status; ↓ Respiratory; ↓ pupil size (miosis).

Remember, heroine and methadone may cause ***pulmonary edema***.

BARBITURATES (e.g. phenobarbitol)

Presentation—**all are ↓**: CNS/Resp system/Pulse/BP/Temp/Reflexes

STIMULANTS (amphetamines; cocaine)

Presentation—↑ BP and Pulse and Pupils (mydriasis); CNS agitation/excitation/seizure/
hallucinations; arrythmias;

SUBSTANCE WITHDRAWAL:

Presentation is as per stimulants above (minus arrythmias) + N/V/abdominal pain

QUICK PEARLS:

❖ Remember, *Naloxone (Narcan)* is used diagnostically in unclear cases to check for opiate
overdose, and is also used therapeutically (e.g. IV Naloxone drip, since the half-life is extremely
short relative to the half-life of the opiates).

▪ Re: ***Anion Gap and Osmolar Gap*** are important in toxicology, since having the results of both can
narrow the cause significantly. Note, for example:

❖ ***Isopropyl alcohol*** (rubbing alcohol) causes an **OG and ketosis, BUT NO AG**.
❖ ***Methanol and ethylene glycol***, on the other hand, **cause BOTH gaps**.

GASTRIC LAVAGE

▪ Before gastric lavage, ***cuffed endotracheal tube*** should be placed if patient has altered mental
status, depressed gag reflex, or seizures, to prevent aspiration.
▪ Activated charcoal treatment of choice for most poisonings (1g/kg)

    o Remember, in *salicylate overdose*, besides activated charcoal:
      ➢ Fluids important to correct losses and promote diuresis;
      ➢ Monitor K+ levels;
      ➢ Alkalinization to increase urinary excretion.

▪ Charcoal is generally ineffective in absorbing ***small ionic compounds***, like Lithium, Mg,
Arsenic, Alcohols (*Hemodialysis* better for these compounds)
▪ Charcoal should not be given for caustic ingestion.

Hemoperfusion-- appropriate for overdoses of phenobarbital; other barbiturates; also theophylline.

✪ **DRUG/TOXIN** → ✪ **ANTIDOTE**

Acetaminophen   N-acetylcysteine (should be given w/in 24h of ingestion: loading dose then q4h x 17 *more* doses)

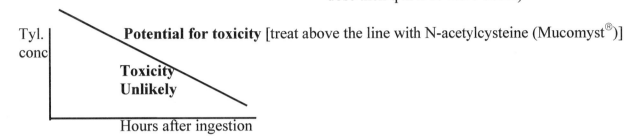

Tyl.
conc | **Potential for toxicity** [treat above the line with N-acetylcysteine (Mucomyst®)]

**Toxicity
Unlikely**

Hours after ingestion

Anticholinergics	Physostigmine
Benzodiazepines	Flumazenil
Beta-blockers	Glucagon
Carbon monoxide	Oxygen
Cyanide	Amyl nitrite, Na+Nitrite, Na+Thiosulfate
Ethylene Glycol	Ethanol
Iron	Deferoxamine
INH	Pyridoxine
Methanol	Ethanol
Narcotics	Naloxone
Nitrites	Methylene Blue
Organophospates	Atropine, Pralidoxime
TCA's	Na+Bicarbonate

SALICYLATES

✓ Remember→*charcoal, fluid diuresis, alkalinize the urine*

✓ Think of OD when you have Resp alkalosis and a High Anion Gap

✓ Progression is from: *Resp Alkalosis→Resp Alkalosis + Metabolic Acidosis→Metabolic Acidosis*

DIGOXIN

✓ Atropine often effective for bradycardias

✓ Lidocaine or Dilantin preferred for Ventricular irritability

✓ Digoxin-specific Fab fragments (Digibind®) *reserved for severe intoxication*—it binds the Digoxin making it incapable of binding at its receptor, the Na+/K+-ATPase.

TRICYCLIC ANTIDEPRESSANT OVERDOSE:

TCA's: Mechanisms →	*Causing:*
1. Quinidine-like effect	↑ PR, QRS, and QT; arrythmias; ↓ BP
2. Anticholinergic	See "Anticholinergic Syndrome" presentation above
3. Block NE reuptake	↓Myocardial contractility; ↓BP and P

TRICYCLIC ANTIDEPRESSANT OVERDOSE

- ✓ One of the most serious types of OD
- ✓ 25% of all deaths due to poisoning
- ✓ Deterioration is rapid
- ✓ Seizures common
- ✓ Activated charcoal
- ✓ Do not induce vomiting
- ✓ Lidocaine and Dilantin may be used for the ventricular arrythmias
- ✓ For hypotension, avoid isuproteronol/Dobutamine/low-dose Dopamine

NEUROLEPTIC MALIGNANT SYNDROME

- ✓ May result from phenothiazene overdose
- ✓ Key clinical manifestations include:
    - o *Altered mental status*
    - o *Autonomic la*bility
    - o *Hyperthermia*
    - o *Rigidity, posturing, and other extrapyramidal symptoms*
- ✓ Bromocryptine and dantrolene are used to treat this potential complication

13. BLOOD GASES, THE EASY WAY:

> **FIRST,** ✓ **the pH for acidosis or alkalosis** ** (see below if pH is normal)

> **SECOND,** ✓ **the pCO$_2$** to see if it's a primary resp disorder (vs metabolic).

Definitions:

o Metabolic Acidosis   — A primary process that causes [HCO$_3^-$] to fall
o Metabolic Alkalosis — A primary process that causes [HCO$_3^-$] to rise
o Respiratory Acidosis— A primary process that causes the pCO$_2$ to rise
o Respiratory Alkalosis— A primary process that causes the pCO$_2$ to fall

> **THIRD,** ✓ **compensation formulas for coexisting** (mixed acid-base) **disorders,** ie....

o **For all METABOLIC ACIDOSIS** → ✓ **serum Anion Gap first;** and ...

> ✓ **Winter's formula** {**pCO$_2$ = 1.5 [HCO$_3$] + 8 $\pm$ 2** } for additional primary resp acidosis or alkalosis. If the pCO$_2$ is greater than expected, there's an additional primary respiratory acidosis. And if the pCO$_2$ is less than expected, there's an additional primary respiratory alkalosis present.

> **IF there's a GAP,** ✓ the **osmolar gap** (essentially for toxic alcohol ingestions—remember, however, isopropyl alcohol will give you osm gap *but not* AG) **AND** always ✓ **delta-delta equation** (change in AG divided by the change in HCO$_3^-$; described later in this handout) to see if the HCO$_3$ is higher or lower than expected, and therefore, if there is an additional primary disorder *as either:*
> o a concealed <u>NON-anion gap METABOLIC ACIDOSIS</u>; or
> o a concealed <u>METABOLIC ALKALOSIS</u>

> **If there's NO GAP,** then ✓ **the UAG** (Urine Anion Gap; described below) to see if the non-anion gap acidosis is due to **GI** losses of bicarb OR insufficient **renal** bicarb/NH$_4^+$production, ie RTAs. (remember the DDx for non-anion gap metabolic acidosis): CRAP...

DDx of Normal or Low Anion Gap Metabolic Acidosis (*CRAP*):

C arbonic anyhydrase inhibitors (eg acetazolamide for glaucoma)
R TAs
A drenal insufficiency, ammonium chloride
P arenteral nutrition (eg TPN), pancreatic fistula, posthypercapnia, parathyroid (hyper)

and, of course, diarrhea (as suggested by the algorithm)

341

URINE ANION GAP:

- It's not always clear whether a non-anion gap metabolic acidosis is due to **defective generation of NH_4^+ in the kidney** (as in RTAs; HCO_3^- is not present in the urine if the urine pH < 6.5) **or** due to **GI loss of HCO_3^-**.

- The urine anion gap **(UAG) can differentiate between these 2** general categories by indirectly testing for urinary NH_4^+. Urinary NH4+, in turn, is indirectly tested for by looking at compensatory moves in the urine Cl^-.

The Urine Anion Gap = $[Na^+ + K^+]_{urine} - [Cl]_{urine}$ (normal UAG = 0 mEq/L)

- In **GI** causes of non-anion gap acidosis, the urine will actually contain ↑ NH_4^+ (the unmeasured cation you're checking for).

- But if there is a tubular defect in the kidneys causing insufficient NH_4^+ production (as in **RTA**), the NH_4^+ will be lower than expected.

- So...a **positive or small negative UAG**→ implies relatively lower urinary Cl^-→ implies lower NH_4^+ present due to tubular dysfunction→ implies renal (usually **RTA)** as the source of the non-anion gap metabolic acidosis.

- And...a **large negative UAG** → implies relatively higher urinary Cl^-→ implies adequate presence/production of NH_4^+→ implies nonrenal source (**GI**)

---

o **For all METABOLIC ALKALOSES** → ✓ **the URINE CHLORIDE** to see if …

the cause is due to **volume loss** (chloride/saline-responsive; U_{Cl^-} < 10) or **mineralcorticoid excess** (chloride/saline-unresponsive; U_{Cl^-} > 10). The first category is associated with volume depletion. The second is associated with *mineralcorticoid excess*, which causes excessive stimulation of Na+ resorption (and H+ excretion) in the distal tubule; thus "saline unresponsive".

➤ With **metabolic alkalosis**, while you may choose to remember the compensatory formula **$pCO_2 = [HCO_3-] + 16$,** you might instead…

just choose to use the surprisingly good **rule of thumb** that states the **pCO_2 should = the last 2 digits of the pH**, there's no mixed disorder present. For example, if a patient has a pH 7.**60**, pO2 95, pCO2 **60**, & HCO3 57, she is appropriately compensated. Similar to the discussion in primary metabolic acidosis, if the pCO_2 is less than expected, then a respiratory alkalosis may also be present. And if the pCO_2 is greater than expected, then a respiratory acidosis may also be present.

○ **For all RESPIRATORY DISORDERS** {acidosis (pH < 7.35, pCO_2 > 40) or alkaloses (pH > 7.35 and pCO_2, < 40)}, then ✓ the **Quick-Chart** ™ for additional primary disorders.

> ➤ **The formulas for <u>respiratory processes</u> are divided into <u>acute</u> (< 8 hours, i.e. uncompensated) and <u>chronic</u> (> 24 hours, i.e. fully compensated) changes and can be used according to the clinical situation. Patients, however, can certainly have an intermediate phase, which values will also fall between the values predicted by the acute and chronic formulas.**
>
> ➤ Knowing the clinical history is critical to to appropriate use of the acute vs. chronic sides of the Quick Chart ™ method. Instead of using hard-to-remember formulas to figure the expected <u>HCO_3^-</u>, here's an easier method:

QUICK-CHART™ METHOD :

	HCO_3^- ↓		HCO_3^- ↓	
ACUTE Respiratory Process		60		**CHRONIC** Respiratory Process
	+1		+4	
		50		
	+1		+4	
Normals →	(24)	40	(24)	
	-2		-5	
		30		
	-2		-5	
		20		
		↑		
		pCO₂		

> ✪ **NOTE that the "+1, -2, +4, and -5" are the amounts that should be added or subtracted** from 24 to calculate the true $HCO3^-$, using compensation formulas, given any pCO_2.
>
> ✪ *If the HCO_3^- is more or less than the expected compensation, then there's <u>another</u> <u>primary</u> process going on.*

HERE'S SOME EXAMPLES TO WORK THROUGH:

> ➢ If a patient is in <u>ACUTE</u> respiratory distress (see the <u>LEFT SIDE</u> of this Winter's formulas quick-chart), and her pCO2 is 20, you see that the bicarb should be 24-2-2more, which=20! If her bicarb is any more or less, there is *another primary* process going on. If her bicarb is 20, then her bicarb is appropriately compensated and the process is straightforward.

> ➢ If a patient is in <u>ACUTE</u> respiratory distress and he becomes lethargic, and his pCO2 is 60, you see that the bicarb should be 24 +1 +1 more, which=26, again if appropriately compensated and assuming no additional contributing process.

> ➢ If a patient is in <u>CHRONIC</u> respiratory distress (see the <u>RIGHT SIDE</u> of the Winter's formulas quick-chart), and his pCO2 is 30, you see that the bicarb should be 24 -5, or 19.

> ➢ If a patient is in <u>CHRONIC</u> respiratory distress, and his pCO2 is 50, you see that the bicarb should be 24 +4, or 28.

✪ **CALCULATING the "** **DELTA-DELTA** **" in Anion Gap Metabolic Acidoses…**

- *Remember*, **delta** also **means "change". The "delta-delta" refers to the change in Anion Gap divided by the change in** HCO_3^- **, or …**

$$\frac{\Delta\ AG}{\Delta\ HCO_3^-}$$

- <u>**It should be calculated whenever you have an ↑AG metabolic acidosis.**</u> <u>**Here's why**</u>: Basically, it's done in order to figure out if there's a second underlying disorder, i.e. a <u>**mixed disorder**</u>. In general, for every ↑ in the AG, there is an equal ↓ in the HCO_3^-, so…

- <u>**If the DELTA-DELTA<1**</u>, that means there's A "<u>CONCEALED</u>" (or additional hidden) *<u>**NON-ANION GAP METABOLIC ACIDOSIS**</u>*. Why? Because < 1 implies that the change in the bicarb was greater than the change in the AG. That means the ↓ in bicarb was more than expected for the anion gap alone.

- <u>**If the DELTA-DELTA is > 1**</u>, that means there's a <u>CONCEALED *METABOLIC ALKALOSIS*</u>. The logic is the same.

✪ <u>**FOR EXAMPLE**</u>, **given the upper limit of a normal AG is 12, if the** patient's AG = 20, the Δ AG therefore = 8, so we'd expect a Δ HCO_3^- to be the same, or (24-X) = 8, so "X", or the measured HCO_3^- we would *expect to be* 16. If it's > 16, the delta-delta will be >1, and there must be a <u>concealed metabolic alkalosis</u>. Perhaps the patient has been vomiting too (losing acid) ? If the measured HCO_3^- <16, the delta-delta <1, so there must be an additional or <u>concealed non-anion gap metabolic acidosis</u>.

> ✪ ****IF the pH is in the NORMAL RANGE (7.35-7.45)...**

…then the *easy* way to go is to **simply look at the bicarb**. There are 2 scenarios based on whether the HCO_3 is < 21 or > 27. In either case, you have a mixed resp + metabolic *disorder*, but the key is that **the metabolic disorder takes the direction of the bicarb (and you simply make the respiratory component opposite)**, so that…

> ➤ If the **HCO_3 < 21**, then there's a mixed **met acidosis** + resp alk; and
> ➤ If the **HCO_3 > 27**, then there's a mixed **met alkalosis** + resp acidosis.

TRIPLE ACID-BASE DISORDERS:

> ➤ The only way a patient can have a triple acid-base disorder is if a mixed disorder coexists with either a respiratory acidosis or a respiratory alkalosis.

> ➤ Typical examples include:
>   - DKA (met acidosis) + dehydration (met alk) + respiratory depression (resp acidosis)
>   - DKA + dehydration + hyperventilation from pneumonia or sepsis (resp alkalosis)

LOW ANION GAPS:

> ➤ Why *multiple myeloma* and other *paraproteinemias* give a low anion gap: protein cations balanced with chloride increase the calculated chloride, thereby reducing the anion gap.

> ➤ *Hypoalbuminemia* is also a cause of low anion gap, since albumin is a negatively charged anion comprising about 75% of the normal anion gap.

> **ADDITIONAL PEARLS:**

> ✪ The #1 cause of hypoxemia is <u>hypoventilation</u>

> ✪ An ↑A-a gradient means <u>abnormal lung!</u>

> ✪ **AGE CORRECTION FOR A-a GRADIENT → Add 4 + ¼(age)** to the calculated A-a gradient. <u>For example</u>, if a 60 yo has a calculated gradient of 16, you'd **add** 4 + 15 =**19** (remember, there is an increase in the gradient with age due to V/Q mismatch) **to the 16** to get your actual age-corrected gradient of 35.

More Important Tips and Rules of Thumb on ABGs:

✪ *Whenever you see a __metabolic ACIDOSIS__, always calculate the* Anion Gap.

✪ *Whenever you see $\downarrow pO_2$ plus $\downarrow pCO_2$, always calculate the* A-a gradient.

✪ An $\uparrow$A-a gradient <u>means</u> *abnormal lung!*

✪ Remember also that as much as 15% of PE cases will have a normal gradient so a normal gradient does *not* rule out PE.

✪ *If a patient's PaO_2 does not $\uparrow$ with an $\uparrow$ in FIO_2, then a __shunt__ is present. (see appendix for more*

✪ *Whenever you see a __metabolic ALKALOSIS__, know* that the next step is to ask for a <u>urine chloride</u>.

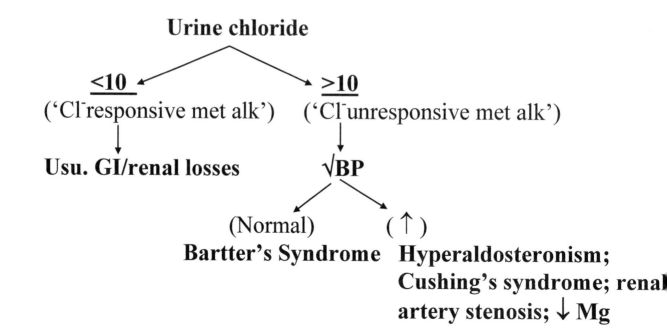

Urine chloride

<u><10</u> ('Cl⁻responsive met alk')   **<u>>10</u>** ('Cl⁻unresponsive met alk')

Usu. GI/renal losses   **√BP**

(Normal)   ($\uparrow$)
Bartter's Syndrome   **Hyperaldosteronism; Cushing's syndrome; renal artery stenosis; $\downarrow$ Mg**

✪   Acidemia ⎯⎯⎯⎯→ Hyperkalemia
      Alkalemia ⎯⎯⎯⎯→ Hypokalemia

✪   The #1 cause of hypoxemia is *hypoventilation*

✪   If you see a ↓PaO_2, ↓sat (lab), normal pulse ox, and patient is non-cyanotic, think→Leukocyte larceny (occurs in the lab)

✪   If you see ↓sat, cyanotic patient, and normal PaO_2, think→Methemoglobinemia (congenital right-shifted hemoglobin)

✪   If you see sat % unusually/inappropriately high for the level of PaO_2, think→Cyanide or carboxyHg (common in firefighters)

Blood Gases APPENDIX
Key Formulas; DDx; & Compensation

Anion Gap: $[Na^+ - (HCO_3 + Cl)] = 8\text{-}12$ (normal range)

- Causes of High Anion Gap (>12) : _**K-U-S-S-M-A-U-L**_ (Ketoacidosis; Uremia; Starvation; Salicylates; Methanol; Alkali loss; Unusual chemicals; Lactate) ; **OR**…

- _**C--M-U-D P-I-L-E-S**_ (Cyanide; Methanol; Uremia; DKA; Paraldehyde/Propylene glycol; INH/Iron; Lactate; Ethylene Glycol; Strychnine/Salicylates/Starvation.)

Osmolar Gap $= 2[Na+] + [Glucose/18] + [BUN/2.8]$. Greater than 10 is abnormal.

- Osmolar Gap= the measured osmolarity (lab) - your calculated osmolarity

- Main causes end in -_**OLS**_: Methan**OL**; Ethan**OL**; Ethylene Glyc**OL**; Isopropyl Alcoh**OL**; Mannit**OL**; and acetone.

✪ A-a Gradient $= pAO_2\text{-}paO_2 = [150 - \dfrac{pCO_2}{0.8}] - paO_2$ (sea level)

DDx of ↑ A-a (Alveolar-arterial) Gradient→Remember, "VSD"

V/Q mismatch
1. PE
2. Airway obstruction (asthma, COPD)
3. Interstitial lung disease
4. Alveolar disease

Shunt
1. Intracardiac (e.g. VSD!)
2. Intrapulmonary shunt (e.g. ARDS or intrapulmonary AVM) and "intraalveolar filling" (pus=pneumonia; water=CHF; protein (AP); blood)
3. Alveolar collapse (atelectasis)

Diffusion defect, e.g.
1. IPF
2. Emphysema

✪ Calculating Compensation

- **Metabolic acidosis** → $pCO_2 = 1.5 (HCO_3^-) + 8$ **± 2**
- **Metabolic alkalosis** → $pCO_2 = HCO3^- + 16$
- **Respiratory acidosis/alkalosis** → HCO_3^- as per our compensation formulas Quick-Chart™

14. STATISTICS

IT'S ALL ABOUT...
- Knowing how to set up your "2 by 2" table
- Knowing the terms and equations
- Knowing the pattern of solving these questions
- Let's walk through it...

ALWAYS SET UP YOUR 2X2 TABLE THIS WAY:

	DISEASE PRESENT	DISEASE ABSENT
DIAGNOSTIC TEST +	True + "a"	False + "b"
DIAGNOSTIC TEST -	False - "c"	True - "d"

IMPORTANT NOTES:

- ✪ *Don't put the headings on the wrong axis !!*
- ✪ **The most important players are "a" and "d"**—remember their position!
- ✪ **Sensitivity** goes **down the 1st column**!
- ✪ **Specificity** goes **down the 2nd column**!
- ✪ **Positive Predictive Value (PPV)** goes **across the 1st row**!
- ✪ **Negative Predictive Value (NPV)** goes **across the 2nd row**!

SO, SETTING IT UP AGAIN spatially MUCH SIMPLER THIS TIME IT GOES LIKE THIS:
{placement of capitals to illustrate relative importance}

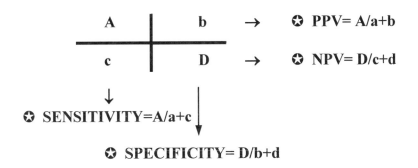

✪ PPV= A/a+b

✪ NPV= D/c+d

✪ SENSITIVITY=A/a+c

✪ SPECIFICITY= D/b+d

✪ And PREVALENCE= a+c/a+b+c+d

SO! Let's Do An <u>EXAMPLE</u> In A Manner Commonly Presented...

- You're given a new diagnostic test that gives abnormal results 80% of patients who have the disease but gives normal results in 95% of patients who are truly disease-free. We also tell you that the prevalence of the disease in the population being tested is 10%. Now let's say you're asked what % of patients who test + actually have the disease (asking Positive Predictive Value).

WE NOW HAVE EVERYTHING WE NEED:

1. Sensitivity = 80%
2. Specificity = 95%
3. Prevalence = 10%

...which is everything we need to set up our 2x2 table and fill in the blanks.

<u>IMPORTANT</u>: *The key to solving these problems is <u>the order in which you proceed</u>. (I've charted the itinerary for you)*

FIRST: <u>Start with the prevalence</u> and arbitrarily assume a population of 100; Well, that means a+b+c+d=100; so 10% of that population the prevalence.

SECOND: That means <u>a+c</u> =10, since those are the ones who actually have the disease.

THIRD: So, we start picking them off one at a time. If a+c=10, and the <u>sensitivity</u> is 80%, that means "<u>a</u>" must = 8; and therefore "<u>c</u>" must =2. Remember, we're setting this all up so we can calculate the PPV in *percent (!) so don't worry.*

FOURTH: <u>100 minus 10 (which was a+c, remember) gives us 90, which must = b+d.</u> Now we punch in the <u>specificity</u>, which is 95%, so d/b+d, or d/90=95%. That means "<u>d</u>"= 85.5 (don't worry that's 855 if you arbitrarily chose a population of 1000), so "<u>b</u>" must = 90-85.5=4.5

FINALLY: <u>So, we now have all the values for "a","b","c", and "d", and we can calculate either PPV or NPV, whatever is asked.</u> Our example asked for PPV, so that's a/a+b, or 8/8+4.5, (or 80/80+45, if you chose to use 1000), so...

<u>PPV=64%</u>, and that's the answer you look for!

RELATIVE RISK

Relative risk (RR), known also as the risk ratio, is the cumulative incidence of disease in exposed persons, divided by the cumulative incidence of disease in unexposed individuals .

$$RR = \frac{A/(A+B)}{C/(C+D)}$$

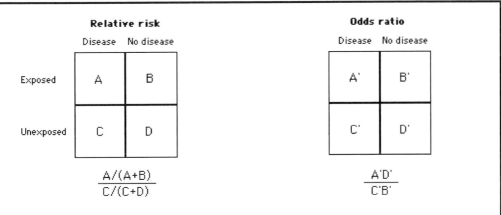

The estimation of relative risk provided by the odds ratio can be illustrated allgebraically. In uncommon diseases A' <<< B' and C' <<< D'. Thus A'/(A' +B') is approximately A'/B' and C'/(C'+D') is approximately C'/D'. Therefore, the risk in exposed versus unexposed is approximately (A'/B')/(C'/D'), or rearranged (A'D')/(C'B')

Relative risk and odds ratio In a cohort study, the relative risk of a disease can be calculated because all patients under study are available for the analysis comparing risk in exposed and unexposed individuals. In contrast, in a case-control study, cases are drawn from a population of patients who have the disease, and controls from a population without the disease. Thus, the relative risk cannot be calculated since the samples do not necessarily reflect the true proportion of patients who have been exposed to a risk factors. Instead, the relative risk can be estimated using the odds ratio.

So, <u>Relative Risk for cohort</u> studies; versus <u>Odds Ratio (aka Odds Risk) for case-control</u> studies, where the OR approximates the RR. The relative risk and odds ratio are *interpreted relative to the number one*. For example, an odds ratio of 0.7 suggests that patients exposed to a variable of interest were 30 % less likely to develop a specific outcome compared to the control group, i.e. exposure conferred some degree of protective benefit. Similarly, an odds ratio of 1.2 suggests that the risk was increased by 20 %.

ODDS RATIO (OR)

The odds-ratio, used for case-control studies to estimate the relative risk, is merely the cross-product of the diagonals in a 2 x 2 table For this reason, it is sometimes called the "cross-product ratio", so that...

$$OR = \frac{AD}{CB}$$

Let's run through an *example*. Let's say that a case-control study is done in the shoe manufacturing industry where thiuram exposure is well known. Staff who present with contact dermatitis and those without contact dermatitis are examined relative to their thiuram exposure.

	CONTACT DERMATITIS	NO CONTACT DERMATITIS	Total
At risk (thiuram exposure)	**235**	465	**700**
Not at risk	**215**	1685	**1900**
Total	450	2150	2600

In this hypothetical example, the odds ratio is (235 x 1685)/(215 x 465) which equals approximately 40. This OR indicates that factory workers with contact dermatitis are approximately forty times more likely to have been exposed to thiuram than their counterparts who do not present with contact dermatitis.

$$OR = \frac{AD}{CB} = \frac{235 \times 1685}{215 \times 465} = \frac{393975}{9675} = \text{approximately } 40$$

RISK DIFFERENCE (RD)

The relative risk and odds ratio provide an understanding of the magnitude of risk *compared with* a standard. However, it is more often desirable to know information about the *absolute* risk. As an example, a 20 % increase in mortality due to a particular exposure does not provide direct insight into the likelihood that exposure in an individual patient will lead to mortality. The ***Risk Difference (also called the "attributable risk") is a measure of absolute risk***. *It reflects the additional incidence of disease related to an exposure taking into account the background rate of the disease*.

In other words, it provides information about the absolute effect of the exposure or excess risk of disease in individuals who are exposed, compared to persons who are not exposed. The attributable risk is *calculated by subtracting the cumulative incidence of a disease in nonexposed persons from the cumulative incidence of disease in exposed persons*.

$$\text{Risk Difference} = CI_{EXPOSED} - CI_{UNEXPOSED}$$

$$= \frac{A}{(A+B)} - \frac{C}{(C+D)}$$

So, using the 2x2 table for assessing risk, we replace "Diagnostic Test +" or "Diagnostic Test –" by "Exposed" or "Unexposed", just like before with Sensitivity, Specificity and predictive values:

	DISEASE	NO DISEASE	Total
EXPOSED	A	B	**A + B**
UNEXPOSED	C	D	**C + D**
Total	A + C	B + D	A + B + C + D

Let's say, *for example*, that a 10-year prospective cohort study is done to chart the development of prostate cancer in two groups, based on their exposure to to a dietary element, say a predominantly high-fat diet, in general:

	PROSTATE CA	NO PROSTATE CA	Total
At risk (high fat diet)	**425**	875	**1300**
Not at risk	**407**	4893	**5300**
Total	832	5768	6600

The cumulative incidence of prostate cancer development in the at-risk group is 435/1300 = .33 and 407/5300 = .08 in the group without risk, making the attributable risk (RD) = .33-.08 = .25. The risk of prostate cancer is increased, therefore, by .25 in individuals who are exposed to a predominantly high-fat diet. Another way to put that would be that, in at-risk patients, the excess occurrence of prostate cancer that is attributable to a predominantly high-fat diet is 250 per 1000. Our RD here then was **.26**. If there were no association between a predominantly high-fat diet and the development of prostate cancer, the RD would have been zero.

ATTRIBUTABLE RISK PERCENT (AR%)

The AR% is an estimate of the proportion of disease in exposed individuals that is attributable to the exposure. *It may be said to represent the % of disease in the exposed or at-risk group that could be eliminated by removing the exposure.*

AR%, as with the RD, is developed from cohort studies and is defined as:

$$AR\% = \frac{RD}{CI_{EXPOSED}} \times 100$$

Using the example provided for RD, $AR\% = \frac{.25}{.33} \times 100 = 76$

So, assuming a causal link existed between high-fat diets and prostate cancer, one could say that high-fat diets account for 76% of prostate cancer in at-risk individuals, and that eliminating that risk by modifying the diet would also eliminate 76% of the prostate cancer in this same group of otherwise exposed individuals with prostate cancer.

E

I

INDEX

INDEX

T

REFERENCES

1.   Harrison's Principles of Internal Medicine 15th edition, McGraw Hill Inc., New York, © 2002 by McGraw Hill Inc.
2.   Cecil Essentials of Medicine, 5th edition, Andreoli, T. et al, W. B. Saunders Company, Philadelphia, PA © 2001.
3.   Frontrunners Internal Medicine Board Review Syllabus, 2002
4.   Frontrunners Internal Medicine Board Review Course, 1996-2002.
5.   Mayo Internal Medicine Board Review, 5th edition, Haberman, T., Lippincott, Williams & Wilkins, © 2002.
6.   ACP Board Review Course, 1996-2002.
7.   Emory University Comprehensive Board Review in Internal Medicine, Stein, S., McGraw-Hill Publishing Co, ©2000.
8.   Medical Knowledge Self Assessment Program VII, VIII, IX, X, XI, and XII, American College of Physicians, Philadelphia, PA.
9.   Heart Disease- A Textbook of Cardiovascular Medicine, edited by Eugene Braunwald, MD, 6th ed, W.B. Saunders Company, © 2001
10. The Sanford Guide to Antimicrobial Therapy 2002, David N. Gilbert, MD, et al, 32nd ed., © 2002.

Quick Order Form

We ALSO provide these additional I.M. board review resources:

☐ *Frontrunners Internal Medicine Q&A Review: Self-Assessement & Board Review*

☐ Frontrunners **Weekend Marathon Review** (for the ABIM Exam): certification & recertification (call **866-MDBOARDS** for dates/details)

☐ Intensive 4 month Internal Medicine Board Review Course (call for dates/details)

ORDER OPTIONS: (check off any of the above; if requesting info only, use this form and just say so ☺)

Fax orders: **516-977-3294**. Fax this form.

Tel. Orders: Call **866-MDBOARDS**. Credit card may be securely left here. V/MC/AmX/Discover only.

E-mail orders: Order details may also be emailed to us at **FRONTRUNNERS@hotmail.com**

Order **by mail**: Frontrunners Board Review, Inc.
Attention: Orders Department
39 Lyon St.
Valley Stream, NY 11580

CUSTOMER: _____

Address: _____

City State Zip: _____

Fax # (to be used for faxback confirmation only!): _____

PAYMENT: ☐ Check ☐ Visa ☐ MC ☐ AmX

Card number: _____

Name on card: _____Exp. Date _____

We ALSO provide these additional I.M. board review resources:

❏ *Frontrunners Internal Medicine Q&A Review: Self-Assessement & Board Review*

❏ Frontrunners **Weekend Marathon Review** (for the ABIM Exam): certification & recertification (call **866-MDBOARDS** for dates/details)

❏ Intensive 4 month Internal Medicine Board Review Course (call for dates/details)

ORDER OPTIONS: (check off any of the above; if requesting info only, use this form and just say so ☺)

Fax orders: **516-977-3294**. Fax this form.

Tel. Orders: Call **866-MDBOARDS**. Credit card may be securely left here. V/MC/AmX/Discover only.

E-mail orders: Order details may also be emailed to us at **FRONTRUNNERS@hotmail.com**

Order **by mail**:   Frontrunners Board Review, Inc.
Attention: Orders Department
39 Lyon St.
Valley Stream, NY 11580

CUSTOMER: _____

Address: _____

City State Zip: _____

Fax # (to be used for faxback confirmation only!): _____

PAYMENT: ☐ Check   ☐ Visa   ☐ MC   ☐ AmX

Card number: _____

Name on card: _____ Exp. Date _____